Bioactive Phytochemicals in Health and Disease

Bioactive Phytochemicals in Health and Disease

Editors

Natália Martins
Célia F. Rodrigues
Marcello Iriti

MDPI • Basel • Beijing • Wuhan • Barcelona • Belgrade • Manchester • Tokyo • Cluj • Tianjin

Editors
Natália Martins
University of Porto
Portugal

Célia F. Rodrigues
University of Porto
Portugal

Marcello Iriti
Milan State University
Italy

Editorial Office
MDPI
St. Alban-Anlage 66
4052 Basel, Switzerland

This is a reprint of articles from the Special Issue published online in the open access journal *Journal of Clinical Medicine* (ISSN 2077-0383) (available at: https://www.mdpi.com/journal/jcm/special_issues/Bioactive_Phytochemicals_heath_disease).

For citation purposes, cite each article independently as indicated on the article page online and as indicated below:

LastName, A.A.; LastName, B.B.; LastName, C.C. Article Title. *Journal Name* **Year**, *Article Number*, Page Range.

ISBN 978-3-03943-138-0 (Hbk)
ISBN 978-3-03943-139-7 (PDF)

Contents

About the Editors vii

Rohit Sharma and Natália Martins
Telomeres, DNA Damage and Ageing: Potential Leads from Ayurvedic Rasayana (Anti-Ageing) Drugs
Reprinted from: *J. Clin. Med.* **2020**, *9*, 2544, doi:10.3390/jcm9082544 1

Jung Sun Min, Dong Eon Kim, Young-Hee Jin and Sunoh Kwon
Kurarinone Inhibits HCoV-OC43 Infection by Impairing the Virus-Induced Autophagic Flux in MRC-5 Human Lung Cells
Reprinted from: *J. Clin. Med.* **2020**, *9*, 2230, doi:10.3390/jcm9072230 9

Artur Adamczak, Marcin Ożarowski and Tomasz M. Karpiński
Antibacterial Activity of Some Flavonoids and Organic Acids Widely Distributed in Plants
Reprinted from: *J. Clin. Med.* **2020**, *9*, 109, doi:10.3390/jcm9010109 23

Min Cheol Kang, Silvia Yumnam, Woo Sung Park, Hae Min So, Ki Hyun Kim, Meong Cheol Shin, Mi-Jeong Ahn and Sun Yeou Kim
Ulmus parvifolia Accelerates Skin Wound Healing by Regulating the Expression of MMPs and TGF-β
Reprinted from: *J. Clin. Med.* **2020**, *9*, 59, doi:10.3390/jcm9010059 41

Daniel Gyingiri Achel, Miguel Alcaraz-Saura, Julián Castillo, Amparo Olivares and Miguel Alcaraz
Radioprotective and Antimutagenic Effects of *Pycnanthus angolensis* Warb Seed Extract against Damage Induced by X rays
Reprinted from: *J. Clin. Med.* **2020**, *9*, 6, doi:10.3390/jcm9010006 53

Vineet Sharma, Rohit Sharma, DevNath Singh Gautam, Kamil Kuca, Eugenie Nepovimova and Natália Martins
Role of Vacha (*Acorus calamus* Linn.) in Neurological and Metabolic Disorders: Evidence from Ethnopharmacology, Phytochemistry, Pharmacology and Clinical Study
Reprinted from: *J. Clin. Med.* **2020**, *9*, 1176, doi:10.3390/jcm9041176 71

Jiansheng Huang, Wenliang Song, Hui Huang and Quancai Sun
Pharmacological Therapeutics Targeting RNA-Dependent RNA Polymerase, Proteinase and Spike Protein: From Mechanistic Studies to Clinical Trials for COVID-19
Reprinted from: *J. Clin. Med.* **2020**, *9*, 1131, doi:10.3390/jcm9041131 117

Bahare Salehi, María L. Del Prado-Audelo, Hernán Cortés, Gerardo Leyva-Gómez, Zorica Stojanović-Radić, Yengkhom Disco Singh, Jayanta Kumar Patra, Gitishree Das, Natália Martins, Miquel Martorell, Marzieh Sharifi-Rad, William C. Cho and Javad Sharifi-Rad
Therapeutic Applications of Curcumin Nanomedicine Formulations in Cardiovascular Diseases
Reprinted from: *J. Clin. Med.* **2020**, *9*, 746, doi:10.3390/jcm9030746 141

Jadwiga Jodynis-Liebert and Małgorzata Kujawska
Biphasic Dose-Response Induced by Phytochemicals: Experimental Evidence
Reprinted from: *J. Clin. Med.* **2020**, *9*, 718, doi:10.3390/jcm9030718 167

Bahare Salehi, Daniela Calina, Anca Oana Docea, Niranjan Koirala, Sushant Aryal, Domenico Lombardo, Luigi Pasqua, Yasaman Taheri, Carla Marina Salgado Castillo, Miquel Martorell, Natália Martins, Marcello Iriti, Hafiz Ansar Rasul Suleria and Javad Sharifi-Rad
Curcumin's Nanomedicine Formulations for Therapeutic Application in Neurological Diseases
Reprinted from: *J. Clin. Med.* **2020**, *9*, 430, doi:10.3390/jcm9020430 . . . . **195**

Md. Jakaria, Shofiul Azam, Song-Hee Jo, In-Su Kim, Raju Dash and Dong-Kug Choi
Potential Therapeutic Targets of Quercetin and Its Derivatives: Its Role in the Therapy of Cognitive Impairment
Reprinted from: *J. Clin. Med.* **2019**, *8*, 1789, doi:10.3390/jcm8111789 . . . . **231**

About the Editor

Natália Martins (Ph.D., Researcher, Professor) has a huge background in dietetics and nutrition, natural product chemistry and biochemistry, drug discovery, phytochemistry, phytopharmacology, functional foods and nutraceuticals. She has been increasingly focused on the use of naturally-occurring bioactives for human health, not only from a point of view of health promotion and disease prevention, but also treatment. Natália has held several specializations in evidence-based medicine, clinical nutrition, and integrative medicine. She has worked as university professor since 2017, was advisor of several MSc and Ph.D. theses, and is a member of the evaluation panel of the College of Nutritionists (Porto, Portugal). She has participated in various research projects, received several grants and awards, and published more than 120 articles in peer-reviewed, highly reputed, international journals (H-index: 21), 8 book chapters, and presented more than 40 communications in national and international conferences. Natália is also a member of the Council for Nutritional and Environmental Medicine (CONEM, Norway), reviewer for more than 50 highly reputed international journals, invited reviewer for several book publishers, and editorial board member of several international journals. She also edited several special issues and research topics in highly reputed journals and is currently editing several books for renowned publishers.

Célia F. Rodrigues (PharmD, Ph.D.). Célia is a *Candida* spp. expert, with extensive know-how working with molecular techniques, susceptibility assays, biofilm development, antimicrobial drugs, *in vivo* assessments, alternative and novel treatments, and biomaterials at LEPABE, Faculty of Engineering, University of Porto. Presently, she is also working in a project related to microorganisms, FISH, and microfluidics, and is an invited assistant professor at CESPU, where she teaches future pharmacists. Célia is a reviewer for more than 40 international journals and has done co-supervision/mentoring of MSc and Ph.D. Students, organized research conferences/seminars, and been a jury of Congress. Finally, Célia has won several grants and awards from Portuguese and international entities. (https://www.researchgate.net/profile/Celia_Rodrigues2; Ciência ID: 5F12-D3E1-E028).

Marcello Iriti (Associate Professor). He has been studying bioactive phytochemicals relevant for human nutrition and health, including melatonin, polyphenols, carotenoids, sterols, sphingolipids and essential oils, focusing on their functional role in planta, as well as on their in vitro/in vivo and human biological activities. He is the author of more than 200 publications with an IF (H-index: 40). He is a member of the Asian Council of Science Editors and Society of African Journal Editors, a founding Member of the Italian Society of Environmental Medicine, and a member of the Working Group 'Pharmacognosy and Phytotherapy' of the Italian Society of Pharmacology. Main Patent: 'Compositions Comprising Rutin Useful for the Treatment of Tumors Resistant to Chemotherapy' (WO2015036875A1; US20160213698; US9757405B2; EP3043821).

Journal of
Clinical Medicine

MDPI

Editorial

Telomeres, DNA Damage and Ageing: Potential Leads from Ayurvedic Rasayana (Anti-Ageing) Drugs

Rohit Sharma [1,*] and Natália Martins [2,3,4,*]

1 Department of Rasashastra and Bhaishajya Kalpana, Faculty of Ayurveda, Institute of Medical Sciences, Banaras Hindu University, Varanasi, Uttar Pradesh 221005, India
2 Faculty of Medicine, University of Porto, Alameda Prof. Hernani Monteiro, 4200-319 Porto, Portugal
3 Institute for research and Innovation in Health (i3S), University of Porto, Rua Alfredo Allen, 4200-135 Porto, Portugal
4 Laboratory of Neuropsychophysiology, Faculty of Psychology and Education Sciences, University of Porto, 4200-319 Porto, Portugal
* Correspondence: rohitsharma@bhu.ac.in or dhanvantari86@gmail.com (R.S.); ncmartins@med.up.pt (N.M.); Tel.: +91-9816724054 (R.S.); +351-22-5512100 (N.M.)

Received: 4 August 2020; Accepted: 5 August 2020; Published: 6 August 2020

Ageing, while a relentless, unidirectional and pleiotropic phenomenon of life, is a key trigger for several age-related disorders, such as cancer, cataract, osteoporosis, hypertension, cardiovascular (CV), metabolic and even neurodegenerative ailments, including Alzheimer's (AD) and Parkinson's (PD) disease [1]. Telomeres shortening has been pointed to as the main factor that speeds up cell ageing and promotes degeneration processes [2]. With each DNA replication, the telomeres are progressively shortened, leading to the appearance of critically shorter telomeres. Telomerase is the key enzyme involved in the chromosomes (telomeres) ends protection and repair from shortening (adding repetitions of TTAGGG) during replication, consequently preventing catastrophic DNA loss and promoting the maintenance of healthy cell function [3]. However, telomerase activity is very low in human cells, and thus, low telomerase activity, leads to the imminent appearance of short telomeres and to a low rate of DNA repair, consequently promoting an accelerated ageing process [4–6]. Briefly, the main sources of telomere shortening or DNA damage can be (i) exogenous, such as radiation, unhealthy diet and lifestyle, mental stress and environmental chemicals, or (ii) endogenous, such as chronic inflammation, chemical instability (purification), spontaneous errors during DNA replication and repair and oxidative stress [7]. Quite recently, and owing to limited efficacy of conventional drugs as anti-ageing modulators, options are being searched from natural products and traditional medicines with potential to arrest or delay ageing.

Ayurvedic medicines, having historical roots more than 5000 years ago, have been increasingly searched for worldwide for multiple purposes. For instance, several Ayurvedic medicinal herbs and formulations, traditionally known as *Rasayana*, have been shown to markedly promote health, immunity, vigor, vitality, and longevity, at same time as protecting from stress. These medicines claim to facilitate healthy ageing, arrest degenerative changes and have rejuvenating potential at cell and tissue levels [8,9]. In this sense, here we briefly discuss the evidence-based perspectives of some of these anti-ageing drugs, considering their role in promoting telomerase activity, telomere length and DNA repair.

There are some Ayurvedic *Rasayana* herbs and formulations with potential telomer protective and DNA repair activities (Figure 1).

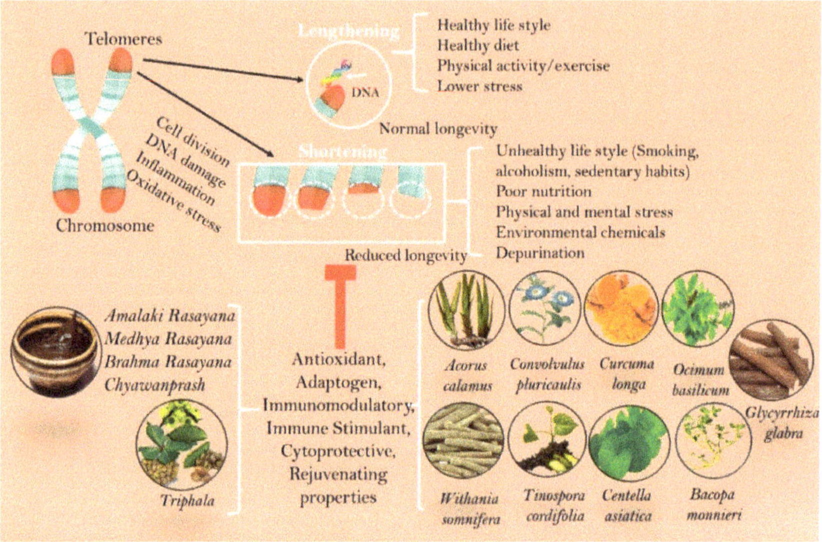

Figure 1. Potential anti-ageing Ayurveda medicines with telomer protective and DNA repair effects.

Ashwagandha [*Withania somnifera* (L.) Dunal], aka Indian ginseng, is a flagship rejuvenating and adaptogen Ayurvedic herb, traditionally used as an anti-ageing agent. Ashwagandha root extract showed ~20% lifespan extension in a nematode model *Caenorhabditis elegans* [10]. Withanolide, a bioactive constituent of Ashwagandha showed a 29.7% extension in the mean lifespan and regulated the insulin/IGF-1 signaling (IIS) pathway and neural activity in *C. elegans* [11]. In human HeLa cell lines, Ashwagandha root extract, tested at various concentrations, led to an enhancement in telomerase activity by ~45% at 10–50 μg (assessed by the Telomerase Rapid Amplification Protocol (TRAP) assay) [12]. Ashwagandha extract also exhibited anti-genotoxic effects against H_2O_2-induced DNA damage in human peripheral blood lymphocytes [13]. Thus, considering the promising achievements in longevity promotion through in vitro and in vivo models, Ashwagandha deserves to be investigated in various degenerative and adult onset health ailments, with more understanding on potential anti-ageing mechanisms.

Guduchi [*Tinospora cordifolia* (Wild) Hook. f. & Thomson] is a celebrated *Rasayana* herb of Ayurveda. It is used at several dosage forms to treat inflammation, arthritis, allergy, diabetes and as an anti-ageing and rejuvenating tonic [14–16]. A study found that extracts from Guduchi markedly enhanced the rate of cell survival and protected against radiation-induced cytotoxicity and DNA damage in PC12 cells [17]. Another study using ethanolic Guduchi stem extracts reported DNA protective ability on sodium arsenite-induced genotoxicity in lymphocytes from Swiss Albino mice using the comet assay [18].

Mandukaparni [*Centella asiatica* (L.) Urban] is another renowned Ayurvedic herb effectively used to improve memory and for rejuvenation in traditional practices. The activity of extracts from this plant has been increasingly investigated on telomerase activity. In a study, the authors found that Mandukaparni extract was able to trigger an almost nine-fold increase in telomerase activity compared to untreated human peripheral blood mononuclear cells [19]. Interestingly, in rodent models, treatment with Mandukaparni extract showed improvement in cognitive functions through improving mitochondrial and antioxidant gene expression in the brain and liver [20]. The plant extracts also have also been shown to promote wound healing (possibly attributed to the presence of triterpenoid saponins) via the facilitation of new skin cell growth, increasing skin tensile strength and resilience, and inhibiting bacterial growth [21]. Castasterone, a Mandukaparni leaf-derived phytoconstituent, was also able to inhibit H_2O_2-induced DNA damage in a single cell gel electrophoresis assay (comet assay) [22].

Brahmi [*Bacopa monnieri* (L.) Wettst. In Eng. & Prantl] is another Ayurvedic plant traditionally used as a nootropic and tonic agent. A study performed on Brahmi extracts reported an extraordinary adaptogenic potential and role in scavenging superoxide anion and hydroxyl radicals and in reducing H_2O_2-induced cytotoxicity and DNA damage in human fibroblast cells [23]. Additionally, in another study, Brahmi methanol extract also demonstrated a marked protective activity against H_2O_2-induced cytotoxicity and DNA damage in human non-immortalized fibroblasts [24]. Furthermore, another investigation reported a significant antioxidant and DNA damage preventive effect (using pRSETA plasmid grown in *E. coli*) in such extracts [25]. In a further investigation, Brahmi extracts displayed protective effects against sodium nitroprusside (SNP)-induced DNA damage [26]. For bacosides, bioactive constituents of Brahmi, remarkable potentialities have been reported in terms of scavenging free radicals and protecting neural cells from cytotoxicity and DNA damage in Alzheimer's disease [27].

Shankhapushpi (*Convolvulus pluricaulis* Choisy) is another Indian traditional plant widely used for its effective nootropic effects [28,29]. A study evaluated the neuroprotective potential of Shankhapushpi ethanol extract, and it was found to possess antioxidant and anti-apoptotic properties and to protect from H_2O_2-induced cytotoxicity and plasmid DNA damage [30].

Yashtimadhu (*Glycyrrhiza glabra* L.), aka Mulethi or Jethimadhu in traditional practice, is rich in glycyrrhizin (a triterpene saponin), and its root extracts have been reported to increase DNA resistance from $CdCl_2$-induced genetic and oxidative damages in human lymphocytes [31]. In vitro, such extracts also protected plasmid pBR322 DNA and microsomal membranes from γ-irradiation-induced strand breaks [32]. In another study, Yashtimadhu ethanol extract used at a concentration of 250 µg/mL, led to a ~33.56% increase in survival rate and 14.28% increase in lifespan in *C. elegans* model [33].

Vacha (*Acorus calamus* Linn.), is another Ayurvedic plant with potent antioxidant and cytoprotective abilities, being able to effectively protect DNA from γ-radiation-induced strand breaks and to enhance DNA repair process *in vitro* [34,35].

Tulsi (*Ocimum basilicum* L.) essential oil has been shown to raise the apparent telomeres length in cell culture and to downregulate the telomeric repeat binding factor 1 (TERF-1) telomere length suppressor [36]. Other authors found that bioactive compounds present in seed extracts from another Tulsi variety, i.e., *Ocimum tenuiflorum* L., exerted a prominent antioxidant potential and conferred DNA protection in a plasmid DNA pBR322 model [37].

Haridra (*Curcuma longa* L.) is also an extensively used medicinal herb and soul of Indian cuisine. Haridra aqueous extracts and its main constituent, curcumin, are found to be protective against lipid peroxide-induced DNA damage [38], twigs-dry leaves smoke condensate-induced DNA damage in calf thymus DNA and human peripheral lymphocytes [39], and fuel smoke condensate-induced DNA damage in human lymphocytes [40], although the mechanism of action has not yet been identified. A recent study in a mouse model with carboplatin-induced myelosuppression suggested that curcumin promotes the DNA repair pathway in bone marrow [41]. In addition, following the curcumin interaction with Kelch-like ECH-associated protein 1 (Keap 1), the nuclear factor E2-related factor 2 (Nrf2) is released, which regulates antioxidant enzymes, anti-inflammatory response proteins, and DNA repair enzymes [42]. In *Drosophila melanogaster* [43] and *C. elegans* [44] models, curcumin led to a 25.8% and 25.0% increase in mean lifespan, respectively.

Several polyherbal Ayurvedic formulations are also being investigated for anti-ageing purposes. Amalaki Rasayana (AR), prepared from Amalaki (*Emblica officinalis* Gaertn.) fruits, is a time-tested Ayurvedic Rasayana drug, widely used for the prevention or even treatment of various age-related health conditions. AR markedly reduces the DNA damage in brain cells and confers genomic stability in neurons and astrocytes [45], and at same time raising the median lifespan and starvation resistance in *D. melanogaster* model [46]. AR has also been revealed to be able to suppress neurodegeneration in fly models of Huntington's and AD [47]. A recent study with humans aged 45 to 60 years reported an increase in telomerase activity with no discernible change in telomere length in peripheral blood mononuclear cells following AR administration, suggesting that AR can avoid the telomeres erosion, promoting healthy ageing [48]. In aged human participants, AR intake maintained, or even enhanced, the DNA strand break repair, with no toxic effects [49]. Amalaki extract also exhibited neuroprotective effects from H_2O_2-induced DNA damage and repair in neuroblastoma cells [50].

Medhya Rasayana, a memory enhancer formulation prepared from a mixture of selected plants and their extracts, has a great ability to promote brain rejuvenation, triggering a marginal but sustained increase in constitutive DNA base excision repair in brain tissues of adult rats [51].

Another preparation, Brahma Rasayana, is a health-promoting formulation with >35 ingredients (*E. officinalis* and *Terminalia chebula* Retz. are the two major), increased constitutive DNA base excision repair and reduced clastogenicity [52].

Chyawanprash is also a popular health supplement traditionally used for rejuvenation, and displays cytoprotective and genoprotective effects [53], though more evidence is required to reinforce its longevity claims related to parameters, such as telomerase activation or telomere lengthening.

Triphala, a preparation of fruits of *Amalaki* (*E. officinalis*), *Bibhitaki* [*Terminalia bellerica* (Gaertn) Roxb.], and *Haritaki* (*T. chebula*), has shown a great ability to prevent and reverse radiation-induced DNA damage in various in vitro and animal models [54].

In short, the multiple Rasayana medicines reported in the Ayurveda literature, while extremely rich sources of key bioactive molecules, such as flavonoids and polyphenols, with remarkable antioxidant, adaptogenic, immunomodulatory, immunostimulant, cytoprotective and rejuvenating properties [8,9], underlines the hope that the ancient literary and experience-based knowledge base of Ayurveda has huge therapeutic potential, and thus can be used to discover and develop new anti-ageing drug candidates with potent telomerase activator, telomer protective and DNA repair properties.

Author Contributions: R.S. conceived the idea and wrote the manuscript. N.M. edited and proofread the document. All authors have read and agreed to published version of the manuscript.

Funding: This research received no external funding.

Acknowledgments: RS kindly acknowledge Banaras Hindu University for the seed grant under IOE for the year 2020-2021. NM acknowledges the Portuguese Foundation for Science and Technology under the Horizon 2020 Program (PTDC/PSI-GER/28076/2017).

Conflicts of Interest: The authors declare no conflict of interest.

References

1. Jin, K.; Simpkins, J.W.; Ji, X.; Leis, M.; Stambler, I. The Critical Need to Promote Research of Aging and Aging-Related Diseases to Improve Health and Longevity of the Elderly Population. *Aging Dis.* **2015**, *6*, 1–5. [CrossRef] [PubMed]
2. Blackburn, E.H. Switching and Signaling at the Telomere. *Cell* **2001**, *106*, 661–673. [CrossRef]
3. Greider, C.W.; Blackburn, E.H. Identification of a Specific Telomere Terminal Transferase Activity in Tetrahymena Extracts. *Cell* **1985**, *43*, 405–413. [CrossRef]
4. Mu, J.; Wei, L.X. Telomere and Telomerase in Oncology. *Cell Res.* **2002**, *12*, 1–7. [CrossRef]
5. Flores, I.; Benetti, R.; Blasco, M.A. Telomerase Regulation and Stem Cell Behaviour. *Curr. Opin. Cell Biol.* **2006**, *18*, 254–260. [CrossRef] [PubMed]
6. Maynard, S.; Fang, E.F.; Scheibye-Knudsen, M.; Croteau, D.L.; Bohr, V.A. DNA Damage, DNA Repair, Aging, and Neurodegeneration. *CSH Perspect. Med.* **2015**, *5*, a025130. [CrossRef]
7. Shammas, M.A. Telomeres, lifestyle, cancer, and aging. *Curr. Opin. Clin. Nutr. Metab. Care* **2011**, *14*, 28–34. [CrossRef] [PubMed]
8. Sharma, R.; Amin, H. Rasayana Therapy: Ayurvedic contribution to improve quality of life. *World J. Pharmacol. Res. Tech.* **2015**, *4*, 23–33.
9. Balasubramani, S.P.; Venkatasubramanian, P.; Kukkupuni, S.K.; Patwardhan, B. Plant-based Rasayana drugs from Ayurveda. *Chin. J. Integr. Med.* **2011**, *17*, 88–94. [CrossRef]
10. Kumar, R.; Gupta, K.; Saharia, K.; Pradhan, D.; Subramaniam, J.R. Withania somnifera root extract extends lifespan of Caenorhabditis elegans. *Ann. Neurosci.* **2013**, *20*, 13. [CrossRef]

11. Akhoon, B.A.; Pandey, S.; Tiwari, S.; Pandey, R. Withanolide A offers neuroprotection, ameliorates stress resistance and prolongs the life expectancy of Caenorhabditis elegans. *Exp. Gerontol.* **2016**, *78*, 47–56. [CrossRef] [PubMed]
12. Raguraman, V.; Subramaniam, J. Withania somnifera Root Extract Enhances Telomerase Activity in the Human HeLa Cell Line. *Adv. Biosci. Biotechnol.* **2016**, *7*, 199–204. [CrossRef]
13. Kumar, N.; Yadav, A.; Gupta, R.; Aggarwal, N. Antigenotoxic effect of Withania somnifera (Ashwagandha) extract against DNA damage induced by hydrogen peroxide in cultured human peripheral blood lymphocytes. *Int. J. Curr. Microbiol. Appl. Sci.* **2016**, *5*, 713–719. [CrossRef]
14. Sharma, R.; Amin, H.; Prajapati, P.; Ruknuddin, G. Therapeutic Vistas of Guduchi (*Tinospora cordifolia*): A medico-historical memoir. *J. Res. Educ. Ind. Med.* **2014**, *20*, 113–128.
15. Sharma, R.; Kumar, V.; Ashok, B.K.; Galib, R.; Prajapati, P.K.; Ravishankar, B. Evaluation of hypoglycaemic and anti-hyperglycaemic activities of Guduchi Ghana in Swiss albino mice. *Int. J. Green Pharm.* **2013**, *7*, 145–148. [CrossRef]
16. Sharma, R.; Kumar, V.; Ashok, B.K.; Galib, R.; Prajapati, P.K.; Ravishankar, B. Hypoglycemic and anti-hyperglycemic activity of Guduchi Satva in experimental animals. *Ayu* **2013**, *34*, 417. [CrossRef]
17. Masuma, R.; Okuno, T.; Kabir Choudhuri, M.S.; Saito, T.; Kurasaki, M. Effect of Tinospora cordifolia on the reduction of ultraviolet radiation-induced cytotoxicity and DNA damage in PC12 cells. *J. Environ. Sci. Health Part B* **2014**, *49*, 416–421. [CrossRef]
18. Ambasta, S.K.; Shashikant, S.U.K. Genoprotective effects of ethanolic stem extracts of Tinospora cordifolia on sodium arsenite-induced DNA damage in swiss mice lymphocytes by comet assay. *Asian J. Pharm. Clin. Res.* **2019**, *12*, 208–212. [CrossRef]
19. Tsoukalas, D.; Fragkiadaki, P.; Docea, A.O.; Alegakis, A.K.; Sarandi, E.; Thanasoula, M.; Spandidos, D.A.; Tsatsakis, A.; Razgonova, M.P.; Calina, D. Discovery of potent telomerase activators: Unfolding new therapeutic and anti-aging perspectives. *Mol. Med. Rep.* **2019**, *20*, 3701–3708. [CrossRef]
20. Gray, N.E.; Harris, C.J.; Quinn, J.F.; Soumyanath, A. *Centella asiatica* modulates antioxidant and mitochondrial pathways and improves cognitive function in mice. *J. Ethnopharmacol.* **2016**, *180*, 78–86. [CrossRef]
21. Somboonwong, J.; Kankaisre, M.; Tantisira, B.; Tantisira, M.H. Wound healing activities of different extracts of Centella asiatica in incision and burn wound models: An experimental animal study. *BMC Complement. Altern. Med.* **2012**. [CrossRef] [PubMed]
22. Sondhi, N.; Bhardwaj, R.; Kaur, S.; Chandel, M.; Kumar, N.; Singh, B. Inhibition of H_2O_2-induced DNA damage in single cell gel electrophoresis assay (comet assay) by castasterone isolated from leaves of Centella asiatica. *Health* **2010**, *2*, 595. [CrossRef]
23. Rai, D.; Bhatia, G.; Palit, G.; Pal, R.; Singh, S.; Singh, H.K. Adaptogenic effect of *Bacopa monniera* (Brahmi). *Pharmacol. Biochem. Behav.* **2003**, *75*, 823–830. [CrossRef]
24. Russo, A.; Izzo, A.A.; Borrelli, F.; Renis, M.; Vanella, A. Free radical scavenging capacity and protective effect of Bacopa monniera L. on DNA damage. *Phytother. Res.* **2003**, *17*, 870–875. [CrossRef]
25. Anand, T.; Naika, M.; Swamy, M.S.; Khanum, F. Antioxidant and DNA Damage Preventive Properties of Bacopa Monniera (L) Wettst. *Free Radic. Antioxid.* **2011**, *1*, 84–90. [CrossRef]
26. Anand, T.; Pandareesh, M.D.; Bhat, P.V.; Venkataramana, M. Anti-apoptotic mechanism of Bacoside rich extract against reactive nitrogen species induced activation of iNOS/Bax/caspase 3 mediated apoptosis in L132 cell line. *Cytotechnology* **2014**, *66*, 823–838. [CrossRef]
27. Singh, H.K.; Srimal, R.C.; Srivastava, A.K.; Garg, N.K.; Dhawan, B.N. Neuropsychopharmacological Effects of Bacosides A and B. In Proceedings of the Fourth Conference on the Neurobiology of Learning and Memory, Irvine, CA, USA, 17–20 October 1990.
28. Amin, H.; Sharma, R.; Vyas, H.; Vyas, M.; Prajapati, P.K.; Dwivedi, R. Nootropic (medhya) effect of Bhāvita Śaṇkhapuṣpī tablets: A clinical appraisal. *Anc. Sci. Life* **2014**, *34*, 109. [CrossRef]
29. Amin, H.; Sharma, R. Nootropic efficacy of Satvavajaya Chikitsa and Ayurvedic drug therapy: A comparative clinical exposition. *Int. J. Yoga* **2015**, *8*, 109. [CrossRef]
30. Rachitha, P.; Krupashree, K.; Jayashree, G.V.; Kandikattu, H.K.; Amruta, N.; Gopalan, N.; Rao, M.K.; Khanum, F. Chemical composition, antioxidant potential, macromolecule damage and neuroprotective activity of Convolvulus pluricaulis. *J. Tradit. Complement. Med.* **2018**, *8*, 483–496. [CrossRef]

31. Dirican, E.; Turkez, H. In vitro studies on protective effect of Glycyrrhiza glabra root extracts against cadmium-induced genetic and oxidative damage in human lymphocytes. *Cytotechnology* **2014**, *66*, 9–16. [CrossRef]
32. Shetty, T.K.; Satav, J.G.; Nair, C.K. Protection of DNA and microsomal membranes in vitro by Glycyrrhiza glabra L. against gamma irradiation. *Phytother. Res.* **2002**, *16*, 576–578. [CrossRef] [PubMed]
33. Reigada, I.; Moliner, C.; Valero, M.S.; Weinkove, D.; Langa, E.; Gómez Rincón, C. Antioxidant and Antiaging Effects of Licorice on the Caenorhabditis elegans Model. *J. Med. Food* **2020**, *23*, 72–78. [CrossRef] [PubMed]
34. Sandeep, D.; Nair, C.K. Protection of DNA and membrane from γ-radiation induced damage by the extract of Acorus calamus Linn.: An in vitro study. *Environ. Toxicol. Pharmacol.* **2010**, *29*, 302–307. [CrossRef] [PubMed]
35. Sharma, V.; Sharma, R.; Gautam, D.S.; Kuca, K.; Nepovimova, E.; Martins, N. Role of Vacha (Acorus calamus Linn.) in Neurological and Metabolic Disorders: Evidence from Ethnopharmacology, Phytochemistry, Pharmacology and Clinical Study. *J. Clin. Med.* **2020**, *9*, 1176. [CrossRef]
36. Plant, J. Effects of essential oils on telomere length in human cells. *Med. Aromat. Plants* **2016**, *5*, 1–6.
37. Kaur, P.; Dhull, S.B.; Sandhu, K.S.; Salar, R.K.; Purewal, S.S. Tulsi (Ocimum tenuiflorum) seeds: In vitro DNA damage protection, bioactive compounds and antioxidant potential. *J. Food Meas. Charact.* **2018**, *12*, 1530–1538. [CrossRef]
38. Shalini, V.K.; Srinivas, L. Lipid peroxide induced DNA damage: Protection by turmeric (Curcuma longa). *Mol. Cell. Biochem.* **1987**, *77*, 3–10. [CrossRef]
39. Srinivas, L.; Shalini, V.K. DNA damage by smoke: Protection by turmeric and other inhibitors of ROS. *Free Radic. Biol. Med.* **1991**, *11*, 277–283. [CrossRef]
40. Shalini, V.K.; Srinivas, L. Fuel smoke condensate induced DNA damage in human lymphocytes and protection by turmeric (Curcuma longa). *Mol. Cell. Biochem.* **1990**, *95*, 21–30. [CrossRef]
41. Chen, X.; Wang, J.; Fu, Z.; Zhu, B.; Wang, J.; Guan, S.; Hua, Z. Curcumin activates DNA repair pathway in bone marrow to improve carboplatin-induced myelosuppression. *Sci. Rep.* **2017**, *7*, 1–11. [CrossRef]
42. Bryan, H.K.; Olayanju, A.; Goldring, C.E.; Park, B.K. The Nrf2 cell defence pathway: Keap1-dependent and-independent mechanisms of regulation. *Biochem. Pharmacol.* **2013**, *85*, 705–717. [CrossRef] [PubMed]
43. Shen, L.R.; Xiao, F.; Yuan, P.; Chen, Y.; Gao, Q.K.; Parnell, L.D.; Meydani, M.; Ordovas, J.M.; Li, D.; Lai, C.Q. Curcumin-supplemented diets increase superoxide dismutase activity and mean lifespan in Drosophila. *Age* **2013**, *35*, 1133–1142. [CrossRef] [PubMed]
44. Cuanalo-Contreras, K.; Park, K.W.; Mukherjee, A.; Peña, L.M.; Soto, C. Delaying aging in Caenorhabditis elegans with protein aggregation inhibitors. *Biochem. Biophys. Res. Commun.* **2017**, *482*, 62–67. [CrossRef]
45. Swain, U.; Sindhu, K.K.; Boda, U.; Pothani, S.; Giridharan, N.V.; Raghunath, M.; Rao, K.S. Studies on the molecular correlates of genomic stability in rat brain cells following Amalaki Rasyana therapy. *Mech. Ageing Dev.* **2012**, *133*, 112–117. [CrossRef] [PubMed]
46. Dwivedi, V.; Anandan, E.M.; Mony, R.S.; Muraleedharan, T.S.; Valiathan, M.S.; Mutsuddi, M.; Lakhotia, S.C. In vivo effects of traditional Ayurvedic formulations in Drosophila melanogaster model relate with therapeutic applications. *PLoS ONE* **2012**, *7*, e37113. [CrossRef]
47. Dwivedi, V.; Tripathi, B.K.; Mutsuddi, M.; Lakhotia, S.C. Ayurvedic Amalaki Rasayana and Rasa-Sindoor suppress neurodegeneration in fly models of Huntington's and Alzheimer's diseases. *Curr. Sci.* **2013**, *104*, 1711–1723.
48. Guruprasad, K.P.; Dash, S.; Shivakumar, M.B.; Shetty, P.R.; Raghu, K.S.; Shamprasad, B.R.; Udupi, V.; Acharya, R.V.; Vidya, P.B.; Nayak, J.; et al. Influence of Amalaki Rasayana on telomerase activity and telomere length in human blood mononuclear cells. *J. Ayurveda Integr. Med.* **2017**, *8*, 105–112. [CrossRef]
49. Vishwanatha, U.; Guruprasad, K.P.; Gopinath, P.M.; Acharya, R.V.; Prasanna, B.V.; Nayak, J.; Ganesh, R.; Rao, J.; Shree, R.; Anchan, S.; et al. Effect of Amalaki rasayana on DNA damage and repair in randomized aged human individuals. *J. Ethnopharmacol.* **2016**, *191*, 387–397. [CrossRef]
50. Ramakrishna, V.; Gupta, K.P.; Setty, H.O.; Kondapi, K.A. Neuroprotective effect of Emblica officinalis extract against H2O2 induced DNA damage and repair in neuroblastoma cells. *J. Homeopath. Ayurvedic Med. Sci.* **2014**, *1*, 1–5.
51. Raghu, K.S.; Shamprasad, B.R.; Kabekkodu, S.P.; Paladhi, P.; Joshi, M.B.; Valiathan, M.S.; Guruprasad, K.P.; Satyamoorthy, K. Age dependent neuroprotective effects of medhya rasayana prepared from Clitoria ternatea Linn. in stress induced rat brain. *J. Ethnopharmacol.* **2017**, *197*, 173–183. [CrossRef]

52. Guruprasad, K.P.; Subramanian, A.; Singh, V.J.; Sharma, R.S.K.; Gopinath, P.M.; Sewram, V.; Varier, P.M.; Satyamoorthy, K. Brahmarasayana protects against Ethyl methanesulfonate or Methyl methanesulfonate induced chromosomal aberrations in mouse bone marrow cells. *BMC Complement. Altern. Med.* **2012**, *12*, 1–9. [CrossRef] [PubMed]
53. Sharma, R.; Martins, N.; Kuca, K.; Chaudhary, A.; Kabra, A.; Rao, M.M.; Prajapati, P.K. Chyawanprash A Traditional Indian Bioactive Health Supplement. *Biomolecules* **2019**, *9*, 161. [CrossRef] [PubMed]
54. Peterson, C.T.; Denniston, K.; Chopra, D. Therapeutic uses of Triphala in Ayurvedic medicine. *J. Altern. Complement. Med.* **2017**, *23*, 607–614. [CrossRef] [PubMed]

Journal of
Clinical Medicine

MDPI

Article

Kurarinone Inhibits HCoV-OC43 Infection by Impairing the Virus-Induced Autophagic Flux in MRC-5 Human Lung Cells

Jung Sun Min [1,2], Dong Eon Kim [1,2], Young-Hee Jin [2,3,*] and Sunoh Kwon [1,2,*]

1 Herbal Medicine Research Division, Korea Institute of Oriental Medicine, Daejeon 34054, Korea; jsmin1019@kiom.re.kr (J.S.M.); ehddjs0@kiom.re.kr (D.E.K.)
2 Center for Convergent Research of Emerging Virus Infection, Korea Research Institute of Chemical Technology, Daejeon 34114, Korea
3 KM Application Center, Korea Institute of Oriental Medicine, Daegu 41062, Korea
* Correspondence: jinohee@kiom.re.kr (Y.-H.J.); sunohkwon@kiom.re.kr (S.K.); Tel.: +82-42-610-8850 (Y.-H.J.); +82-42-868-9675 (S.K.)

Received: 20 May 2020; Accepted: 9 July 2020; Published: 14 July 2020

Abstract: Kurarinone is a prenylated flavonone isolated from the roots of *Sophora flavescens*. Among its known functions, kurarinone has both anti-apoptotic and anti-inflammatory properties. Coronaviruses (CoVs), including HCoV-OC43, SARS-CoV, MERS-CoV, and SARS-CoV-2, are the causative agents of respiratory virus infections that range in severity from the common cold to severe pneumonia. There are currently no effective treatments for coronavirus-associated diseases. In this report, we examined the anti-viral impact of kurarinone against infection with the human coronavirus, HCoV-OC43. We found that kurarinone inhibited HCoV-OC43 infection in human lung fibroblast MRC-5 cells in a dose-dependent manner with an IC_{50} of 3.458 ± 0.101 μM. Kurarinone inhibited the virus-induced cytopathic effect, as well as extracellular and intracellular viral RNA and viral protein expression. Time-of-addition experiments suggested that kurarinone acted at an early stage of virus infection. Finally, we found that HCoV-OC43 infection increased the autophagic flux in MRC-5 cells; kurarinone inhibited viral replication via its capacity to impair the virus-induced autophagic flux. As such, we suggest that kurarinone may be a useful therapeutic for the treatment of diseases associated with coronavirus infection.

Keywords: kurarinone; coronavirus; HCoV-OC43; autophagy; infection; MRC-5 cell; LC3; p62/SQSTM1 protein

---

1. Introduction

Infection with human coronavirus HCoV-OC43 was first described in the 1960s; this virus is a representative and prototype of the virus family *Coronaviridae*. HCoV-OC43 is typically associated with mild respiratory tract infections. By contrast, the emergence of Severe Acute Respiratory Syndrome–associated coronavirus (SARS-CoV) in 2002 and the Middle East respiratory syndrome coronavirus (MERS-CoV) in 2012 proved that coronavirus pathogens can initiate cross-species infections and create significant healthcare risks [1]. Indeed, the novel SARS-CoV-2 pathogen has generated a global pandemic severe respiratory infection known as Coronavirus Disease 2019 (COVID-19). Although the antiviral agent, remdesivir, was recently authorized for emergency use for treatment for severely ill COVID-19 patients [2], the clinical utility and safety of remdesivir remains under investigation [3,4].

Viruses utilize various cellular processes to promote intracellular replication. Cellular autophagy is a particularly important feature promoting viral replication due to the fact that vesicle formation is critical to formation of autophagosomes and for transport of viral components [5]. The influenza A virus (IAV) [6], human immunodeficiency virus (HIV) [7,8], zikavirus (ZIKV) [9], and herpes simplex virus (HSV) [10] all use autophagy to promote viral replication and virion production [11]. Likewise, the hepatitis C virus (HCV) induces autophagy and can escape autophagic destruction [12] and treatment with an autophagy inhibitor-inhibited replication of the influenza A virus H3N2 [13]. Conversely, host cells also use autophagy as a means to inhibit viral replication to eliminate viral particles and to stimulate the immune response in order to prevent virus-induced disease. Autophagic processes can stimulate production of interferon and thereby promote innate immune signaling that ultimately results in degradation of the viral RNA genome and viral proteins (i.e., virophagy) [12,14,15]. The highly pathogenic avian influenza virus H5N1, Coxsackievirus B3, and HSV-1 were all reported to include mechanisms that facilitate escape from the autophagic degradation [12,16,17]. In the case of coronaviruses, SARS-CoV and the murine hepatitis virus (MHV) were reported to induce the formation of double-membrane-bound replication complexes that served to enhance viral replication [18]. Similarly, autophagic processes were critical features supporting the replication of the transmissible gastroenteritis virus (TGEV); furthermore, virus infection resulted in an increase in the autophagic flux [19].

Kurarinone is a prenylated flavonone isolated from the roots of the Asian shrub, *Sophora flavescens*; it is used as an analgesic in traditional Asian medicine. Kurarinone has been identified as an agent capable of inducing cell death by the activation of pro-apoptotic proteins and via the caspase-dependent pathway [20]; kurarinone also sensitizes TRAIL-induced tumor cell apoptosis via suppression of NF-κB-dependent cFLIP expression [21]. In other studies, kurarinone inhibited the development of chronic inflammatory dermatitis via suppression of $CD4^+$ T cell differentiation [22]; combined administration of kurarinone and IFNα-1b promotes a positive response in patients with chronic hepatitis B [23]. Interestingly, kurarinone was shown to induce autophagic cell death via activation of autophagy-related proteins in human hepato-carcinoma cells [20]. However, to the best of our knowledge, there are no experimental reports directed at elucidating the antiviral impact of kurarinone.

In this study, we demonstrated that kurarinone inhibited HCoV-OC43 infection by interfering with virus-induced autophagy in the human lung cell MRC-5 line. As such, this study features a therapeutic approach to inhibit coronavirus infection by targeting virus-induced autophagy. Our work suggests that kurarinone may be useful as a novel therapeutic drug for the treatment of coronavirus disease.

2. Experimental Section

2.1. Preparation of Compounds

Kurarinone (PubChem CID: 10812923) was purchased from ChemFace (Wuhan, China), and remdesivir (PubChem CID: 121304016) was purchased from LALPharm Co., Ltd. (Beijing, China). Compounds were dissolved in dimethyl sulfoxide (DMSO), and stored as 20 mM stock solutions at −80°C. The stock solutions were diluted in serum-free culture medium prior to use. The final concentration of DMSO did not exceed 0.05%.

2.2. Cells and Virus Infection

The MRC-5 cell line was obtained from American Type Culture Collection (ATCC, Manassas, VA, USA). MRC-5 cells were cultured in Modified Eagle's medium (MEM; Corning Incorporated, Corning, NY, USA) containing 10% fetal bovine serum (FBS; Gibco, Carlsbad, CA, USA) and 1% penicillin/streptomycin at 37 °C in 5% CO_2. Human coronavirus-OC43 (HCoV-OC43) was obtained from ATCC and propagated and titrated, as previously described [24]. The titer of the purified HCoV-OC43 was $10^{6.5}$ $TCID_{50}$ units (median tissue culture infectious dose)/100 μL. MRC-5 cells were seeded in 96-well plates at 5×10^3 cells/well, infected with HCoV-OC43 ($10^{3.5}$ $TCID_{50}$/100 μL) and then incubated for 4 days at 33 °C.

2.3. MTS Assay

Cell viability was determined using the colorimetric 3-(4,5-dimethylthiazol-2-yl)-5-(3-carboxymethoxyphenyl)-2-(4-sulfophenyl)-2H-tetrazolium (MTS) assay (Promega Corporation, Madison, WI, USA) according to the manufacturer's instructions. Absorbance was detected at 490 nm using a GloMax Microplate Reader (Promega).

2.4. Quantification of HCoV-OC43 RNA Copy Number

The viral RNA in the culture supernatants was isolated using a viral RNA purification QiaAMP kit (Qiagen, Hilden, Germany). Viral RNA in cell lysates were isolated using an RNeasy RNA purification kit (Qiagen) according to the manufacturer's instructions. Quantitative reverse transcription PCR (qRT-PCR) was performed using the One Step SYBR® PrimeScriptTM RT-PCR Kit (Takara Bio Inc., Shiga, Japan) according to the manufacturer's protocol using primer pairs to amplify the HCoV-OC43 Nucleoprotein (NP) gene that included a sense primer, 5′-AGCAACCAGGCTGATGTCAATACC-3′, and an antisense primer, 5′-AGCAGACCTTCCTGAGCCTTCAAT-3′. The copy number was calculated using a standard curve of known concentrations of HCoV-OC43 RNA.

2.5. Western Blot Assay

MRC-5 cells were seeded in 24-well plates. Cells were harvested and lysed in Glo Lysis buffer (Promega). Proteins were separated on the SDS-PAGE gel and transferred to a nitrocellulose filter membrane (Bio-Rad Laboratories, Hercules, CA, USA). The membranes were blocked with 5% skim milk in tris-buffered saline with 0.5% Tween (TBST) for 30 min at room temperature (RT). The membranes were then rinsed with TBST and incubated with specific antibodies, including anti-viral-Spike protein (CusaBio Technology LLC, Houston, TX, USA), anti-LC3 protein (Abcam, Cambridge, United Kingdom), anti-p62/SQSTM1 protein (Abcam) or anti-β-actin (Cell Signaling Technology Inc., Danvers, MA, USA) at 4 °C overnight. Membranes were then incubated with horseradish peroxidase (HRP)-conjugated secondary antibodies (Abcam) for 1 h at RT and then developed with ECL solution (Thermo) using Chemidoc (Bio-Rad).

2.6. Quantification of Cytokine mRNA by qRT-PCR

Total RNA was isolated with the RNeasy® Mini kit (Qiagen) according to the manufacturer's instructions, and was used to synthesize complementary DNA (cDNA) using the One Step SYBR® PrimeScript™ RT-PCR Kit (Takara Bio) according to the manufacturer's instructions. The following specific primers used for qRT-PCR were the following: for IFN-β1, sense primer 5′-ACCAACAAGTGTCTCCTCCA-3′ and antisense primer 5′-GTAGTGGAGAAGCACAACAGG-3; for β-Actin, sense primer 5′-GGAAATCGTGCGTGACATCA-3′ and antisense primer 5′-ATCT CCTGCTCGAAGTCCAG-3′.

2.7. Immunofluorescence Assay

MRC-5 cells were grown on coverslips; cells were fixed with 4% para-formaldehyde for 10 min and washed with phosphate-buffered saline (PBS). Cells were permeabilized with PBS containing 0.2% Triton X-100 for 10 min and blocked with 3% bovine serum albumin (BSA) for 30 min. After blocking, cells were incubated with anti-HCoV-OC43 S protein antibody (CusaBio) and/or anti-p62/SQSTM1 protein antibody (Abcam) at 4 °C overnight, followed by AlexaFluor555 goat-anti-rabbit IgG (ThermoFisher, Waltham, MA, USA) and/or AlexaFluor488 goat-anti-mouse IgG (ThermoFisher) at room temperature for 1 h. The labeled cells were mounted on slides with SlowFade Gold anti-fade reagent with DAPI (Invitrogen) and visualized by fluorescence microscopy (Olympus Corporation, Tokyo, Japan). Immunofluorescence data were quantified using ImageJ software (NIH).

2.8. Time-of-Addition Assay

MRC-5 cells (5×10^3) were seeded in 96-well plates overnight. For the pretreatment assay, the cells were pre-treated with the compounds at concentrations indicated. After 24 h, the media were removed, and cells were washed and infected with HCoV-OC43 for 4 days at 33 °C. For the co-treatment and post-treatment assays, the compounds were added to the MRC-5 cell cultures during inoculation of the virus (co-treatment) or at 24 h after the virus was removed (post-treatment). At 4 dpi, the cell viability was determined using the MTS assay described above.

2.9. Statistical Analysis

The data were presented as the mean ± SEM. Statistical comparison by two-way analysis of variance (ANOVA) followed by Bonferroni's multiple comparison's test and non-linear regression analysis of IC_{50} and CC_{50} were conducted using GraphPad Prism® Software V.6.05 for Windows (GraphPad Software Inc., San Diego, CA, USA). P values of less than 0.05 indicated statistical significance.

3. Results

3.1. Kurarinone Inhibited HCoV-OC43 Infection in MRC-5 Cells

Kurarinone is a flavonoid isolated from the roots of *Sophora flavescens* (Figure 1A). To examine its inhibitory activity with respect to HCoV-OC43 infection, we added kurarinone to uninfected or HCoV-OC43-infected MRC-5 cells for a period of 4 days. We determined the cytotoxic concentration $(CC)_{50}$ of kurarinone for MRC-5 cells at 7.953 ± 0.148 μM by MTS assay (Figure 1B). We found that administration of kurarinone inhibited the virus-induced cytopathic effect (CPE) in a dose-dependent manner. As a positive control, 5 μM remdesivir was used (Figure 1C). An inhibitory concentration $(IC)_{50}$ for kurarinone was calculated at 3.458 ± 0.101 μM by nonlinear regression analysis (Figure 1D). As such, we confirmed that kurarinone had antiviral activity against HCoV-OC43; we used 5 μM kurarinone for all further experiments. We then evaluated the impact of kurarinone on cell growth and morphology; we treated HCoV-OC43-infected MRC-5 cells with 5 μM kurarinone for 4 days and examined the morphology of cells by light microscopy. As shown in Figure 1E, HCoV-OC43 induced a clear cytopathic effect (CPE) that was detected in infected cells at 4 days post-infection (dpi); by contrast, cells treated with kurarinone had no virus-induced CPE and were indistinguishable from uninfected cells.

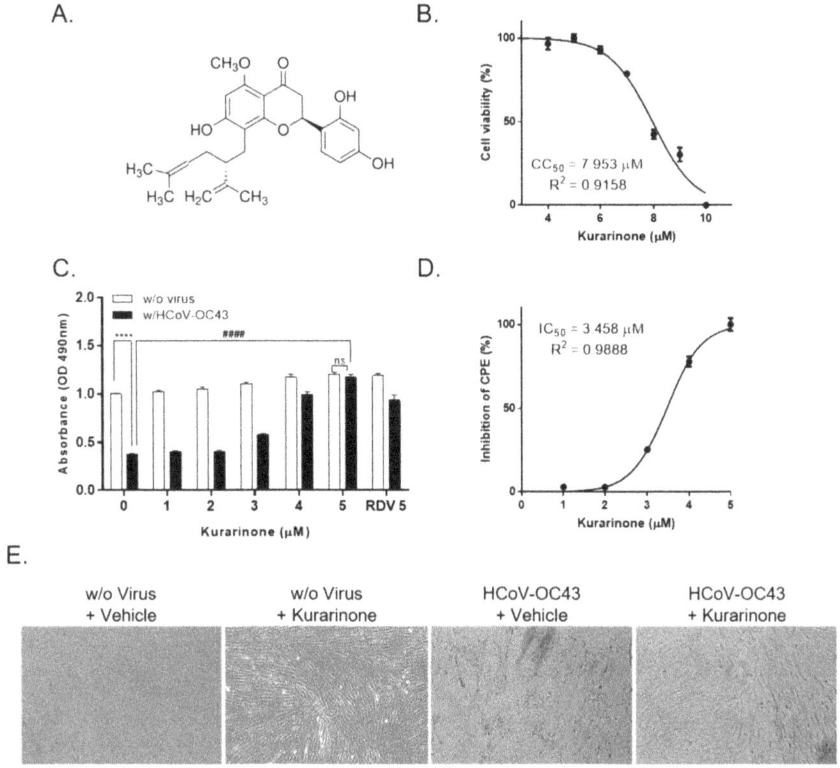

Figure 1. Chemical structure of kurarinone and antiviral activities in MRC-5 cells. (**A**) Chemical structure of kurarinone; (**B**) cytotoxicity associated with kurarinone. MRC-5 cells were incubated with increasing concentrations of kurarinone for 4 days; cell viability was measured by MTS assay (vehicle-treated cell as 100% of viability, 20% DMSO treated cell as 0% of viability). Cytotoxic concentration (CC_{50}) of kurarinone was calculated after 4 days by nonlinear regression analysis; (**C**) Antiviral impact of kurarinone determined by degree of virus-induced cytopathic effect (CPE). MRC-5 cells were infected with HCoV-OC43 and incubated with various concentrations of kurarinone, or positive control, remdesivir (RDV) 5 μM for 4 days; cell viability was measured by MTS assay; (**D**) Inhibitory concentration (IC_{50}) of kurarinone was calculated at 4 days post-infection (dpi) by nonlinear regression analysis. (vehicle-treated virus-infected cell as 0% of inhibition, vehicle-treated non-virus infected cell as 100% of inhibition); (**E**) Images of virus-infected MRC-5 cells at 4 dpi. Data were presented as means ± SEM of three independent experiments, and analyzed by two-way ANOVA with Bonferroni's multiple comparisons test and nonlinear regression analysis. Virus effect, $F(1, 36) = 1522$; dose effect, $F(5, 36) = 238.6$; virus × dose interaction, $F(5, 36) = 93.39$; n.s., not significant; **** $p < 0.0001$; #### $p < 0.0001$.

3.2. *Kurarinone Inhibited HCoV-OC43 Replication and Viral Protein Expression in MRC-5 Cells*

To examine the impact of kurarinone on virus replication, MRC-5 cells were infected with HCoV-OC43. Culture supernatants and cells pellet were harvested separately on days 1, 2, 3, and 4 post-infection; viral RNA levels were evaluated by qRT-PCR. As shown in Figure 2A, the level of HCoV-OC43 RNA in cell culture supernatant, which is the released viral RNA increased over time in cells treated with vehicle alone; the level of viral RNA in the supernatants of kurarinone-treated cells was significantly reduced. Consistent with the findings from cell culture supernatants, intracellular viral RNA was detected in MRC-5 lysates from vehicle-treated cells and at decreased levels in cells treated with kurarinone (Figure 2B).

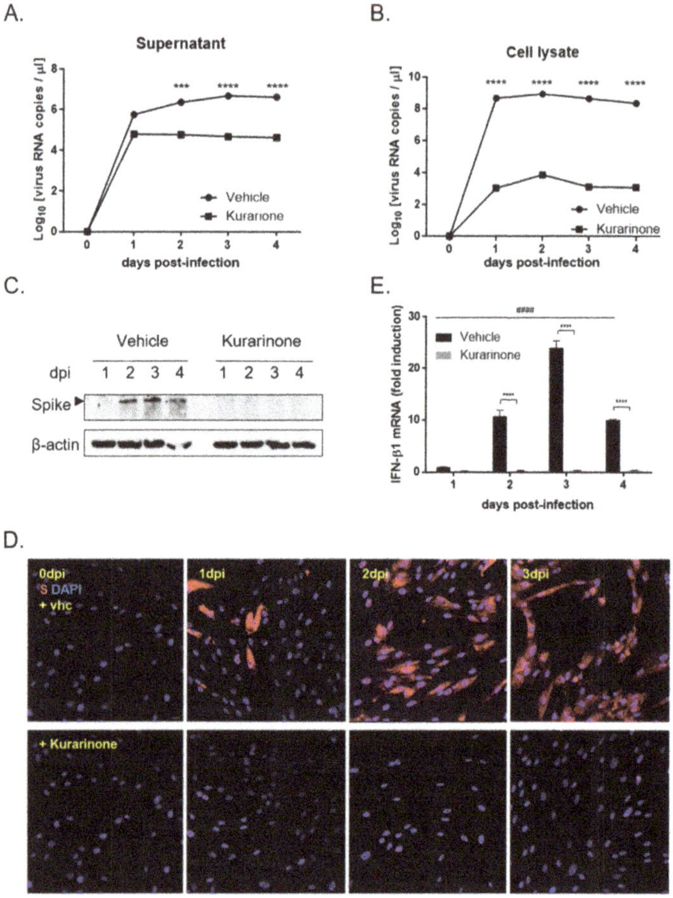

Figure 2. Detection of viral RNA and virus Spike protein in cell cultures treated with kurarinone. Viral RNA was purified from (**A**) culture supernatants or (**B**) cell lysates for quantification of HCoV-OC43 virus replication. RNA copy numbers were measured by qRT-PCR; (**C**) Western blot of the lysates of HCoV-OC43-infected MRC-5 cells treated with kurarinone or vehicle and evaluated at 1, 2, 3, and 4 dpi. The HCoV-OC43 Spike protein was detected and indicated by an arrowhead as shown; β-actin was used as a loading control. (**D**) Immunofluorescence analysis of HCoV-OC43-infected MRC-5 cells treated with vehicle (vhc) or kurarinone; cells were probed with an anti-viral Spike protein-specific antibody (red) and mounted with DAPI (blue) at 0, 1, 2, and 3 dpi. Scale bar is 50 µm. (**E**) Quantification of mRNA encoding interferon (IFN)-β1 by qRT-PCR in vehicle and kurarinone-treated MRC-5 cells; probes targeting the β-actin gene were used for data normalization. Data were presented as means ± SEM of three independent experiments, and analyzed by two-way ANOVA with Bonferroni's multiple comparisons test. In (A), treatment effect, $F(1, 8) = 218.7$; dpi effect, $F(4, 8) = 36.31$; treatment × dpi interaction, $F(4, 8) = 36.1$; in (B), treatment effect, $F(1, 8) = 2766$; dpi effect, $F(4, 8) = 338.5$; treatment × dpi interaction, $F(4, 8) = 338.5$; *** $p < 0.001$, **** $p < 0.0001$ versus vehicle-treated group; in (E), treatment effect, $F(1, 8) = 617.4$; dpi effect, $F(3, 8) = 112.7$; treatment × dpi interaction, $F(3, 8) = 112.0$; **** $p < 0.0001$ versus virus-infected and vehicle-treated group, #### $p < 0.0001$ versus virus-infected vehicle-treated group at 1 dpi.

We also evaluated HCoV-OC43 Spike protein expression in infected MRC-5 cells both with and without kurarinone treatment via Western blot analysis (Figure 2C). Viral Spike protein was first detected at 2 dpi in vehicle-treated cells; no S protein was detected in virus-infected and kurarinone-treated cells during the entire time period evaluated. Similarly, HCoV-OC43 Spike protein was detected in the cytoplasm of virus-infected cells examined by immunofluorescence at 1, 2, and 3 dpi; no Spike protein was detected in virus-infected and kurarinone-treated cells at this time point (Figure 2D).

To evaluate the impact of kurarinone treatment on the induction of the host antiviral response, we examined expression of the host antiviral gene, IFN-β1, in response to virus infection. IFN-β1 mRNA was induced prominently and time-dependently in MRC-5 cells during the 3 days after infection with HCoV-OC45, and then reduced at 4 dpi; by contrast, no IFN-β1 mRNA was detected in virus-infected cells that were treated with kurarinone (Figure 2E). These data suggested that the antiviral impact of kurarinone may not be related to its capacity to induce the host antiviral immune response.

3.3. Kurarinone Inhibits HCoV-OC43 Infection at the Early Stage of Virus Infection

In an effort to identify the stage of the HCoV-OC43 life cycle that is affected by the administration of kurarinone, we designed pre-treatment (kurarinone added for a period of 24 h prior to infection), co-treatment (kurarinone together with virus for the full 96 h), and post-treatment experiments (kurarinone added for 24 h after virus was introduced; Figure 3A). As shown in Figure 3B, when kurarinone was added to the cell culture before virus infection (pre-treatment), no protection against virus-induced CPE was observed. By contrast, the addition of kurarinone for a period of 24 h post-infection (post-treatment) resulted in up to 70% protection against virus-induced CPE, while co-treatment with kurarinone at a 5 μM concentration completely abolished virus-induced CPE (Figure 3B). These data suggested that the antiviral effect of kurarinone was focused on the early stages of virus infection; kurarinone was clearly most effective when added within 24 h of initial HCoV-OC43 infection.

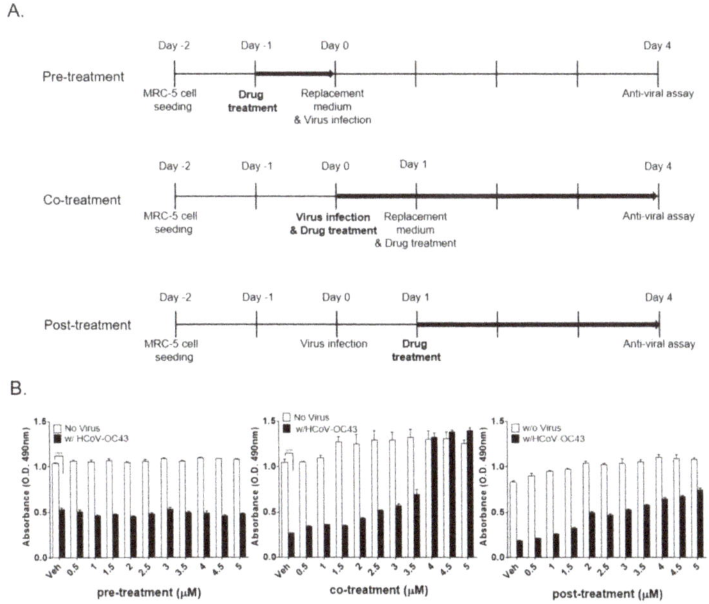

Figure 3. Time-of-addition assay to evaluate the impact of kurarinone. (**A**) Overall scheme for time-of-addition assay. The bold arrows denote the duration of kurarinone treatment. Kurarinone was

added to MRC-5 cultures 24 h before infection, for 96 h during infection, or 24 h after virus infection; (**B**) Virus-induced cytopathic effect (CPE) was determined by MTS-based assay at 4 dpi. Data were presented as means ± SEM of three independent experiments, and analyzed by two-way ANOVA with Bonferroni's multiple comparisons test; pre-treatment virus effect, $F(1, 50) = 6494$, $p < 0.0001$; dose effect, $F(10, 50) = 1.695$, $p = 0.1081$; virus × dose interaction, $F(10, 50) = 2.478$, $p = 0.0170$; co-treatment virus effect, $F(1, 50) = 568.6$, $p < 0.0001$; dose effect, $F(10, 50) = 52.08$, $p < 0.0001$; virus × dose interaction, $F(10, 50) = 28.85$, $p < 0.0001$; post-treatment virus effect, $F(1, 50) = 3631$, $p < 0.0001$; dose effect, $F(10, 50) = 101.9$, $p < 0.0001$; virus × dose interaction, $F(10, 50) = 16.00$, $p < 0.0001$; n.s., not significant; **** $p < 0.0001$ versus virus-infected vehicle-treated group.

3.4. Kurarinone Inhibits the HCoV-OC43 Infection by Modulating the Autophagy

Earlier reports indicate that infection with the MHV coronavirus-induced autophagy was required for effective virus replication [25]; kurarinone was also reported to modulate the expression of autophagy-associated protein [20]. As such, we proceeded to explore whether kurarinone was capable of modulating autophagy in HCoV-OC43-infected cells. To monitor autophagy, expression of LC3-I and LC3-II was examined in virus–infected cells by Western blot in cultures both with and without kurarinone (Figure 4A); the relative intensities of the protein bands are as shown in Figure 4B.

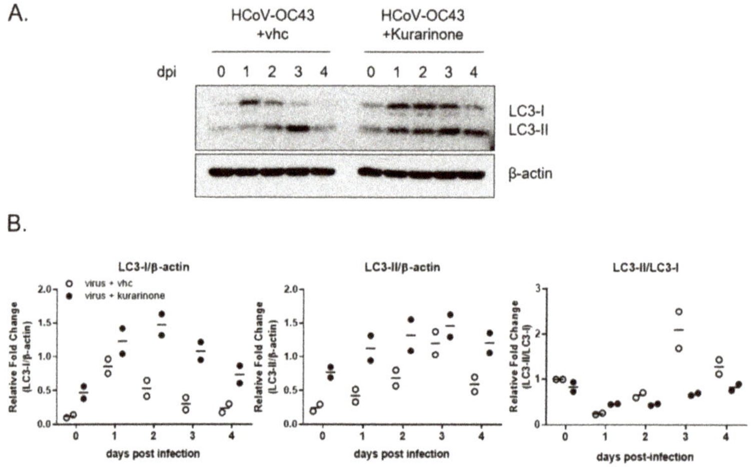

Figure 4. Autophagy induced by HCoV-OC43 infection was impaired by administration of kurarinone; (**A**) MRC-5 cells were infected with HCoV-OC43, treated with kurarinone or vehicle (vhc), and evaluated post-infection (dpi) on days 0, 1, 2, 3, and 4 by Western blot probed with anti-LC3 protein antibody; β-actin was used as the internal loading control. (**B**) The protein band intensities of LC3-I and LC3-II were quantified. Data were presented as means of two independent experiments.

LC3-I expression increases at day 1 of HCoV-OC43 infection, and then falls thereafter, beginning on 2 dpi. Levels of phosphatidylethanolamine (PE)-conjugated LC3-I, LC3-II gradually increase until 3 dpi, and then decrease thereafter. The LC-3-I/II transversion (LC3-II/LC3-I ratio), an indicator of autophagy activity, increases steadily until 3 dpi and then decreases at day 4; these results suggest that autophagy increases for 3 dpi and that LC3-II undergoes autophagic degradation, beginning at 4 dpi [26]. Taken together, these data confirm that HCoV-OC43 induced cellular autophagy in infected MRC-5 cells; these findings are consistent with those reported previously for infection with other coronaviruses [27]. However, expression of both LC3-I and LC3-II proteins increased simultaneously for 2 dpi in response to administration of kurarinone to levels that were higher than those of either untreated infected cells or cells treated with vehicle alone. The level of LC3-I protein decreased, starting at 3 dpi; levels of LC3-II remained high for 3 dpi and were not degraded at 4 dpi, as were those detected in virus-infected cells and cells treated with vehicle alone. Finally, LC-3-I/II transversion was lower in virus-infected cells treated with kurarinone than in those of vehicle-treated and virus-infected cells alone; this was largely due to persistently high levels of LC3-I. Taken together, these results suggest that kurarinone has an impact on cellular autophagy induced by HCoV-OC43 infection.

Finally, we examined expression of p62/SQSTM1 protein, a recognized indicator of autophagic flux together with the expression of LC3 protein and viral Spike protein (Figure 5A). Expression p62/SQSTM1 protein was time-dependently reduced during virus infection (Supplementary Figure S1A); these results indicate that the autophagy flux was increased in response to virus infection. Interestingly, p62/SQSTM1 protein levels were increased at days 2 and 3 in those that were kurarinone-treated, including those both infected and uninfected by HCoV-OC43. Furthermore, we determined the time to kurarinone-mediated induction of p62/SQSTM1 at 3, 6, 24, and 48 hpi. Levels of p62/SQSTM1 protein increased from 6 h of treatment, reaching a maximum at 48 h and remaining sustained throughout the period of virus infection (Figure 5B). Moreover, the immunofluorescence assay showed that HCoV-OC43-infected and kurarinone-treated cells exhibited a higher level of p62/SQSTM1 protein than those of HCoV-OC43 infected cells at 1, 2, and 3 dpi (Figure 5C). Some cells showed the increased level of p62/SQSTM1 protein without Spike protein expression. It may be the transiently increased p62/SQSTM1 protein in cells where there is an increase in autophagy flux at initial stage of virus infection, before Spike protein is expressed. We also confirmed that autophagy inhibitors, NH_4Cl, and Chloroquine induced the p62/SQSTM1 proteins, which were known to inhibit the coronavirus infection (Supplementary Figure S1B). As such, these data suggest that kurarinone can inhibit HCoV-OC43 infection by inducing expression of p62/SQSTM1 protein and thereby impairing the autophagic flux.

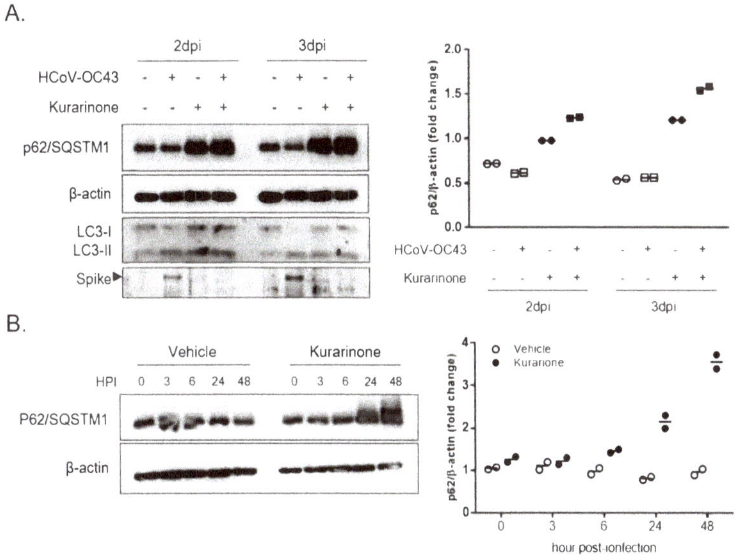

Figure 5. *Cont.*

C.

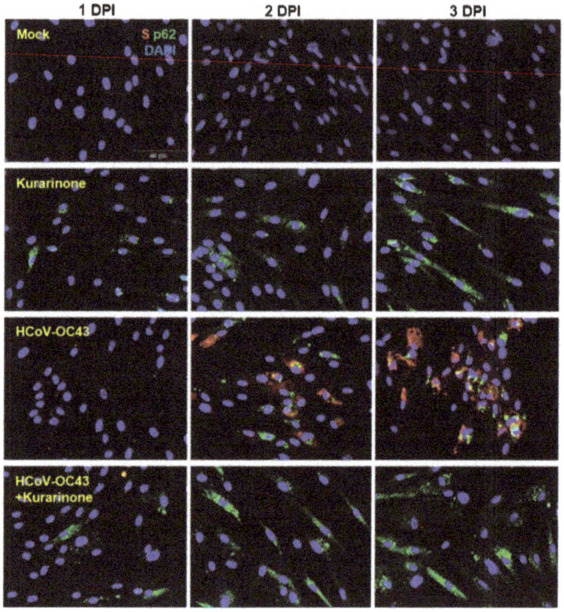

Figure 5. Expression of p62/SQSTM1 protein in response to administration of kurarinone; (**A**) HCoV-OC43-infected MRC-5 cells were treated with kurarinone or vehicle for 2 or 3 days; Western blot was performed with anti-p62/SQSTM1, -LC3, and -viral Spike antibodies at 2 or 3 dpi. (**B**) Virus-infected MRC-5 cells treated with kurarinone or vehicle alone were harvested at 3, 6, 24 or 48 h post-infection (hpi); cell lysates were analyzed by Western blot. Data were presented as means of two independent experiments. (**C**) Immunofluorescence analysis of HCoV-OC43-infected MRC-5 cells treated with vehicle (vhc) or kurarinone; cells were probed with an anti-viral Spike protein-specific antibody (red), p62/SQSTM1 protein-specific antibody (green) and DAPI (blue) at 1, 2, and 3 dpi. Scale bar is 50 μm.

4. Discussion

In this study, we explored mechanisms underlying the anti-viral activity of kurarinone on coronavirus HCoV-OC43 infection in human lung MRC-5 cells. Kurarinone is a prenylated flavonone isolated from the roots of *S. flavescens* that has well-characterized pro-apoptotic and anti-inflammatory effects. However, to the best of our knowledge, there are no published reports documenting the antiviral activities of kurarinone, save for one clinical report suggested that the combination of kurarinone and IFNα-1b might be used to treat patients with chronic hepatitis B [23].

In our first set of experiments, we found that kurarinone treatment inhibited HCoV-OC43 infection in MRC-5 cells in a dose-dependent manner with an IC_{50} 3.458 ± 0.101 μM (Figure 1C,D). Kurarinone treatment resulted in diminished levels of extracellular and intracellular viral RNA and diminished expression of the virus Spike protein compared to the virus-infected and vehicle-treated controls (Figure 2). Pre-treatment with kurarinone prior to virus infection did not protect against virus-induced CPE. Kurarinone treatment at 24 h post-infection resulted in partial protection against virus-induced CPE; as such, our results suggest that kurarinone may have a primary antiviral effect at the early stages of infection (Figure 3). To determine whether kurarinone has the capacity to modulate cytokine expression in HCoV-OC43-infected cells, we examined the kinetics of the antiviral cytokine, IFN-β1. The mRNA encoding IFN-β1 was significantly upregulated by virus infection but could not be detected at all in virus-infected and kurarinone-treated cells (Figure 2E). These data indicated that the antiviral response by kurarinone was not related to the induction of this antiviral cytokine.

Autophagy is a metabolic process that involves the intracellular membrane transport pathway and promotes recycling of proteins and organelles. Autophagy is also a critical factor with respect to virus infection and virion propagation [6–10]. During the stage of viral entry, HCoV-OC43 entered the cells by 9-O-acetylated sialic acids-mediated endocytosis, which is the determinant of host and tissue tropism [28]. Some viruses induced the early wave of autophagy induction upon virus infection, which may have contributed to viral entry [29]. Moreover, the coronavirus required the autophagy process for the formation of double-membrane-bound MHV replication complexes, which can significantly enhance the efficiency of replication [25]. As reported in a previous publication, treatment with the autophagy inhibitor, NH_4Cl, which alters lysosomal pH, limited the extent of HCoV-OC43 infection [29]. These results suggested that HCoV-OC43 infection induced autophagic processes, a finding that is consistent with observations associated with other coronavirus infections [18,28]. To verify the cellular status of autophagy and to monitor autophagic flux during HCoV-OC43 infection, we evaluated the expression of LC3 and p62/SQSTM1 proteins [19] (Figures 4 and 5). In HCoV-OC43-infected cells, we detected autophagy up to and including 3 dpi, as documented by the LC-3-I/II transversion.

Interestingly, treatment with kurarinone resulted in increased expression of LC-3-I and LC-3-II for 2 dpi; the LC-3-I/II transversion detected in kurarinone-treated cells was lower than that identified in vehicle-treated cells due to the comparatively high levels of LC3-I expression. These results suggested that kurarinone might disturb the HCoV-OC43-induced autophagy process. Consistent with this hypothesis, levels of the autophagic degradation substrate, p62/SQSTM1, were decreased in HCoV-OC43 infected cells; these results suggest that HCoV-OC43 infection induced the autophagic flux. However, kurarinone treatment induced the accumulation of p62/SQSTM1 protein in HCoV-OC43-infected cells starting at 6 h post-infection; p62/SQSTM1 protein-bound ubiquitinated protein is incorporated and degraded in the autophagosome, which indicates an autophagic degradation [30]. During the early stages of HSV-1 infection, down-regulation of p62/SQSTM1 protein is important for viral gene expression; exogenous overexpression of p62/SQSTM1 protein decreased the viral load, suggesting that p62/SQSTM1 protein has an antiviral function [31,32]. Our data also suggested that the increased expression of p62/SQSTM1 protein induced by kurarinone may have an important role in inhibiting HCoV-OC43 infection in MRC-5 cells. Therefore, kurarinone could not block the viral entry, as indicated by no antiviral effect of 24 h pre-treatment. The induced p62/SQSTM1 protein and disturbed autophagy flux within 24 h post-infection were important for the antiviral effect of kurarinone, and the weakened antiviral effect of 24 h post-infection treatment suggests that the benefits of kurarinone treatment may be optimal at the initial infection stages.

In conclusion, our results indicate that kurarinone can inhibit the progression of coronavirus infection by interrupting virus-induced autophagy. Therefore, this study outlines a therapeutic approach that may be used to inhibit coronavirus infection by targeting the virus-induced autophagy. These data suggested that kurarinone may be considered to be the basis of a novel and useful prophylaxis for high-risk exposure groups and therapeutic regiment for the treatment of diseases associated with coronavirus infection at the initial infection stage. Although we found the therapeutic potentials of kurarinone against HCoV-OC43 infection, the proof of concept (POC) was executed only in vitro, and the selectivity index was only 2.29 folds, which may have acted as a hurdle of its application in the clinic. Therefore, pharmacokinetic study and an in vivo toxicity test should be executed to determine its biostability and biosafety, and in vivo POC should also be confirmed in further study.

Supplementary Materials: The following are available online at http://www.mdpi.com/2077-0383/9/7/2230/s1, Figure S1: Expression of p62/SQSTM1 protein in response to administration of kurarinone and autophagy inhibitors (NH_4Cl and Chloroquine).

Author Contributions: Conceptualization, Y.-H.J. and S.K.; Data curation, D.E.K., J.S.M., Y.-H.J., and S.K.; Formal analysis, J.S.M., Y.-H.J., and S.K.; Funding acquisition, S.K.; Investigation, J.S.M., Y.-H.J., and S.K.; Methodology, D.E.K., J.S.M., and Y.-H.J.; Project administration, Y.-H.J. and S.K.; Resources, S.K.; Supervision, Y.-H.J. and S.K.; Validation, Y.-H.J. and S.K.; Visualization, J.S.M., Y.-H.J. and S.K.; Writing—original draft preparation, J.S.M. and Y.-H.J.; Writing—review and editing, Y.-H.J. and S.K. All authors have read and agreed to the published version of the manuscript.

Funding: This study was supported by the National Research Council of Science & Technology (NST) grant [grant numbers CRC-16-01-KRICT and NSN1621350] funded by the Korea government (MSIT). J.S.M. and D.E.K. were supported by the 'National Research Council of Science & Technology (NST)–Korea Institute of Oriental Medicine (KIOM)' Postdoctoral Research Fellowship for Young Scientists at the Korea Institute of Oriental Medicine in South Korea.

Conflicts of Interest: The authors declare no conflict of interest. The funders had no role in the design of the study; in the collection, analyses, or interpretation of data; in the writing of the manuscript, or in the decision to publish the results.

References

1. Reusken, C.B.; Raj, V.S.; Koopmans, M.P.; Haagmans, B.L. Cross host transmission in the emergence of MERS coronavirus. *Curr. Opin. Virol.* **2016**, *16*, 55–62. [CrossRef] [PubMed]
2. Food and Drug Administration. *Coronavirus (COVID-19) Update: FDA Issues Emergency Use Authorization for Potential COVID-19 Treatment*; FDA: Silver Spring, MD, USA, 2020.
3. Grein, J.; Ohmagari, N.; Shin, D.; Diaz, G.; Asperges, E.; Castagna, A.; Feldt, T.; Green, G.; Green, M.L.; Lescure, F.-X. Compassionate use of remdesivir for patients with severe Covid-19. *N. Engl. J. Med.* **2020**, *382*, 2327–2336. [CrossRef]
4. Wang, Y.; Zhang, D.; Du, G.; Du, R.; Zhao, J.; Jin, Y.; Fu, S.; Gao, L.; Cheng, Z.; Lu, Q. Remdesivir in adults with severe COVID-19: A randomised, double-blind, placebo-controlled, multicentre trial. *Lancet* **2020**, *395*, 1569–1578. [CrossRef]
5. Ahmad, L.; Mostowy, S.; Sancho-Shimizu, V. Autophagy-Virus Interplay: From Cell Biology to Human Disease. *Front. Cell Dev. Biol.* **2018**, *6*, 155. [CrossRef] [PubMed]
6. Law, A.H.; Lee, D.C.; Yuen, K.Y.; Peiris, M.; Lau, A.S. Cellular response to influenza virus infection: A potential role for autophagy in CXCL10 and interferon-alpha induction. *Cell. Mol. Immunol.* **2010**, *7*, 263–270. [CrossRef] [PubMed]
7. Nardacci, R.; Amendola, A.; Ciccosanti, F.; Corazzari, M.; Esposito, V.; Vlassi, C.; Taibi, C.; Fimia, G.M.; Del Nonno, F.; Ippolito, G.; et al. Autophagy plays an important role in the containment of HIV-1 in nonprogressor-infected patients. *Autophagy* **2014**, *10*, 1167–1178. [CrossRef]
8. Liu, Z.; Xiao, Y.; Torresilla, C.; Rassart, E.; Barbeau, B. Implication of Different HIV-1 Genes in the Modulation of Autophagy. *Viruses* **2017**, *9*, 389. [CrossRef]
9. Cao, B.; Parnell, L.A.; Diamond, M.S.; Mysorekar, I.U. Inhibition of autophagy limits vertical transmission of Zika virus in pregnant mice. *J. Exp. Med.* **2017**, *214*, 2303–2313. [CrossRef]
10. Katzenell, S.; Leib, D.A. Herpes Simplex Virus and Interferon Signaling Induce Novel Autophagic Clusters in Sensory Neurons. *J. Virol.* **2016**, *90*, 4706–4719. [CrossRef] [PubMed]
11. Judith, D.; Mostowy, S.; Bourai, M.; Gangneux, N.; Lelek, M.; Lucas-Hourani, M.; Cayet, N.; Jacob, Y.; Prevost, M.C.; Pierre, P.; et al. Species-specific impact of the autophagy machinery on Chikungunya virus infection. *EMBO Rep.* **2013**, *14*, 534–544. [CrossRef]
12. Choi, Y.; Bowman, J.W.; Jung, J.U. Autophagy during viral infection—A double-edged sword. *Nat. Rev. Microbiol.* **2018**, *16*, 341–354. [CrossRef] [PubMed]
13. Zhu, H.Y.; Han, L.; Shi, X.L.; Wang, B.L.; Huang, H.; Wang, X.; Chen, D.F.; Ju, D.W.; Feng, M.Q. Baicalin inhibits autophagy induced by influenza A virus H3N2. *Antivir. Res.* **2015**, *113*, 62–70. [CrossRef] [PubMed]
14. Sagnier, S.; Daussy, C.F.; Borel, S.; Robert-Hebmann, V.; Faure, M.; Blanchet, F.P.; Beaumelle, B.; Biard-Piechaczyk, M.; Espert, L. Autophagy restricts HIV-1 infection by selectively degrading Tat in CD4+ T lymphocytes. *J. Virol.* **2015**, *89*, 615–625. [CrossRef] [PubMed]
15. Kim, N.; Kim, M.-J.; Sung, P.S.; Bae, Y.; Shin, E.-C.; Yoo, J.-Y. Interferon-inducible protein SCOTIN interferes with HCV replication through the autolysosomal degradation of NS5A. *Nat. Commun.* **2016**, *7*, 10631. [CrossRef]

16. Ma, J.; Sun, Q.; Mi, R.; Zhang, H. Avian influenza A virus H5N1 causes autophagy-mediated cell death through suppression of mTOR signaling. *J. Genet. Genom.* **2011**, *38*, 533–537. [CrossRef]
17. Tallóczy, Z.; Jiang, W.; Virgin, H.W.; Leib, D.A.; Scheuner, D.; Kaufman, R.J.; Eskelinen, E.-L.; Levine, B. Regulation of starvation- and virus-induced autophagy by the eIF2α kinase signaling pathway. *Proc. Natl. Acad. Sci. USA* **2002**, *99*, 190. [CrossRef]
18. Maier, H.J.; Britton, P. Involvement of autophagy in coronavirus replication. *Viruses* **2012**, *4*, 3440–3451. [CrossRef]
19. Guo, L.; Yu, H.; Gu, W.; Luo, X.; Li, R.; Zhang, J.; Xu, Y.; Yang, L.; Shen, N.; Feng, L.; et al. Autophagy Negatively Regulates Transmissible Gastroenteritis Virus Replication. *Sci. Rep.* **2016**, *6*, 23864. [CrossRef]
20. Soon Jin, K.; Jae Su, C. Induction of Apoptosis via Autophagy on SK-Hep1 Human Hepatocellular Carcinoma Cells by Kurarinone Isolated from Sophora flavescens. *J. Cancer Prev.* **2012**, *17*, 87–94.
21. Seo, O.W.; Kim, J.H.; Lee, K.S.; Lee, K.S.; Kim, J.H.; Won, M.H.; Ha, K.S.; Kwon, Y.G.; Kim, Y.M. Kurarinone promotes TRAIL-induced apoptosis by inhibiting NF-kappaB-dependent cFLIP expression in HeLa cells. *Exp. Mol. Med.* **2012**, *44*, 653–664. [CrossRef]
22. Kim, B.H.; Na, K.M.; Oh, I.; Song, I.H.; Lee, Y.S.; Shin, J.; Kim, T.Y. Kurarinone regulates immune responses through regulation of the JAK/STAT and TCR-mediated signaling pathways. *Biochem. Pharmacol.* **2013**, *85*, 1134–1144. [CrossRef] [PubMed]
23. Pan, Z.S.; Yu, Q.H.; Yan, H.; Zhang, Y. Clinical study on treatment of chronic hepatitis B by kurarinone combined with interferon alpha-1b. *Chin. J. Integr. Tradit. West. Med.* **2005**, *25*, 700–703.
24. Kim, D.E.; Min, J.S.; Jang, M.S.; Lee, J.Y.; Shin, Y.S.; Song, J.H.; Kim, H.R.; Kim, S.; Jin, Y.H.; Kwon, S. Natural Bis-Benzylisoquinoline Alkaloids-Tetrandrine, Fangchinoline, and Cepharanthine, Inhibit Human Coronavirus OC43 Infection of MRC-5 Human Lung Cells. *Biomolecules* **2019**, *9*, 696. [CrossRef] [PubMed]
25. Prentice, E.; Jerome, W.G.; Yoshimori, T.; Mizushima, N.; Denison, M.R. Coronavirus replication complex formation utilizes components of cellular autophagy. *J. Biol. Chem.* **2004**, *279*, 10136–10141. [CrossRef] [PubMed]
26. Galluzzi, L.; Green, D.R. Autophagy-Independent Functions of the Autophagy Machinery. *Cell* **2019**, *177*, 1682–1699. [CrossRef] [PubMed]
27. Chen, X.; Wang, K.; Xing, Y.; Tu, J.; Yang, X.; Zhao, Q.; Li, K.; Chen, Z. Coronavirus membrane-associated papain-like proteases induce autophagy through interacting with Beclin1 to negatively regulate antiviral innate immunity. *Protein Cell* **2014**, *5*, 912–927. [CrossRef]
28. Owczarek, K.; Szczepanski, A.; Milewska, A.; Baster, Z.; Rajfur, Z.; Sarna, M.; Pyrc, K. Early events during human coronavirus OC43 entry to the cell. *Sci. Rep.* **2018**, *8*, 7124. [CrossRef]
29. Joubert, P.E.; Meiffren, G.; Gregoire, I.P.; Pontini, G.; Richetta, C.; Flacher, M.; Azocar, O.; Vidalain, P.O.; Vidal, M.; Lotteau, V.; et al. Autophagy induction by the pathogen receptor CD46. *Cell Host Microbe* **2009**, *6*, 354–366. [CrossRef]
30. Yang, N.; Shen, H.M. Targeting the Endocytic Pathway and Autophagy Process as a Novel Therapeutic Strategy in COVID-19. *Int. J. Biol. Sci.* **2020**, *16*, 1724–1731. [CrossRef]
31. Klionsky, D.J.; Abdelmohsen, K.; Abe, A.; Abedin, M.J.; Abeliovich, H.; Acevedo Arozena, A.; Adachi, H.; Adams, C.M.; Adams, P.D.; Adeli, K.; et al. Guidelines for the use and interpretation of assays for monitoring autophagy (3rd edition). *Autophagy* **2016**, *12*, 1–222. [CrossRef]
32. Waisner, H.; Kalamvoki, M. The ICP0 Protein of Herpes Simplex Virus 1 (HSV-1) Downregulates Major Autophagy Adaptor Proteins Sequestosome 1 and Optineurin during the Early Stages of HSV-1 Infection. *J. Virol.* **2019**, *93*. [CrossRef] [PubMed]

Journal of
Clinical Medicine

MDPI

Article

Antibacterial Activity of Some Flavonoids and Organic Acids Widely Distributed in Plants

Artur Adamczak [1], Marcin Ożarowski [2] and Tomasz M. Karpiński [3,*]

1 Department of Botany, Breeding and Agricultural Technology of Medicinal Plants, Institute of Natural Fibres and Medicinal Plants, Kolejowa 2, 62-064 Plewiska, Poland; artur.adamczak@iwnirz.pl
2 Department of Biotechnology, Institute of Natural Fibres and Medicinal Plants, Wojska Polskiego 71b, 60-630 Poznań, Poland; marcin.ozarowski@iwnirz.pl
3 Department of Medical Microbiology, Poznań University of Medical Sciences, Wieniawskiego 3, 61-712 Poznań, Poland
* Correspondence: tkarpin@ump.edu.pl

Received: 21 November 2019; Accepted: 27 December 2019; Published: 31 December 2019

Abstract: Among natural substances widespread in fruits, vegetables, spices, and medicinal plants, flavonoids and organic acids belong to the promising groups of bioactive compounds with strong antioxidant and anti-inflammatory properties. The aim of the present work was to evaluate the antibacterial activity of 13 common flavonoids (flavones, flavonols, flavanones) and 6 organic acids (aliphatic and aromatic acids). The minimal inhibitory concentrations (MICs) of selected plant substances were determined by the micro-dilution method using clinical strains of four species of pathogenic bacteria. All tested compounds showed antimicrobial properties, but their biological activity was moderate or relatively low. Bacterial growth was most strongly inhibited by salicylic acid (MIC = 250–500 µg/mL). These compounds were generally more active against Gram-negative bacteria: *Escherichia coli* and *Pseudomonas aeruginosa* than Gram-positive ones: *Enterococcus faecalis* and *Staphylococcus aureus*. An analysis of the antibacterial effect of flavone, chrysin, apigenin, and luteolin showed that the presence of hydroxyl groups in the phenyl rings A and B usually did not influence on the level of their activity. A significant increase in the activity of the hydroxy derivatives of flavone was observed only for *S. aureus*. Similarly, the presence and position of the sugar group in the flavone glycosides generally had no effect on the MIC values.

Keywords: kaempferol; naringin; orientin; rutin; vitexin; chlorogenic acid; citric acid; malic acid; quinic acid; rosmarinic acid

1. Introduction

Screening biological studies of chemical compounds of natural origin allow for assessment of their activity and determine further research stages in order to search for new therapeutic solutions based on active compounds known in plants. This is especially important during the observed increasing resistance of bacteria and fungi to antibiotics. Multidrug resistance (MDR) is a serious threat to human health, but also to crops and animals. MDR is a growing challenge in medicine. Recently, several multinational studies have been carried out to determine the prevalence of herbal medicine use in infections due to pathogenic microorganisms [1,2]. It is considered that extracts of medicinal plants can be an alternative source of resistance modifying substances [2]. It is well known that plant extracts and other herbal products are complex mixtures containing the wide variety of primary and secondary metabolites, and their action may be the result of the synergy of different chemical components. Moreover, these extracts may show various mechanisms of biological and pharmacological activity, i.e., ability to bind to protein domains, modulation of the immune response, mitosis, apoptosis, and signal transduction [2]. However, it should be noted that plants interact with the environment and other organisms, therefore their chemical composition and the level of active substances can be very diverse [3,4]. In addition, the manufacturing process of herbal medicinal products is very complex because it encompasses non-standardized processes like the cultivation of plants, obtaining the vegetable raw material from various parts of the world, preparing of extract, and producing a product in accordance with local guidelines of the good manufacturing practice. Therefore, it can be concluded that using pure chemical compounds of natural origin would be an interesting complementary option due to their easier therapeutic dosage, the study of mechanisms of the pharmacological action and monitoring of their side effects.

A lot of widespread plant substances, including alkaloids, organosulfur compounds, phenolic acids, flavonoids, carotenoids, coumarins, terpenes, tannins, and some primary metabolites (amino acids, peptides, organic acids) exhibit antimicrobial properties [1,5–8]. Among them, flavonoids are a promising group of bioactive substances with low systemic toxicity. Natural flavonols, flavones, flavanones, and other compounds of this class belong to the common secondary metabolites found in various fruits, vegetables, and medicinal plants [9] showing strong antioxidant and anti-inflammatory properties [10,11]. Dietary polyphenols such as flavonoids and phenolic acids, consumed in large quantities in foods of plant origin, exhibit a number of beneficial effects and play an important role in the prevention of chronic and degenerative diseases. Not only their antioxidant and anti-inflammatory activities, but also neuroprotective, anticancer, immunomodulatory, antidiabetic, and anti-adipogenic properties have been shown [12,13]. Biological availability of dietary polyphenols is low as compared with micro- and macronutrients. Their absorption in the small intestine amounts only about 5–10%. However, recent studies showed that these phytochemicals exhibit prebiotic properties and antimicrobial activity against pathogenic intestinal microflora [13].

Flavonoids selected for our microbiological tests are presented in Figure 1. In the large quantities, they occur in stems and leaves, flowers as well as fruits of the species from the families of Apiaceae, Asteraceae, Betulaceae, Brassicaceae, Ericaceae, Fabaceae, Hypericaceae, Lamiaceae, Liliaceae, Passifloraceae, Polygonaceae, Primulaceae, Ranunculaceae, Rosaceae, Rubiaceae, Rutaceae, Scrophulariaceae, Tiliaceae, and Violaceae. Two flavonols: quercetin, kaempferol, and flavones: apigenin, luteolin belong to the most ubiquitous plant flavonoids [14]. A glycoside form of quercetin—rutin (sophorin, rutoside) is present in the highest concentrations in buckwheat (*Fagopyrum esculentum* Moench), rue (*Ruta graveolens* L.), flower buds of *Styphnolobium japonicum* (L.) Schott (*Sophora japonica* L.), apricots, peaches, and citrus fruits [15,16]. Apigenin derivatives, such as vitexin, isovitexin, and vitexin 2″-*O*-rhamnoside constitute the main bioactive compounds of leaves and flowers of hawthorn (*Crataegus* spp.) [17]. The 8- and 6-*C*-glucosides of luteolin: orientin and isoorientin are reported from different crop plants, including buckwheat, corn silk (*Zea mays* L.), acai fruits (*Euterpe oleracea* Mart., *E. precatoria* Mart.), and Moso bamboo leaves (*Phyllostachys edulis*/Carrière/J.Houz.) [18,19]. In turn, passion fruits (*Passiflora* spp.), skullcap roots (*Scutellaria* spp.) as well as honey and propolis are the main natural sources of chrysin [20–23]. Naringin is a flavanone glycoside isolated from grapes and citrus fruits, and it imparts a bitter taste to grapefruit juice [24].

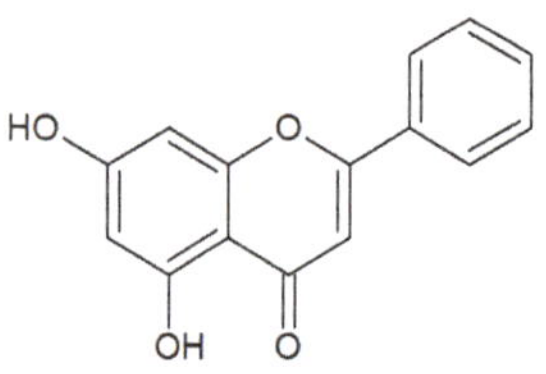

Chrysin

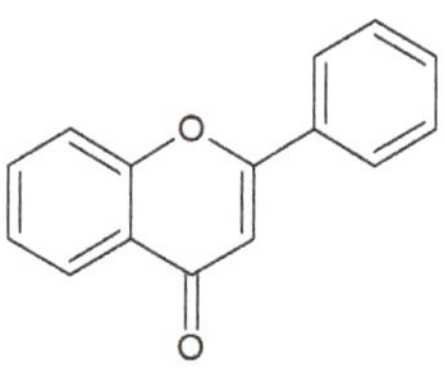

Flavone

Figure 1. *Cont.*

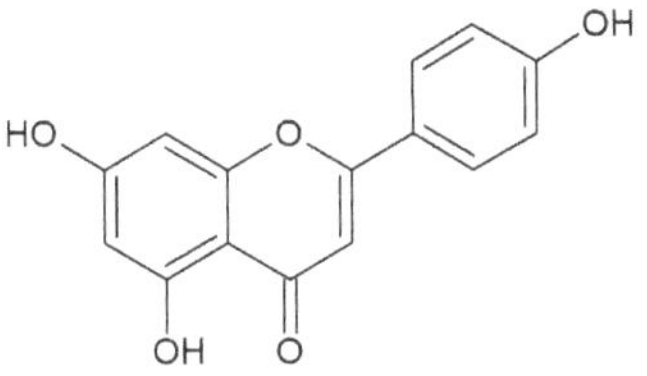

Apigenin

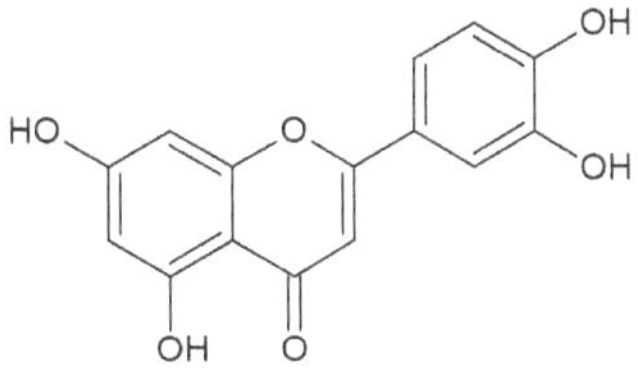

Luteolin

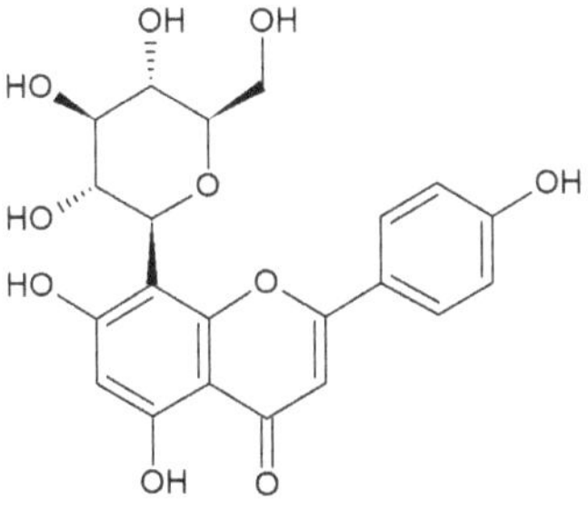

Vitexin

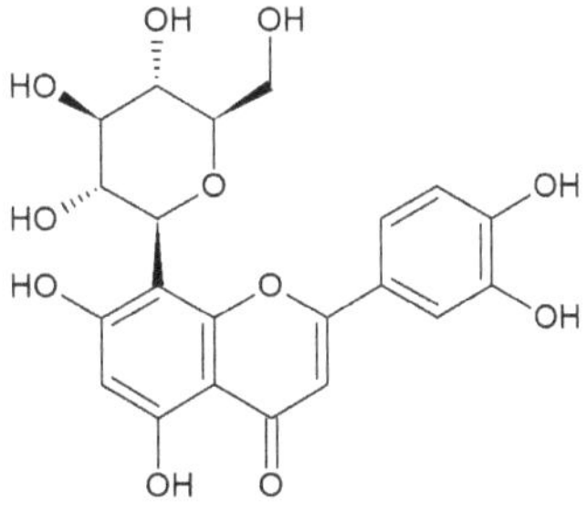

Orientin

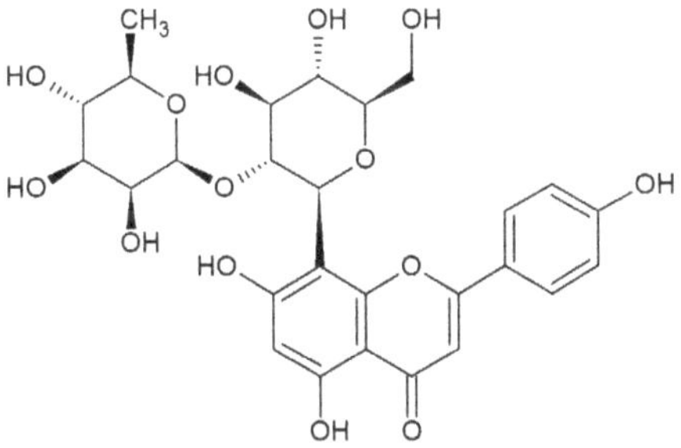

Vitexin 2″-*O*-rhamnoside

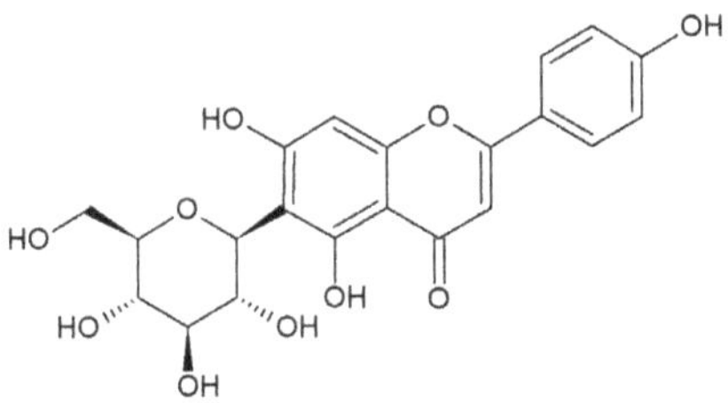

Isovitexin

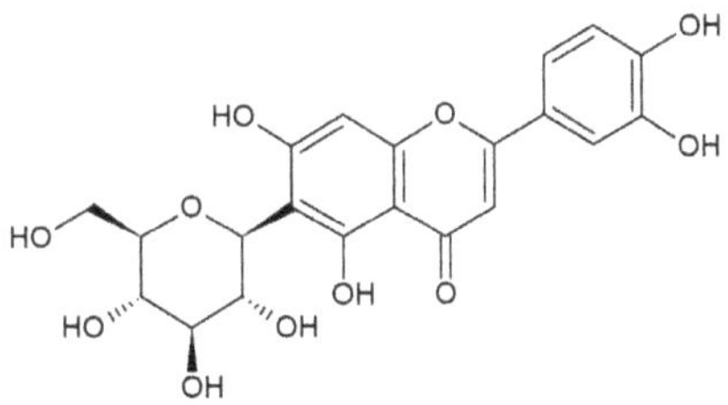

Isoorientin

Figure 1. *Cont.*

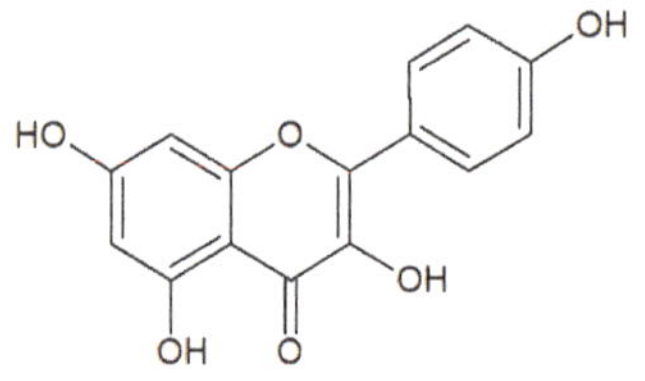

Kaempferol

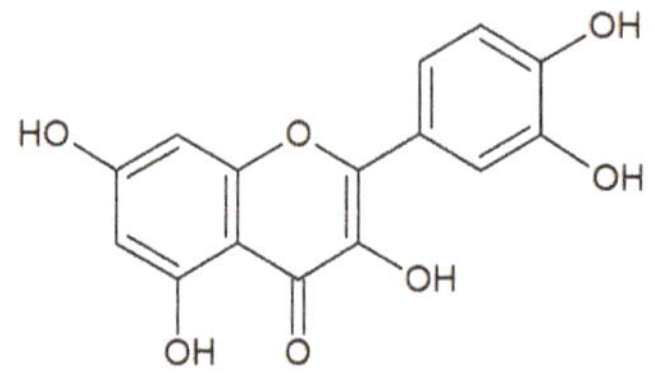

Quercetin

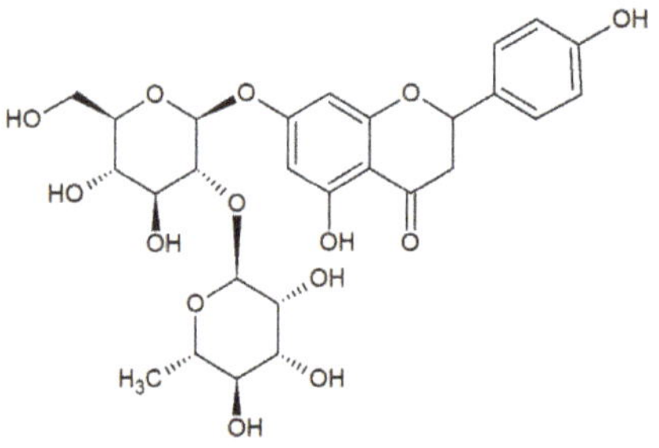

Naringin

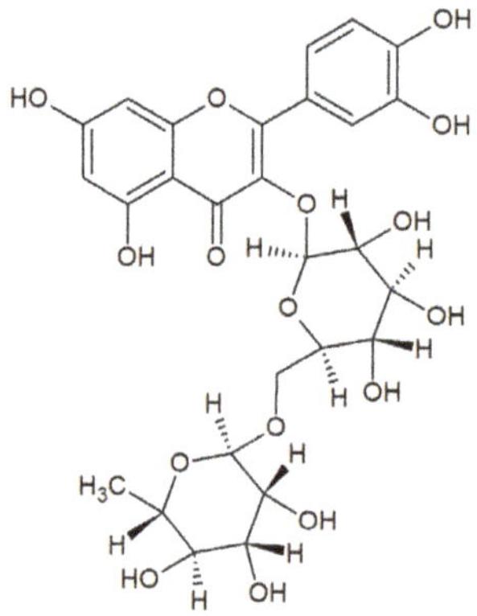

Rutin

Figure 1. Chemical structures of flavonoids tested in the present research.

In addition to flavonoids, a lot of organic acids: both aliphatic and aromatic ones, especially phenolics are the important bioactive compounds of edible and medicinal plants (Figure 2). Among non-aromatic, short-chain hydroxy acids, malic, citric, and quinic acids belong to the most abundant substances with a key role in plant metabolism and physiology. Malic and citric acids are mainly produced in the tricarboxylic acid cycle (Krebs cycle) and, to a lesser degree, in the glyoxylate cycle, while quinic acid is a byproduct of the shikimic acid pathway [4]. High accumulation of these compounds is observed in various berry fruits of wild and cultivated plants from the Ericaceae, Rosaceae, and Grossulariaceae families, including cranberry (*Vaccinium macrocarpon* Aiton and *V. oxycoccos* L.), bilberry (*V. myrtillus* L.), blueberry (*V. corymbosum* L.), blackberry (*Rubus* spp.), raspberry (*Rubus idaeus* L.), black chokeberry (*Aronia melanocarpa*/Michx./Elliott), red currant (*Ribes rubrum* L.), black currant (*Ribes nigrum* L.), and many others [25–30]. For example, the total content of citric, malic, and quinic acids in fruits of European cranberry can reach almost 37% of dry matter [31].

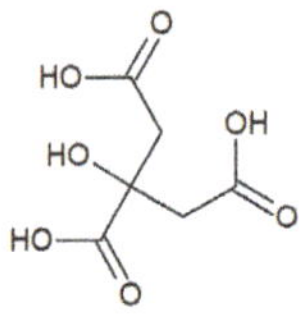

Citric acid

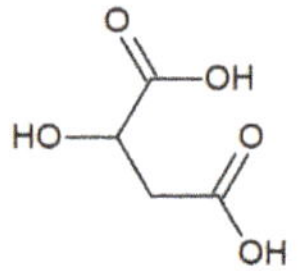

Malic acid

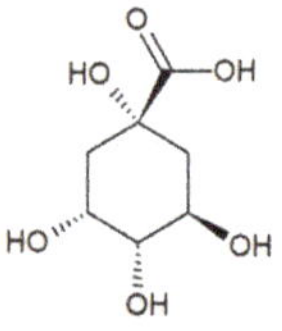

Quinic acid

Figure 2. *Cont.*

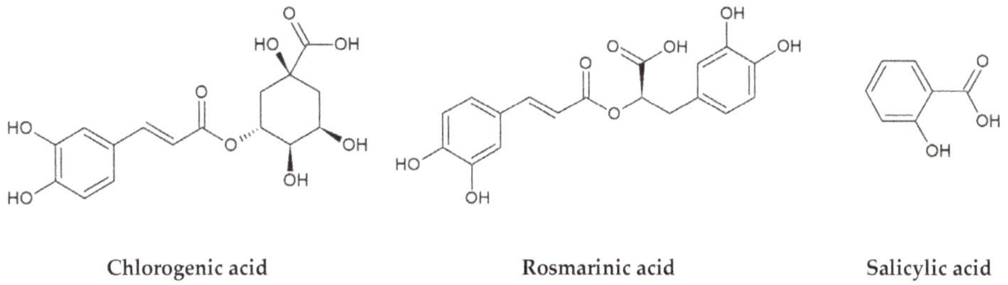

Figure 2. Chemical structures of organic acids tested in the present research.

Berries are also a rich source of hydroxycinnamic acids and their derivatives, including chlorogenic (5-*O*-caffeoylquinic) and neochlorogenic (3-*O*-caffeoylquinic) acids, which are the esters formed between caffeic (3,4-dihydroxycinnamic) and quinic acids [32,33]. A great amount of chlorogenic acid isomers has been found, among others, in yerba mate (*Ilex paraguariensis* A.St-Hil.), coffee (*Coffea* spp.), and tea plant (*Camellia sinensis*/L./Kuntze) [34]. In turn, rosmarinic acid, an ester of caffeic and 3,4-dihydroxyphenyllactic acids, was isolated for the first time from the rosemary leaves (*Rosmarinus officinalis* L.). It commonly occurs in many aromatic and medicinal plants of the Lamiaceae family, especially mint (*Mentha* spp.) and thyme (*Thymus* spp.) species, lemon balm (*Melissa officinalis* L.), common sage (*Salvia officinalis* L.), oregano (*Origanum vulgare* L.), and sweet basil (*Ocimum basilicum* L.) [35–37]. Another well-known secondary metabolite, the phytohormone salicylic acid (SA), is a key signaling compound that participates in the plant response to pathogens, herbivores, and abiotic stress [38]. Natural salicylates such as salicylic acid and salicin (salicyl alcohol glucoside) were found in large amounts in the willow bark (*Salix* spp.), the buds of black poplar (*Populus nigra* L.), elm leaves (*Ulmus* spp.), and meadowsweet herb (*Filipendula ulmaria*/L./Maxim.) [39,40].

Our studies were focused on the estimation of antibacterial activity of selected flavonoids and organic acids widespread in fruits, vegetables, spices, and popular medicinal plants which are very often used for the prevention and treatment of various diseases. For example, many herbal preparations utilized as natural diuretics, and plant extracts with other main pharmacological activities (i.e., drugs against cardiovascular diseases, sedatives, anti-inflammatory agents) exhibit additional beneficial effects by the antimicrobial action [41,42]. Recent data show that flavonoids have protective potential against cutaneous inflammatory reactions and affect wound healing [43,44]. In addition, organic acids (especially citric acid) seem to be of significant importance in the antimicrobial activity and health of the skin [45,46]. In the present studies, we tested the biological activity of chosen flavonoids and organic acids against four widespread pathogens: *Staphylococcus aureus*, *Enterococcus faecalis*, *Pseudomonas aeruginosa*, and *Escherichia coli*. These Gram-positive and Gram-negative bacteria can cause many diseases in humans, including opportunistic infections and belong to the most common etiological factors of the skin and wound infections [47,48].

Microbiological screening tests included 19 plant metabolites from the various flavonoid classes: flavones, flavonols, flavanones, and simple organic acids: aliphatic and aromatic ones. The chosen flavonoids differed in the number of hydroxyl groups on the aromatic rings as well as the presence and position of the sugar group, which gave the opportunity to test the effect of these parameters on the biological activity of the natural compounds.

2. Materials and Methods

2.1. Chemicals

Chemicals used in this study were purchased from Merck (Sigma-Aldrich, Supelco, Poland). Plant compounds selected for the microbiological tests are presented in Table 1. All substances were dissolved in 20% water solution of dimethyl sulfoxide DMSO (Sigma-Aldrich, Poland) in a final concentration of

1 mg/mL. Additionally, DMSO was used as a negative control, while two antibiotics, ciprofloxacin (Sigma, cat. no. 17850) and gentamicin sulfate (Sigma-Aldrich, cat. no. G1914) as positives.

Table 1. Plant pure substances used in the microbiological assays.

No	Merck (Sigma-Aldrich, Supelco)	CAS No	PubChem CID	Purity
1	Apigenin	520-36-5	5280443	≥95.0% (HPLC)
2	Chrysin	480-40-0	5281607	≥98.0% (HPLC)
3	Flavone	525-82-6	10680	≥99.0%
4	Isoorientin	4261-42-1	114776	≥98.0% (HPLC)
5	Isovitexin	38953-85-4	162350	≥98.0% (HPLC)
6	Kaempferol	520-18-3	5280863	≥97.0% (HPLC)
7	Luteolin	491-70-3	5280445	≥97.0% (HPLC)
8	Naringin	10236-47-2	442428	≥95.0% (HPLC)
9	Orientin	28608-75-5	5281675	≥98.0% (HPLC)
10	Quercetin	117-39-5	5280343	≥95.0% (HPLC)
11	Rutin	153-18-4	5280805	≥95.0% (HPLC)
12	Vitexin	3681-93-4	5280441	≥95.0% (HPLC)
13	Vitexin 2″-*O*-rhamnoside	64820-99-1	5282151	≥98.0% (HPLC)
14	Chlorogenic acid	327-97-9	1794427	≥95.0% (HPLC)
15	Citric acid	77-92-9	311	≤100%
16	Malic acid	6915-15-7	525	≤100%
17	Quinic acid	77-95-2	6508	analytical standard
18	Rosmarinic acid	20283-92-5	5281792	≥98.0% (HPLC)
19	Salicylic acid	69-72-7	338	≥99.0%

2.2. Bacterial Strains and Antimicrobial Activity

In the in vitro tests, there were investigated clinical isolates of two Gram-positive (*Staphylococcus aureus, Enterococcus faecalis*) and Gram-negative bacteria (*Escherichia coli, Pseudomonas aeruginosa*). For each species, four strains obtained from the collection of the Department of Medical Microbiology at Poznań University of Medical Sciences (Poland) were tested. None of them were multidrug-resistant. The species of bacteria were grown at 35 °C for 24 h, in tryptone soy agar (TSA; Graso, Poland).

The minimal inhibitory concentrations (MICs) of selected plant substances were determined by the micro-dilution method using the 96-well plates (Nest Scientific Biotechnology). Studies were conducted according to the Clinical and Laboratory Standards Institute (CLSI) [49], European Committee on Antimicrobial Susceptibility Testing (EUCAST) recommendations [50], and as described in our previous publications [48,51]. Primarily, 90 μL of Mueller–Hinton broth (Graso, Poland) was placed in each well. Serial dilutions of each of the substances were performed so that concentrations in the range of 15.6–1000 μg/mL were obtained. In the initial tests of antibacterial activity of phytochemicals, the lowest concentration amounted to 1.95 μg/mL (Figure 3), while for positive controls (antibiotics) it was 0.98 μg/mL. The inoculums were adjusted to contain approximately 10^8 CFU/mL bacteria. 10 μL of the proper inoculums were added to the wells, obtaining concentration 10^5 CFU/mL. The plates were incubated at 35 °C for 24 h, then 20 μL of 1% MTT water solution (3-(4,5-Dimethyl-2-thiazolyl)-2,5-diphenyl-2H-tetrazolium bromide, Sigma-Aldrich) was added to the wells. Next, the plates were incubated 2–4 h at 37 °C. This assay is based on the reduction of yellow tetrazolium salt (MTT) to a soluble purple formazan product [48]. The MIC value was taken as the lowest concentration of the substance that inhibited any visible bacterial growth. The analyses were repeated three times.

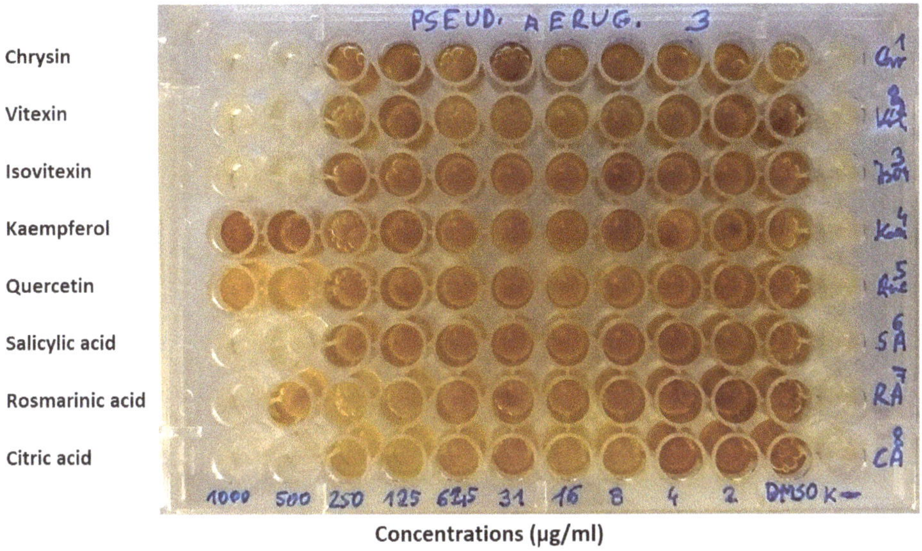

Figure 3. The minimal inhibitory concentrations (MICs) of selected plant substances against *Pseudomonas aeruginosa* strain according to the micro-dilution method.

In our investigations, we adopted the range of tested concentrations of phytochemicals for the MICs between 15.6 and 1000 µg/mL, although some authors determine the antimicrobial activity of natural compounds at the level of 2000–4000 µg/mL or more [52–54]. However, in our opinion, such high values indicate a very weak effect of these substances. During the description of the results, it was taken that the MIC = 250 µg/mL shows a relatively high antibacterial activity of plant chemicals, while the MICs = 500 and 1000 µg/mL mean moderate and low effects, respectively.

3. Results

Our research exhibited antibacterial properties of all tested flavonoids and organic acids, but their activity was quite diverse. These compounds were generally more active against Gram-negative than Gram-positive bacteria. The following tendency of microbial sensitivity to plant substances was observed: *E. coli* > *P. aeruginosa* > *E. faecalis* > *S. aureus* (Table 2). Salicylic acid showed the highest biological effect on all bacterial species (MIC = 250–500 µg/mL). However, other chemicals demonstrated a similar activity, especially against *E. coli* and *P. aeruginosa* (MIC = 500 µg/mL). Among 19 investigated phytochemicals, only three: kaempferol, quercetin, and chlorogenic acid had no significant influence on *P. aeruginosa*, while up to 10 compounds were relatively inactive against *S. aureus* (MIC > 1000 µg/mL). It was interesting that the individual strains of a given bacterial species most often did not show differences in the sensitivity to one plant substance. Only salicylic acid, rosmarinic acid, and apigenin exhibited differentiating effects on individual strains.

Table 2. Antibacterial activity of selected plant substances against Gram (+) and Gram (−) bacteria.

Plant Substance	Tested Bacteria			
	Staphylococcus aureus	*Enterococcus faecalis*	*Escherichia coli*	*Pseudomonas aeruginosa*
	MIC (µg/mL)			
Kaempferol	>1000	>1000	500	>1000
Quercetin	>1000	>1000	500	>1000
Rutin	1000	1000	500	500
Naringin	>1000	1000	500	500
Flavone	>1000	500	500	500
Chrysin	500	1000	500	500
Apigenin	500, 1000 (3x)	1000	500	500
Vitexin	>1000	1000	500	500
Isovitexin	>1000	1000	500	500
Vitexin 2″-*O*-rhamnoside	>1000	1000	500	500
Luteolin	500	1000	500	500
Orientin	500	1000	500	500
Isoorientin	500	1000	500	500
Citric acid	>1000	1000	500	500
Malic acid	1000	1000	500	500
Quinic acid	>1000	1000	500	500
Chlorogenic acid	1000	1000	500	>1000
Rosmarinic acid	>1000	1000	500	500 (2x), 1000 (2x)
Salicylic acid	250 (2x), 500 (2x)	500	250 (3x), 500	500
Median	>1000	1000	500	500
20% DMSO (negative control)	>1000	>1000	>1000	>1000
Ciprofloxacin (positive)	<1	<1	<1	<1
Gentamicin sulfate (positive)	<1	<1–62.5	<1–3.9	<1

Although flavonol aglycones kaempferol and quercetin displayed a moderate activity only against *E. coli*, quercetin glycoside rutin demonstrated influence on all strains tested (MIC = 500–1000 µg/mL). A similar activity level was found for the glycosides from the other classes of flavonoids: flavanones (naringin) and flavones (vitexin, isovitexin, vitexin 2″-*O*-rhamnoside, orientin, isoorientin). Differences were determined only in the case of *S. aureus*. Naringin, vitexin and its derivatives showed no significant activity, while orientin and isoorientin were clearly stronger antibacterial agents than rutin.

Among organic acids, the highest variability in the microbiological effect was found against *S. aureus* and *P. aeruginosa*. Some metabolites such as citric, quinic, and rosmarinic acids for *S. aureus*, and also chlorogenic acid for *P. aeruginosa* were relatively inactive. The aliphatic acids: citric, malic and quinic ones showed the same level of activity within individual species of *E. faecalis*, *E. coli*, and *P. aeruginosa* (MIC = 500–1000 µg/mL). In turn, phenolic compounds: chlorogenic, rosmarinic, and salicylic acids exhibited variation within all bacterial species with the MIC values from 250 to above 1000 µg/mL.

4. Discussion

In recent years, a rapid increase in the number of studies concerning the antibacterial properties of plant extracts rich in phenolic compounds, including flavonoids and phenolic acids has been observed. However, due to the enormous wealth of species and natural substances, the degree of their examination is very diverse and still insufficient. Particularly, works on the antibacterial activity of individual pure compounds are relatively few. There is a small number of microbiological investigations describing the effects of some common flavonoid glycosides such as vitexin [55–58], isovitexin [59,60], vitexin 2″-*O*-rhamnoside [61], orientin [62,63], and isoorientin [56,60,62].

In addition, literature data are difficult to compare due to the use of various methods for assessing antibacterial activity, different solvents, and the origin and purity of test compounds, often isolated from various plant extracts [55,57,59,60,62–65]. Antimicrobial properties of natural chemicals were described not only by the minimum inhibitory concentration (MIC) [33,54,57,62,64,66–72] and by the minimum bactericidal concentration (MBC) [72], but also by the agar well or disc-diffusion methods [59,60,63,65]. Some authors expressed results as the IC_{50} or MIC_{80} values [33,67,73]. Moreover, the plant substances were tested in various concentrations. The kind of solvent used for the dissolution of pure compounds is the next important point in the assessment of in vitro activity. Although most authors utilized dimethyl sulfoxide, sometimes they did not give its concentration [59,62,63,65] or it is 100% DMSO [54], which may affect the level of antimicrobial activity of the tested solutions. The other solvents used were, for example, acetone [67], chloroform [59], Mueller Hinton II broth [68], and water [71]. In several cases, there was no information about dissolving procedures [57,58,60]. In this context, there is still a need for extensive screening studies that would compare the activity of a large number of plant metabolites against the same bacterial strains by a standardized method.

Our investigations exhibited moderate antibacterial properties of tested flavonoids and organic acids against clinical strains of Gram-negative pathogens: *E. coli* and *P. aeruginosa* (MIC = 500 μg/mL). Among 19 selected plant substances, only three: kaempferol, quercetin, and chlorogenic acid were inactive against *P. aeruginosa* at all concentrations tested (15.6–1000 μg/mL). However, for up to 10 compounds, no significant activity was found against the Gram-positive bacteria *S. aureus*. Additionally, another microorganism from this group *E. faecalis* showed low sensitivity (MIC = 1000 μg/mL) to most analyzed metabolites (Table 2). The above-described observations confirm the results of works which indicate a higher activity of natural plant substances, including flavonoids, against some Gram-negative bacteria than Gram-positive ones, although it is usually considered that this regularity is the opposite [48,55]. The general tendency of bacterial sensitivity to selected plant substances was observed as follows: *E. coli* > *P. aeruginosa* > *E. faecalis* > *S. aureus* (Table 2). Some screening studies showed the greater activity of alkaloids, flavonoids, and phenolic acids especially against *P. aeruginosa*, and also *E. coli* than *S. aureus* [5,55]. However, this relationship seems to have significant limitations and requires further detailed research. For example, all strains of *S. aureus*, *E. coli*, and *P. aeruginosa* tested by us had the same level of sensitivity to flavones chrysin, luteolin, orientin, isoorientin, and some clinical isolates of them to apigenin and salicylic acid. No differences in the inhibitory potency of bacterial growth of above-mentioned species were previously reported, among others, for luteolin, orientin, isoorientin [62], and in the case of *S. aureus* and *E. coli* for chrysin [67], luteolin [74], and glycosides of quercetin hyperoside and rutin [72].

Numerous studies allow to state that in antibacterial mechanisms of flavonoids are included mainly: inhibition of synthesis of nucleic acid, inhibition of cytoplasmic membrane function by influence the biofilm formation, porins, permeability, and by interaction with some crucial enzymes [6,8,75,76]. It was shown that apigenin inhibits the DNA gyrase of *E. coli* [77], and has inhibitory effects on the formation of *E. coli* biofilm [78]. Recently, a liposomal formulation of apigenin was examined, and it was observed increasing of its antibacterial property by the interaction of apigenin liposomes with the membrane of tested bacteria resulted in the lysis of the bacterial cells. Comparison of results exhibited much greater efficiency of liposomal apigenin against both Gram-positive and Gram-negative bacteria: *B. subtilis* (MIC = 4 μg/mL), *S. aureus* (MIC = 8 μg/mL), and *E. coli* (MIC = 16 μg/mL), *P. aeruginosa* (MIC = 64 μg/mL) [68]. Other flavones, including apigenin *C*-glucosides such as vitexin and isovitexin, have also been tested in order to study their effect on bacterial surface hydrophobicity and biofilm formation [57–59]. Das et al. [58] reported that vitexin reduces the hydrophobicity of cell surface and membrane permeability of *S. aureus* at the sub-MIC dose of 126 μg/mL. This flavone down-regulated the *ica*AB and *agr*AC gene expression showing antibiofilm activity and bactericidal effect. In similar work, Das et al. [57] demonstrated that vitexin exerts the MIC of 260 μg/mL against *P. aeruginosa*, and exhibits moderate antibiofilm activity. In turn, isovitexin (200–500 μg/mL) decreased the adhesion of methicillin-sensitive *S. aureus* ATCC 29213, and simultaneously increased the adhesion of two strains of *E. coli* [59]. Currently, it was shown that isovitexin has the potent antibacterial properties described as the diameter of the zone of growth inhibition (ZOI) for *B. subtilis* (19.5 mm), *P. aeruginosa* (17.5 mm), *E. coli* (14.1 mm), and *Staphylococcus aureus* (12.8 mm). The even stronger activity was found for isoorientin (luteolin C-glucoside), and it was as follows: *B. subtilis* (20.1 mm), *P. aeruginosa* (19.1 mm), *S. aureus* (18.7 mm), and *E. coli* (14.8 mm) [60].

Microbiological literature provides interesting data on the mechanism of action of two main flavonols: kaempferol and quercetin. It was shown that quercetin increases the cytoplasmic membrane permeability of *S. pyogenes* which resulted in the inhibitory influence on this Gram-positive bacterium at the MIC value of 128 μg/mL [79]. Moreover, in this study, the synergistic effect of quercetin with antibiotic ceftazidime was observed. Barbieri et al. [6] concluded that this flavonol is active not only against Gram-positive pathogens: *S. aureus*, *S. haemolyticus*, and *S. pyogenes*, but also against Gram-negative ones: *E. coli* and *K. pneumoniae*. Additionally, Betts et al. [80] showed a strongly inhibiting effect against methicillin-resistant *S. aureus*, which was significantly increased in the presence of epigallocatechin gallate. Studies of the mechanism of antimicrobial action allowed to state that quercetin diacyl glycosides show dual inhibition of DNA gyrase and topoisomerase IV [81]. In turn, our investigations exhibited the moderate effect of these plant metabolites against *E. coli* (MIC = 500 μg/mL), and lack of significant activity in the case of *S. aureus* (MIC > 1000 μg/mL). Research of Chen and Huang [82] concerning quercetin and kaempferol reported inhibition of the interaction of DNA B helicase of *K. pneumoniae* with deoxynucleotide triphosphates (dNTPs). Further study showed that the ATPase activity of this helicase *Kp*DnaB was decreased to 75% and 65% in the presence of quercetin and kaempferol, respectively [83]. In the next work, Huang et al. [84] observed that kaempferol inhibits the DNA PriA helicase of *S. aureus*, and these results showed that the concentration of phosphate from ATP hydrolysis by this DNA helicase was decreased to 37% in the presence of 35 μM kaempferol. Thus, it was summarized that kaempferol can bind to DNA helicase and then inhibit its ATPase activity and this is a new mechanism of action for this chemical compound. According to the results, this flavonol may be taken into consideration as an active natural molecule in the development of new antibiotics against *S. aureus* [84]. Currently, Huang [73] demonstrated the inhibitory effect of kaempferol on the activity of a dihydropyrimidinase from *P. aeruginosa* with the IC_{50} value of 50 ± 2 μM.

Nowadays, it is believed that the structure-activity relationship in the antimicrobial effect of flavonoids should be further examined because it is a very large group of compounds, and many issues have not yet been clarified. Xie et al. [75] concluded that hydroxyl groups at special positions on the aromatic rings of flavonoids improve the antibacterial effect. Flavonoids have the C_6-C_3-C_6 carbon structure consisting of two phenyl rings (A and B) and a heterocyclic ring (C). Generally, it was observed that at least one hydroxyl group in the ring A (especially at C-7) is vital for the antibacterial activity of flavones, and in another position such as C-5 and C-6 can increase this biological effect [85]. In this context, it is interesting to compare our results regarding the antibacterial activity of flavones with the hydroxyl groups at C-5 and C-7 (chrysin, apigenin, luteolin, and their glycosides) and flavone devoid of them. Just like other chemicals from this flavonoid class, flavone showed moderate inhibitory influence on the growth of *E. coli* and *P. aeruginosa* (MIC = 500 μg/mL). The same level of flavone activity was found against *E. faecalis*, and it was the highest value among the flavonoids tested. Only against *S. aureus*, the above-mentioned substance was inactive at concentrations tested (15.6–1000 μg/mL). Furthermore, we observed that a number of hydroxyl groups at two aromatic rings do not correspond with higher antimicrobial activity of flavonoids, i.e., quercetin has five hydroxyl groups, but it was not active against *E. faecalis*, *S. aureus*, and *P. aeruginosa*. In addition, some studies displayed a low effect of quercetin on *B. subtilis*, *E. cloacae*, *E. coli*, and *K. pneumoniae* [86]. The structure-activity relationships of flavonoids were discussed by Xie et al. [87], and it was summarized that two hydroxyl substituents on C-5 and C-7 of ring A of quercetin, rutin, and naringenin lead to their antibacterial activities. Moreover, it was found that the saturation of the C_2=C_3 double bond (in naringin) increased the antibacterial activity. However, in our study naringin was the most active against *P. aeruginosa* only in comparison with kaempferol and quercetin. On the other side, a recent study showed that the presence of glycosyl conjugated groups to polyphenols may reduce antibacterial activity [88]. We showed that glycosides of flavonoids (vitexin, vitexin 2″-*O*-rhamnoside, isovitexin, orientin, isoorientin, naringin, rutin) have some antibacterial effects (Table 2). The aglycone apigenin exhibited higher activity against *S. aureus* in comparison with its glycosides vitexin, isovitexin, and vitexin 2″-*O*-rhamnoside, however the aglycon luteolin had the same antibacterial effects on all bacterial strains as its *C*-glucosides orientin and isoorientin.

According to the literature, the level of sensitivity of the bacterial species studied by us to plant substances is very diverse and strongly depends not only on the type of active compound but also on the selected strains, as shown by comparative analyses in this regard [5,53]. It may also affect large discrepancies in the results between individual investigations. Some literature data suggest that standard strains are generally much more sensitive to antibiotics and natural plant compounds than current clinical isolates. For example, the MIC values of quercetin, apigenin, naringin, chlorogenic, and quinic acids for *E. coli* ATCC 35218, *P. aeruginosa* ATCC 10145, *S. aureus* ATCC 25923, and *E. faecalis* ATCC 29212 reached 2–16 μg/mL, while for the clinical strains it ranged between 32 and 128 μg/mL or above this [5]. In turn, research conducted by Su et al. [53] showed a slightly higher sensitivity of some clinical isolates of methicillin-resistant *S. aureus* to luteolin and quercetin (MIC = 31.2–62.5 μg/mL) than methicillin-sensitive strains (MIC = 125 μg/mL). In the study of Morimoto et al. [89], quinolone-resistant *S. aureus* Mu50 was much more sensitive to apigenin (MIC = 4 μg/mL) than quinolone-susceptible *S. aureus* strain FDA 209P (MIC > 128 μg/mL). Compared to the above-cited works [5,89], it was interesting that apigenin and chlorogenic acid were practically inactive (MIC > 4000 μg/mL) against all 34 strains of *S. aureus* tested by Su et al. [53]. Our investigations exhibited the moderate or weak activity of these two compounds against *S. aureus* (MIC = 500–1000 μg/mL). A recent review of the literature [33] showed that chlorogenic acid has a broad spectrum of antimicrobial activity, but its effect is very diverse. This phenolic acid strongly inhibited the growth of *E. faecalis* (MIC = 64 μg/mL), while it was inactive against *P. aeruginosa* (MIC_{80} = 10,000 μg/mL). For *S. aureus* and *E. coli*, its MIC values ranged from 40–80 to 10,000 μg/mL. The above data are largely consistent with the results of the current work (Table 2). We exhibited the moderate activity of chlorogenic acid against *E. coli* (MIC = 500 μg/mL) and confirmed the lack of significant influence of this substance on *P. aeruginosa* at the concentrations tested (MIC > 1000 μg/mL).

In addition to chlorogenic acid, we also studied the biological influence of other phenolic acids: rosmarinic and salicylic ones. In addition, their antibacterial activity was compared with some aliphatic acids: citric, malic, and quinic. Generally, there were no clear differences in the activity of these two groups of substances. However, the simple phenolic compound salicylic acid showed the highest activity with the MIC values of 250–500 μg/mL. Many studies proved that rosmarinic acid has an antimicrobial effect on Gram-positive and Gram-negative bacteria [65,71,90]. Sometimes, the level of this activity was not high. Recently, Akhtar et al. [65] indicated the moderate growth inhibition zones of clinical isolates of *P. aeruginosa* (13 mm in diameter), *S. aureus* (12 mm), *Proteus vulgaris* (11 mm), and *E. coli* (10 mm) at 1 μg/mL concentration of rosmarinic acid. Similarly, Matejczyk et al. [71] observed a not very strong antibacterial effect of this phenolic acid on *E. coli* (MIC > 250 μg/mL), *Bacillus* sp. (MIC > 500 μg/mL), *S. epidermidis* (MIC > 500 μg/mL), and *S. pyogenes* (MIC > 500 μg/mL) in comparison with an antibiotic kanamycin (MIC > 100 μg/mL). In turn, Ekambaram et al. [69] demonstrated the MIC values of rosmarinic acid against *S. aureus* and MRSA on the level of 800 and 10,000 μg/mL, respectively. Blaskovich et al. [54] carried out experimental research and made a critical review of the antimicrobial activity of salicylic acid. Results of these studies demonstrated that salicylic acid was practically inactive against various bacterial strains, including *B. subtilis* ATCC 6633, *E. faecalis* ATCC 29212, *S. aureus*, MSSA ATCC 25923, and *S. pneumoniae* ATCC 33400 (MIC = 32,000 μg/mL). The antibacterial properties are relatively well known for small aliphatic molecules tested by us: citric, malic, and quinic acids [91–93]. Investigations concerning the effect of quinic acid on cellular functions of *S. aureus* demonstrated that this organic acid could significantly decrease the intracellular pH and ATP concentration, and also reduce the DNA content [93]. Citric acid was previously shown to have the MICs of 900 μg/mL for *S. aureus* and 1500 μg/mL for *E. coli*, and to be very effective in the treatment of chronic wound infections in a dose of 3 g of citric acid dissolved in 100 mL of distilled water [91]. In turn, Gao et al. [85] demonstrated no clear activity of citric and malic acids against *E. coli* (MIC = 1667 and 2000 μg/mL, respectively) *B. subtilis* (MIC = 2000 μg/mL), and *S. suis* (MIC = 8000 and 6667 μg/mL). However, Jensen et al. [92] exhibited that cranberry juice and its main compounds (citric, malic, quinic, and shikimic acids) reduce *E. coli* colonization of the bladder. These organic acids decreased bacterial levels when they were administered together or in a combination of malic acid and citric or quinic ones. Our research confirmed the antibacterial activity of citric, malic, and quinic acids not only against *E. coli* (MIC = 500 μg/mL), but also against *P. aeruginosa* and *E. faecalis* (Table 2).

5. Conclusions

Our research confirmed the antibacterial activity of all tested plant compounds. With the exception of kaempferol and quercetin, they showed a biological effect against clinical strains of 3–4 bacterial species. Microbiological screening of flavonoids and organic acids allowed to exhibit some interesting details and relationships. First of all, these metabolites were generally more potent against Gram-negative bacteria: *E. coli* and *P. aeruginosa* than Gram-positive ones: *E. faecalis* and *S. aureus*. On the other hand, the comparative study of antibacterial activity of flavone, chrysin, apigenin, and luteolin demonstrated that the presence of hydroxyl groups in the phenyl rings A (C-5, C-7) and B (C-3′, C-4′) usually did not affect the activity level of flavones. Only in the case of *S. aureus*, a clear increase in the activity of the hydroxy derivatives of flavone was observed. Similarly, the presence and position of the sugar group in the flavone glycosides generally had no effect on the MIC values.

A comparison of our results with the literature data exhibited that the level of sensitivity of the bacterial species to plant substances is very diverse, and strongly depends not only on the type of active compounds but also on the strains tested. Moreover, it seems that current clinical isolates are generally much less sensitive to the natural plant metabolites than standard strains. Numerous standard strains have been isolated many years ago, therefore, with the currently growing resistance of bacteria, their use for the screening microbiological tests is limited. In our investigations, we found the moderate or even low activity of flavonoids and organic acids compared to the traditional antibiotics and some plant substances. However, examples of the use of natural compounds with a relatively low in vitro activity in the treatment of urinary tract infections, chronic wound infections, etc. or as food additives show that widely distributed flavonoids and organic acids could find broad practical applications.

Author Contributions: Conceptualization, A.A. and T.M.K.; methodology, A.A. and T.M.K.; reagents and investigation, A.A., M.O., and T.M.K.; visualization of chemical structures, T.M.K.; literature search, A.A., and M.O.; writing—original draft preparation, A.A., and M.O.; writing—review and editing, A.A., and M.O. All authors have read and agreed to the published version of the manuscript.

Funding: This research was funded from the budget of the Department of Medical Microbiology, Poznań University of Medical Sciences and the Polish Multiannual Programme entitled 'Creating the scientific basis of the biological progress and conservation of plant genetic resources as a source of innovation to support sustainable agriculture and food security of the country'.

Conflicts of Interest: The authors declare no conflict of interest.

References

1. Chandra, H.; Bishnoi, P.; Yadav, A.; Patni, B.; Mishra, A.P.; Nautiyal, A.R. Antimicrobial resistance and the alternative resources with special emphasis on plant-based antimicrobials–A review. *Plants* **2017**, *6*, 16. [CrossRef] [PubMed]
2. Gupta, P.D.; Birdi, T.J. Development of botanicals to combat antibiotic resistance. *J. Ayur. Integr. Med.* **2017**, *8*, 266–275. [CrossRef] [PubMed]
3. Mate, A. (Ed.) *Medicinal and Aromatic Plants of the World. Scientific, Production, Commercial and Utilization Aspects*; Springer Science + Business Media: Dordrecht, The Netherlands, 2015; Volume 1.
4. Zheng, J.; Huang, C.; Yang, B.; Kallio, H. Regulation of phytochemicals in fruits and berries by environmental variation—Sugars and organic acids. *J. Food Biochem.* **2019**, *43*, e12642. [CrossRef] [PubMed]

5. Özçelik, B.; Kartal, M.; Orhan, I. Cytotoxicity, antiviral and antimicrobial activities of alkaloids, flavonoids, and phenolic acids. *Pharm. Biol.* **2011**, *49*, 396–402. [CrossRef]
6. Barbieri, R.; Coppo, E.; Marchese, A.; Daglia, M.; Sobarzo-Sánchez, E.; Nabavi, S.F.; Nabavi, S.M. Phytochemicals for human disease: An update on plant-derived compounds antibacterial activity. *Microbiol. Res.* **2017**, *196*, 44–68. [CrossRef]
7. Fialova, S.; Rendekova, K.; Mucaji, P.; Slobodnikova, L. Plant natural agents: Polyphenols, alkaloids and essential oils as perspective solution of microbial resistance. *Curr. Org. Chem.* **2017**, *21*, 1875–1884. [CrossRef]
8. Khameneh, B.; Iranshahy, M.; Soheili, V.; Bazzaz, B.S.F. Review on plant antimicrobials: A mechanistic viewpoint. *Antimicrob. Resist. Infect. Control* **2019**, *8*, 118. [CrossRef]
9. Gutiérrez-Grijalva, E.P.; Picos-Salas, M.A.; Leyva-López, N.; Criollo-Mendoza, M.S.; Vazquez-Olivo, G.; Heredia, J.B. Flavonoids and phenolic acids from oregano: Occurrence, biological activity and health benefits. *Plants* **2018**, *7*, 2. [CrossRef]
10. Jungbauer, A.; Medjakovic, S. Anti-inflammatory properties of culinary herbs and spices that ameliorate the effects of metabolic syndrome. *Maturitas* **2012**, *71*, 227–239. [CrossRef]
11. Goncalves, S.; Moreira, E.; Grosso, C.; Andrade, P.B.; Valentao, P.; Romano, A. Phenolic profile, antioxidant activity and enzyme inhibitory activities of extracts from aromatic plants used in mediterranean diet. *J. Food Sci. Technol.* **2017**, *54*, 219–227. [CrossRef]
12. Mileo, A.M.; Nisticò, P.; Miccadei, S. Polyphenols: Immunomodulatory and therapeutic implication in colorectal cancer. *Front. Immunol.* **2019**, *10*, 729. [CrossRef] [PubMed]
13. Singh, A.K.; Cabral, C.; Kumar, R.; Ganguly, R.; Rana, H.K.; Gupta, A.; Lauro, M.R.; Carbone, C.; Reis, F.; Pandey, A.K. Beneficial effects of dietary polyphenols on gut microbiota and strategies to improve delivery efficiency. *Nutrients* **2019**, *11*, 2216. [CrossRef] [PubMed]
14. Wang, M.; Firrman, J.; Liu, L.S.; Yam, K. A review on flavonoid apigenin: Dietary intake, ADME, antimicrobial effects, and interactions with human gut microbiota. *BioMed Res. Int.* **2019**, *2019*, 7010467. [CrossRef]
15. Chua, L.S. A review on plant-based rutin extraction methods and its pharmacological activities. *J. Ethnopharmacol.* **2013**, *150*, 805–817. [CrossRef] [PubMed]
16. Enogieru, A.B.; Haylett, W.; Hiss, D.C.; Bardien, S.; Ekpo, O.E. Rutin as a potent antioxidant: Implications for neurodegenerative disorders. *Oxid. Med. Cell Longev.* **2018**, *2018*, 6241017. [CrossRef] [PubMed]
17. Edwards, J.E.; Brown, P.N.; Talent, N.; Dickinson, T.A.; Shipley, P.R. A review of the chemistry of the genus *Crataegus*. *Phytochemistry* **2012**, *79*, 5–26. [CrossRef]
18. Yamaguchi, K.K.L.; Pereira, L.F.R.; Lamarão, C.V.; Lima, E.S.; da Veiga-Junior, V.F. Amazon acai: Chemistry and biological activities: A review. *Food Chem.* **2015**, *179*, 137–151. [CrossRef]
19. Yuan, L.; Wang, J.; Wu, W.; Liu, Q.; Liu, X. Effect of isoorientin on intracellular antioxidant defence mechanisms in hepatoma and liver cell lines. *Biomed. Pharmacother.* **2016**, *81*, 356–362. [CrossRef]
20. Mani, R.; Natesan, V. Chrysin: Sources, beneficial pharmacological activities, and molecular mechanism of action. *Phytochemistry* **2018**, *145*, 187–196. [CrossRef]
21. Ożarowski, M.; Piasecka, A.; Paszel-Jaworska, A.; Chaves, D.S.; Romaniuk, A.; Rybczyńska, M.; Gryszczynska, A.; Sawikowska, A.; Kachlicki, P.; Mikolajczak, P.L.; et al. Comparison of bioactive compounds content in leaf extracts of *Passiflora incarnata*, *P. caerulea* and *P. alata* and in vitro cytotoxic potential on leukemia cell lines. *Rev. Bras. Farmacogn.* **2018**, *28*, 79–191. [CrossRef]
22. Naz, S.; Imran, M.; Rauf, A.; Orhan, I.E.; Shariati, M.A.; Haq, I.U.; Yasmin, I.; Shahbaz, M.; Qaisrani, T.B.; Shah, Z.A.; et al. Chrysin: Pharmacological and therapeutic properties. *Life Sci.* **2019**, *235*, 116797. [CrossRef]
23. Przybyłek, I.; Karpiński, T.M. Antibacterial properties of propolis. *Molecules* **2019**, *24*, 2047. [CrossRef] [PubMed]
24. Alam, M.A.; Subhan, N.; Rahman, M.M.; Uddin, S.J.; Reza, H.M.; Sarker, S.D. Effect of *Citrus* flavonoids, naringin and naringenin, on metabolic syndrome and their mechanisms of action. *Adv. Nutr.* **2014**, *5*, 404–417. [CrossRef] [PubMed]
25. Viljakainen, S.; Visti, A.; Laakso, S. Concentrations of organic acids and soluble sugars in juices from Nordic berries. *Acta Agric. Scand. Sect. B Soil Plant Sci.* **2002**, *52*, 101–109. [CrossRef]
26. Pande, G.; Akoh, C.C. Organic acids, antioxidant capacity, phenolic content and lipid characterisation of Georgia-grown underutilized fruit crops. *Food Chem.* **2010**, *120*, 1067–1075. [CrossRef]
27. Nour, V.; Trandafir, I.; Ionica, M.E. Ascorbic acid, anthocyanins, organic acids and mineral content of some black and red currant cultivars. *Fruits* **2011**, *66*, 353–362. [CrossRef]

28. Kaume, L.; Howard, L.R.; Devareddy, L. The blackberry fruit: A review on its composition and chemistry, metabolism and bioavailability, and health benefits. *J. Agric. Food Chem.* **2012**, *60*, 5716–5727. [CrossRef]
29. Wang, Y.; Johnson-Cicalese, J.; Singh, A.P.; Vorsa, N. Characterization and quantification of flavonoids and organic acids over fruit development in American cranberry (*Vaccinium macrocarpon*) cultivars using HPLC and APCI-MS/MS. *Plant Sci.* **2017**, *262*, 91–102. [CrossRef]
30. Denev, P.; Kratchanova, M.; Petrova, I.; Klisurova, D.; Georgiev, Y.; Ognyanov, M.; Yanakieva, I. Black chokeberry (*Aronia melanocarpa* (Michx.) Elliot) fruits and functional drinks differ significantly in their chemical composition and antioxidant activity. *J. Chem.* **2018**, *2018*, 9574587. [CrossRef]
31. Adamczak, A.; Buchwald, W.; Kozłowski, J. Variation in the content of flavonols and main organic acids in the fruit of European cranberry (*Oxycoccus palustris* Pers.) growing in peatlands of North-Western Poland. *Herba Pol.* **2011**, *57*, 5–15.
32. Jurikova, T.; Mlcek, J.; Skrovankova, S.; Sumczynski, D.; Sochor, J.; Hlavacova, I.; Snopek, L.; Orsavova, J. Fruits of black chokeberry *Aronia melanocarpa* in the prevention of chronic diseases. *Molecules* **2017**, *22*, 944. [CrossRef] [PubMed]
33. Santana-Gálvez, J.; Cisneros-Zevallos, L.; Jacobo-Velázquez, D.A. Chlorogenic Acid: Recent advances on its dual role as a food additive and a nutraceutical against metabolic syndrome. *Molecules* **2017**, *22*, 358. [CrossRef]
34. Meinhart, A.D.; Damin, F.M.; Caldeirao, L.; Silveira, T.F.F.; Filho, J.T.; Godoy, H.T. Chlorogenic acid isomer contents in 100 plants commercialized in Brazil. *Food Res. Int.* **2017**, *99*, 522–530. [CrossRef] [PubMed]
35. Shekarchi, M.; Hajimehdipoor, H.; Saeidnia, S.; Gohari, A.R.; Hamedani, M.P. Comparative study of rosmarinic acid content in some plants of Labiatae family. *Pharmacogn. Mag.* **2012**, *8*, 37–41. [PubMed]
36. Ożarowski, M.; Mikołajczak, P.; Bogacz, A.; Gryszczyńska, A.; Kujawska, M.; Jodynis-Libert, J.; Piasecka, A.; Napieczynska, H.; Szulc, M.; Kujawski, R.; et al. *Rosmarinus officinalis* L. leaf extract improves memory impairment and affects acetylcholinesterase and butyrylcholinesterase activities in rat brain. *Fitoterapia* **2013**, *91*, 261–271. [CrossRef] [PubMed]
37. Ożarowski, M.; Mikolajczak, P.L.; Piasecka, A.; Kachlicki, P.; Kujawski, R.; Bogacz, A.; Bartkowiak-Wieczorek, J.; Szulc, M.; Kaminska, E.; Kujawska, M.; et al. Influence of the *Melissa officinalis* leaf extract on long-term memory in scopolamine animal model with assessment of mechanism of action. *Evid. Based Complem. Alternat. Med.* **2016**, *2016*, 9729818. [CrossRef] [PubMed]
38. Balcke, G.U.; Handrick, V.; Bergau, N.; Fichtner, M.; Henning, A.; Stellmach, H.; Tissier, A.; Hause, B.; Frolov, A. An UPLC-MS/MS method for highly sensitive high-throughput analysis of phytohormones in plant tissues. *Plant Methods* **2012**, *8*, 47. [CrossRef]
39. Toiu, A.; Vlase, L.; Oniga, I.; Benedec, D.; Tămaş, M. HPLC analysis of salicylic derivatives from natural products. *Farmacia* **2011**, *59*, 106–112.
40. Bijttebier, S.; van der Auwera, A.; Voorspoels, S.; Noten, B.; Hermans, N.; Pieters, L.; Apers, S. A first step in the quest for the active constituents in *Filipendula ulmaria* (meadowsweet): Comprehensive phytochemical identification by liquid chromatography coupled to quadrupole-orbitrap mass spectrometry. *Planta Med.* **2016**, *82*, 559–572. [CrossRef]
41. Nabavi, S.F.; Habtemariam, S.; Ahmed, T.; Sureda, A.; Daglia, M.; Sobarzo-Sánchez, E.; Nabavi, S.M. Polyphenolic composition of *Crataegus monogyna* Jacq.: From chemistry to medical applications. *Nutrients* **2015**, *7*, 7708–7728. [CrossRef]
42. Kerasioti, E.; Apostolou, A.; Kafantaris, I.; Chronis, K.; Kokka, E.; Dimitriadou, C.; Tzanetou, E.N.; Priftis, A.; Koulocheri, S.D.; Haroutounian, S.; et al. Polyphenolic composition of *Rosa canina, Rosa sempervivens* and *Pyrocantha coccinea* extracts and assessment of their antioxidant activity in human endothelial cells. *Antioxidants* **2019**, *8*, 92. [CrossRef] [PubMed]
43. Cho, J.W.; Cho, S.Y.; Lee, S.R.; Lee, K.S. Onion extract and quercetin induce matrix metalloproteinase-1 in vitro and in vivo. *Int. J. Mol. Med.* **2010**, *25*, 347–352. [PubMed]
44. Chuang, S.Y.; Lin, Y.K.; Lin, C.F.; Wang, P.W.; Chen, E.L.; Fang, J.Y. Elucidating the skin delivery of aglycone and glycoside flavonoids: How the structures affect cutaneous absorption. *Nutrients* **2017**, *9*, 1304. [CrossRef]
45. Nagoba, B.S.; Suryawanshi, N.M.; Wadher, B.; Selkar, S. Acidic environment and wound healing: A review. *Wounds* **2015**, *27*, 5–11.

46. Nagoba, B.; Davane, M.; Gandhi, R.; Wadher, B.; Suryawanshi, N.; Selkar, S. Treatment of skin and soft tissue infections caused by *Pseudomonas aeruginosa*—A review of our experiences with citric acid over the past 20 years. *Wound Med.* **2017**, *19*, 5–9. [CrossRef]
47. Bessa, L.J.; Fazii, P.; Di Giulio, M.; Cellini, L. Bacterial isolates from infected wounds and their antibiotic susceptibility pattern: Some remarks about wound infection. *Int. Wound J.* **2013**, *12*, 47–52. [CrossRef]
48. Karpiński, T.M. Efficacy of octenidine against *Pseudomonas aeruginosa* strains. *Eur. J. Biol. Res.* **2019**, *9*, 135–140.
49. CLSI. *Performance Standards for Antimicrobial Disk Susceptibility Tests. Approved Standard*, 12th ed.; CLSI document M02-A12; Clinical and Laboratory Standards Institute: Wayne, PA, USA, 2015; Volume 35, no 1.
50. EUCAST. *MIC Determination of Non-Fastidious and Fastidious Organisms*. Available online: http://www.eucast.org/ast_of_bacteria/mic_determination (accessed on 26 July 2019).
51. Karpiński, T.M.; Adamczak, A. Fucoxanthin—An antibacterial carotenoid. *Antioxidants* **2019**, *8*, 239. [CrossRef] [PubMed]
52. Gao, Z.; Shao, J.; Sun, H.; Zhong, W.; Zhuang, W.; Zhang, Z. Evaluation of different kinds of organic acids and their antibacterial activity in Japanese Apricot fruits. *Afr. J. Agric. Res.* **2012**, *7*, 4911–4918. [CrossRef]
53. Su, Y.; Ma, L.; Wen, Y.; Wang, H.; Zhang, S. Studies of the in vitro antibacterial activities of several polyphenols against clinical isolates of methicillin-resistant *Staphylococcus aureus*. *Molecules* **2014**, *19*, 12630–12639. [CrossRef]
54. Blaskovich, M.A.; Elliott, A.G.; Kavanagh, A.M.; Ramu, S.; Cooper, M.A. In vitro antimicrobial activity of acne drugs against skin-associated bacteria. *Sci. Rep.* **2019**, *9*, 14658. [CrossRef] [PubMed]
55. Basile, A.; Giordano, S.; López-Sáez, J.A.; Cobianchi, R.C. Antibacterial activity of pure flavonoids isolated from mosses. *Phytochemistry* **1999**, *52*, 1479–1482. [CrossRef]
56. Afifi, F.U.; Abu-Dahab, R. Phytochemical screening and biological activities of *Eminium spiculatum* (Blume) Kuntze (family Araceae). *Nat. Prod. Res.* **2012**, *26*, 878–882. [CrossRef] [PubMed]
57. Das, M.C.; Sandhu, P.; Gupta, P.; Rudrapaul, P.; De, U.C.; Tribedi, P.; Akhter, Y.; Bhattacharjee, S. Attenuation of *Pseudomonas aeruginosa* biofilm formation by vitexin: A combinatorial study with azithromycin and gentamicin. *Sci. Rep.* **2016**, *6*, 23347. [CrossRef] [PubMed]
58. Das, M.C.; Das, A.; Samaddar, S.; Dawarea, A.V.; Ghosh, C.; Acharjee, S.; Sandhu, P.; Jawed, J.J.; De Utpal, C.; Majumdar, S.; et al. Vitexin alters *Staphylococcus aureus* surface hydrophobicity to interfere with biofilm 2 formation. *bioRxiv* **2018**. [CrossRef]
59. Awolola, G.V.; Koorbanally, N.A.; Chenia, H.; Shode, F.O.; Baijnath, H. Antibacterial and anti-biofilm activity of flavonoids and triterpenes isolated from the extracts of *Ficus sansibarica* Warb. subsp. *Sansibarica* (*Moraceae*) extracts. *Afr. J. Tradit. Complem. Altern. Med.* **2014**, *11*, 124–131. [CrossRef]
60. Rammohan, A.; Bhaskar, B.V.; Venkateswarlu, N.; Rao, V.L.; Gunasekar, D.; Zyryanov, G.V. Isolation of flavonoids from the flowers of *Rhynchosia beddomei* Baker as prominent antimicrobial agents and molecular docking. *Microb. Pathog.* **2019**, *136*, 103667. [CrossRef]
61. Aderogba, M.A.; Akinkunmi, E.O.; Mabusela, W.T. Antioxidant and antimicrobial activities of flavonoid glycosides from *Dennettia tripetala* G. Baker leaf extract. *Nig. J. Nat. Prod. Med.* **2011**, *15*, 49–52. [CrossRef]
62. Cottiglia, F.; Loy, G.; Garau, D.; Floris, C.; Casu, M.; Pompei, R.; Bonsignore, L. Antimicrobial evaluation of coumarins and flavonoids from the stems of *Daphne gnidium* L. *Phytomedicine* **2001**, *8*, 302–305. [CrossRef]
63. Ali, H.; Dixit, S. In vitro antimicrobial activity of flavanoids of *Ocimum sanctum* with synergistic effect of their combined form. *Asian Pac. J. Trop. Dis.* **2012**, *2*, S396–S398. [CrossRef]
64. Celiz, G.; Daz, M.; Audisio, M.C. Antibacterial activity of naringin derivatives against pathogenic strains. *J. Appl. Microbiol.* **2011**, *111*, 731–738. [CrossRef] [PubMed]
65. Akhtar, M.S.; Hossain, M.A.; Said, S.A. Isolation and characterization of antimicrobial compound from the stem-bark of the traditionally used medicinal plant *Adenium obesum*. *J. Tradit. Complem. Med.* **2017**, *7*, 296–300. [CrossRef] [PubMed]
66. Singh, M.; Govindarajan, R.; Rawat, A.K.S.; Khare, P.B. Antimicrobial flavonoid rutin from *Pteris vittata* L. against pathogenic gastrointestinal microflora. *Am. Fern J.* **2008**, *98*, 98–103. [CrossRef]
67. Liu, H.; Mou, Y.; Zhao, J.; Wang, J.; Zhou, L.; Wang, M.; Wang, D.; Han, J.; Yu, Z.; Yang, F. Flavonoids from *Halostachys caspica* and their antimicrobial and antioxidant activities. *Molecules* **2010**, *15*, 7933–7945. [CrossRef] [PubMed]

68. Banerjee, K.; Banerjee, S.; Das, S.; Mandal, M. Probing the potential of apigenin liposomes in enhancing bacterial membrane perturbation and integrity loss. *J. Colloid Interface Sci.* **2015**, *453*, 48–59. [CrossRef] [PubMed]
69. Ekambaram, S.P.; Perumal, S.S.; Balakrishnan, A.; Marappan, N.; Gajendran, S.S.; Viswanathan, V. Antibacterial synergy between rosmarinic acid and antibiotics against methicillin-resistant *Staphylococcus aureus*. *J. Intercult. Ethnopharmacol.* **2016**, *5*, 358–363. [CrossRef] [PubMed]
70. Smiljkovic, M.; Stanisavljevic, D.; Stojkovic, D.; Petrovic, I.; Vicentic, M.J.; Popovic, J.; Golic Grdadolnik, S.; Markovic, D.; Sankovic-Babice, S.; Glamoclija, J.; et al. Apigenin-7-O-glucoside versus apigenin: Insight into the modes of anticandidal and cytotoxic actions. *EXCLI J.* **2017**, *16*, 795–807.
71. Matejczyk, M.; Swisłocka, R.; Golonko, A.; Lewandowski, W.; Hawrylik, E. Cytotoxic, genotoxic and antimicrobial activity of caffeic and rosmarinic acids and their lithium, sodium and potassium salts as potential anticancer compounds. *Adv. Med. Sci.* **2018**, *63*, 14–21. [CrossRef]
72. Ren, G.; Xue, P.; Sun, X.; Zhao, G. Determination of the volatile and polyphenol constituents and the antimicrobial, antioxidant, and tyrosinase inhibitory activities of the bioactive compounds from the by-product of *Rosa rugosa* Thunb. var. *plena* Regal tea. *BMC Complem. Altern. Med.* **2018**, *18*, 307. [CrossRef]
73. Huang, C.Y. Inhibition of a putative dihydropyrimidinase from *Pseudomonas aeruginosa* PAO1 by flavonoids and substrates of cyclic amidohydrolases. *PLoS ONE* **2015**, *10*, e0127634. [CrossRef]
74. Bustos, P.S.; Deza-Ponzio, R.; Páez, P.L.; Cabrera, J.L.; Virgolini, M.B.; Ortega, M.G. Flavonoids as protective agents against oxidative stress induced by gentamicin in systemic circulation. Potent protective activity and microbial synergism of luteolin. *Food Chem. Toxicol.* **2018**, *118*, 294–302. [CrossRef] [PubMed]
75. Xie, Y.; Yang, W.; Tang, F.; Chen, X.; Ren, L. Antibacterial activities of flavonoids: Structure-activity relationship and mechanism. *Curr. Med. Chem.* **2015**, *22*, 132–149. [CrossRef] [PubMed]
76. Górniak, I.; Bartoszewski, R.; Króliczewski, J. Comprehensive review of antimicrobial activities of plant flavonoids. *Phytochem. Rev.* **2019**, *18*, 241–272. [CrossRef]
77. Ohemeng, K.A.; Schwender, C.F.; Fu, K.P.; Barrett, J.F. DNA gyrase inhibitory and antibacterial activity of some flavones. *Bioorg. Med. Chem. Lett.* **1993**, *3*, 225–230. [CrossRef]
78. Lee, J.H.; Regmi, S.C.; Kim, J.A.; Cho, M.H.; Yun, H.; Lee, C.S.; Lee, J. Apple flavonoid phloretin inhibits *Escherichia coli* O157:H7 biofilm formation and ameliorates colon inflammation in rats. *Infect. Immun.* **2011**, *79*, 4819–4827. [CrossRef]
79. Siriwong, S.; Thumanu, K.; Hengpratom, T.; Eumkeb, G. Synergy and mode ofaction of ceftazidime plus quercetin or luteolin on *Streptococcus pyogenes*. *Evid. Based Complem. Altern. Med.* **2015**, *2015*, 759459. [CrossRef]
80. Betts, J.W.; Sharili, A.S.; Phee, L.M.; Wareham, D.W. In vitro activity of epigallocatechin gallate and quercetin alone and in combination versus clinical isolates of methicillin-resistant *Staphylococcus aureus*. *J. Nat. Prod.* **2015**, *78*, 2145–2148. [CrossRef]
81. Hossion, A.M.; Zamami, Y.; Kandahary, R.K.; Tsuchiya, T.; Ogawa, W.; Iwado, A. Quercetin diacylglycoside analogues showing dual inhibition of DNA gyrase and topoisomerase IV as novel antibacterial agents. *J. Med. Chem.* **2011**, *54*, 3686–3703. [CrossRef]
82. Chen, C.C.; Huang, C.Y. Inhibition of *Klebsiella pneumoniae* DnaB helicase by the flavonol galangin. *Protein J.* **2011**, *30*, 59–65. [CrossRef]
83. Lin, H.H.; Huang, C.Y. Characterization of flavonol inhibition of DnaB helicase: Real-time monitoring, structural modeling, and proposed mechanism. *J. Biomed. Biotechnol.* **2012**, *2012*, 735368. [CrossRef]
84. Huang, Y.H.; Huang, C.C.; Chen, C.C.; Yang, K.; Huang, C.Y. Inhibition of *Staphylococcus aureus* PriA helicase by flavonol kaempferol. *Protein J.* **2015**, *34*, 169–172. [CrossRef] [PubMed]
85. Farhadi, F.; Khameneh, B.; Iranshahi, M.; Iranshahy, M. Antibacterial activity of flavonoids and their structure-activity relationship: An update review. *Phytother. Res.* **2019**, *33*, 13–40. [CrossRef] [PubMed]
86. Echeverría, J.; Opazo, J.; Mendoza, L.; Urzúa, A.; Wilkens, M. Structure-activity and lipophilicity relationships of selected antibacterial natural flavones and flavanones of chilean flora. *Molecules* **2017**, *22*, 608. [CrossRef] [PubMed]
87. Xie, Y.; Chen, J.; Xiao, A.; Liu, L. Antibacterial activity of polyphenols: Structure-activity relationship and influence of hyperglycemic condition. *Molecules* **2017**, *22*, 1913. [CrossRef] [PubMed]

88. Bouarab-Chibane, L.; Forquet, V.; Lantéri, P.; Clément, Y.; Léonard-Akkari, L.; Oulahal, N.; Degraeve, P.; Bordes, C. Antibacterial properties of polyphenols: Characterization and QSAR (Quantitative Structure–Activity Relationship) models. *Front. Microbiol.* **2019**, *10*, 829. [CrossRef] [PubMed]
89. Morimoto, Y.; Baba, T.; Sasaki, T.; Hiramatsu, K. Apigenin as an anti-quinolone-resistance antibiotic. *Int. J. Antimicrob. Agents.* **2015**, *46*, 666–673. [CrossRef]
90. Amin, A.; Vincent, R.; Séverine, M. Rosmarinic acid and its methyl ester as antimicrobial components of the hydromethanolic extract of *Hyptis atrorubens* Poit. (*Lamiaceae*). *Evid. Based Complem. Alternat. Med.* **2013**, *2013*, 604536.
91. Nagoba, B.S.; Gandhi, R.C.; Wadher, B.J.; Potekar, R.M.; Kolhe, S.M. Microbiological, histopathological and clinical changes in chronic infected wounds after citric acid treatment. *J. Med. Microbiol.* **2008**, *57*, 681–682. [CrossRef]
92. Jensen, H.D.; Struve, C.; Christensen, S.B.; Krogfelt, K.A. Cranberry juice and combinations of its organic acids are effective against experimental urinary tract infection. *Front. Microbiol.* **2017**, *8*, 542. [CrossRef]
93. Bai, J.; Wu, Y.; Zhong, K.; Xiao, K.; Liu, L.; Huang, Y.; Wang, Z.; Gao, H. A comparative study on the effects of quinic acid and shikimic acid on cellular functions of *Staphylococcus aureus*. *J. Food Prot.* **2018**, *81*, 1187–1192. [CrossRef]

Journal of
Clinical Medicine

MDPI

Article

Ulmus parvifolia Accelerates Skin Wound Healing by Regulating the Expression of MMPs and TGF-β

Min Cheol Kang [1,†], Silvia Yumnam [1,†], Woo Sung Park [2], Hae Min So [3], Ki Hyun Kim [3], Meong Cheol Shin [2], Mi-Jeong Ahn [2] and Sun Yeou Kim [1,4,*]

1 College of Pharmacy, Gachon University 191, Hambakmoero, Yeonsu-gu, Incheon 21936, Korea; mincjf07@gmail.com (M.C.K.); silviayumnam@gmail.com (S.Y.)

2 College of Pharmacy and Research Institute of Pharmaceutical Sciences, Gyeongsang National University, Jinju 52828, Korea; pws8822@gmail.com (W.S.P.); shinmc@gnu.ac.kr (M.C.S.); mjahn07@gmail.com (M.-J.A.)

3 School of Pharmacy, Sungkyunkwan University, Suwon 16419, Korea; haemi9312@naver.com (H.M.S.); khkim83@skku.edu (K.H.K.)

4 Gachon Institute of Pharmaceutical Science, Gachon University, Yeonsu-gu, Incheon 21936, Korea

* Correspondence: sunnykim@gachon.ac.kr; Tel.: +82-32-820-4931

† These authors contributed equally to this work.

Received: 14 November 2019; Accepted: 23 December 2019; Published: 26 December 2019

Abstract: *Ulmus parvifolia* is one of the medicinal plants used traditionally for treatment of wounds. We intended to investigate the wound healing effect of the powder of *Ulmus parvifolia* (UP) root bark in a mouse wound healing model. We also determined the mechanisms of effects of *U. parvifolia* in skin and skin wound healing effects using a keratinocyte model. Animal experiments showed that the wound lesions in the mice decreased with 200 mesh *U. parvifolia* root bark powder and were significantly reduced with treatment by UP, compared with those treated with *Ulmus macrocarpa* (UM). Results from in vitro experiments also revealed that UP extract promoted the migration of human skin keratinocytes. UP powder treatment upregulated the expression of the matrix metalloproteinase-2 and -9 protein and significantly increased transforming growth factor (TGF)-β levels. We confirmed that topical administration of the bark powder exerted a significant effect on skin wound healing by upregulating the expression of MMP and transforming growth factor-β. Our study suggests that *U. parvifolia* may be a potential candidate for skin wound healing including epidermal skin rejuvenation.

Keywords: *Ulmus parvifolia*; wound healing; matrix metalloproteinase; transforming growth factor; skin rejuvenation

1. Introduction

Skin is composed of the dermis and epidermis layers. Skin protects our body against environmental factors such as harmful ultraviolet (UV) rays and pathogens and prevents water loss from the body [1]. When skin is injured, skin repairs itself. The wound healing process in a complex multistep which includes blood clot formation, wound inflammation, and skin tissue proliferation and remodeling [2]. Wounds begin to heal immediately after an injury to release various clotting factors. During the inflammatory phase, neutrophils and macrophages are activated by the release of proinflammatory cytokines including Interleukin (IL)-1β, IL-6, IL-8, Tumor necrosis factor (TNF)-α, and growth factors such as platelet-derived factors (PDGF), transforming growth factors (TGF), Insulin-like growth factor (IGF)-1, and fibroblast growth factors (FGF). In the proliferative phase, these factors stimulate proliferation and migration of cells to move to the injured site for extracellular matrix (ECM) formation. Finally, fibroblast and vascular density decrease during the remodeling phase, old collagen fibers of the initial scar are replaced with matrix, and new collagen fibers are synthesized to form new tissue [3–6].

Because the skin healing process is very complex, there can be limits to fully overcoming wound injury with a single compound. Thus, the development of wound healing agents with natural products may be an option for cutaneous wound treatment. The use of natural products as wound healing materials can have some advantage such as low cost and high safety in comparison to other synthetic agents. For thousands of years, many natural resources have been reported to be used for skin injury. Over the last 10 years, many studies have reported evidence that natural products can improve skin wounds [7]. As part of such research, this study was conducted to demonstrate the pharmacological function of elm tree for skin wounds.

The elm tree is widely distributed in Asia and its stem and root barks have use in traditional oriental medicine to treat gastric disorders and intestinal inflammation [8]. Particularly, it has long been used in regenerating stomach or skin epithelial cells. Korea elms are also known for their effects on blood circulation, the protection of cartilage degeneration, and damaged tissue regeneration [9]. With regard to topical use, elms have been administered for the treatment of minor skin irritations, cold sores, ulcers, abscesses, and boils [10]. Bioactivities of various Ulmus species have been reported. *Ulmus davidiana* var. *japonica* has antioxidant, anti-inflammatory, and immune-modulating effects [11]. Recent studies on *U. parvifolia* Jacq. (UP), a species of elm native to China, Korea, and Japan, have shown that its leaves and stems have anti-inflammatory and antioxidant effects [12]. *U. parvifolia* bark, which contains phenolic compounds and steroidal glucosides, is used for the treatment of eczema and edema [13]. Water-soluble extracts of the root bark of *U. parvifolia* showed anti-inflammatory properties, and cotreatment with the mycelia of mushroom protected against allergic asthma in mice [14,15]. Interestingly, the powder of the original *U. parvifolia* material itself has also been used in oriental medicine, rather than being used only as an extract for a clinical purpose. Therefore, our study aimed to check the possibility of *U. parvifolia* as a candidate for skin wound healing. Firstly, we investigated the influence of dorsal treatment with *U. parvifolia* in the animal model of cutaneous wounds according to the particle size of the *U. parvifolia* root bark power. Furthermore, we performed a comparative study of species differences, such as *U. parvifolia* and *U. macrocarpa*, on potential efficacy in skin wound models.

2. Materials and Methods

2.1. Sample Preparation

Ulmus parvifolia was collected from Busan and Jinju, provided by Prof. MJ Ahn at Gyeongsang National University, Jinju 52828, Korea, in April 2018. The root barks were washed with water, dried, and pulverized using a grinder. Each powder was sieved through 20, 50, 100, and 200 mesh sieves (pore sizes: 0.85, 0.35, 0.15, and 0.075 mm, respectively), to obtain 4 grades of root bark powder. UP powder was extracted twice in 80% methanol for 24 h with 1 h sonication. The solution was filtered through Whatman No. 1 filter paper (GE Healthcare, Cleveland, OH, USA), concentrated using a rotary vacuum evaporator under reduced pressure. The extract was dissolved in dimethyl sulfoxide (DMSO) for in vitro use.

2.2. Measurement of the Angle of Repose of the Powder

The angle of repose (θ) for the root bark powder was measured using the cone height method. Briefly, a funnel was fixed at a height of 30 cm (H) above ground level, and different sizes of the powder were allowed to gently flow through it until the tip of the powder cone touched the outlet of the funnel. The diameter (2R) of the cone was measured for each powder type. The angle of repose (θ) was calculated as follows:

$$\theta = \tan - 1 \times (h/r) \quad (1)$$

This test was performed in triplicate for each sample.

2.3. Wound Healing Model

Specific, pathogen-free, 5-week-old male SKH-1 hairless mice were purchased (Orient Bio; Gyeonggi-do, Korea) and acclimatized for 1 week in a temperature- and humidity-controlled room (23 °C and 60% humidity), under a 12 h light–dark cycle, before the start of the experiments. All experimental protocol for animal experiments was reviewed and approved by the animal care committee of the Center of Animal Care and Use (CACU, LCDI-2018-0007) at the Lee Gil Ya Cancer and Diabetes Institute, Gachon University, Korea. Set A: The mice were randomly divided into 5 groups ($n = 7$). The mice were anesthetized using 5% isoflurane, and the skin was cleaned with 70% ethanol. Two excision wounds were created in the posterior dorsal area of each mouse using a 6 mm biopsy punch (0.28 cm^2), Each wound was (1) untreated; or (2) treated with 50 mesh (12 mg); (3) 100 mesh (12 mg); or (4) 200 mesh (12 mg) root bark powder of UP; and (5) Madecassol® (12 mg, positive control, Dongkook Co.; Korea) topically applied. The wounds were covered with a commercial dressing Tegaderm (3M) to prevent wound infection. The wound was treated once daily for 6 days until the day of sacrifice. Set B (large scale wounds): The mice were randomly divided into 4 groups ($n = 8$). The mice were anesthetized using 5% isoflurane, and the skin was cleaned with 70% ethanol. An excision wound was created on the dorsal by cutting out a circular region, 20 mm in diameter, with surgical scissors. Each wound was (1) untreated; or (2) treated with UP 200 mesh (20 mg); (3) *U. macrocarpa* (UM) 200 mesh (20 mg); and (4) Madecassol® (20 mg, positive control) topically applied. The wounds were covered with a commercial dressing (Tegaderm, 3M, MN, USA) to prevent wound infection. The wound was treated once daily for 15 days until the day of sacrifice.

2.4. Wound Analysis and Histological Assessment

Digital photographs of the wounds were captured on each day of treatment or at day 0, 3, 7, 10, and 14, using a digital camera (Olympus, Tokyo, Japan), and ImageJ software (version 1.5a; Bethesda, MD, USA) was used to measure the wound sizes. Mice were sacrificed at the end of experiments after grafting for histological assessment. The harvested wound areas, including a border of normal tissue, were immediately fixed in 10% neutral-buffered formalin. The specimens were embedded in paraffin, sectioned, and stained with hematoxylin and eosin (H and E) and Masson's trichrome (MT). ImageJ software (version 1.5a) was used for the quantification of collagen in tissue sections.

2.5. Western Blotting

The harvested skin tissues were homogenized in Pro-prep solution (iNtRON Biotechnology; Seoul, Korea), and their lysates were centrifuged at 12,000× *g* for 30 min. The proteins were separated by SDS-PAGE and transferred onto a polyvinylidene difluoride (PVDF) membrane (Millipore, MA, USA). The membranes were blocked with 5% nonfat milk for 2 h and washed with Tris-Buffered Saline containing 0.05% Tween-20 (TBST) buffer. The membranes were incubated with primary antibodies of Matrix metalloproteinase (MMP)-1 (ab137332, 1:1000, abcam, Cambridge, UK) -2, -9, and TGF-β1 (sc-13595, sc-393859, sc-130348, 1:1000, Santa Cruz, CA, USA), at 4 °C overnight. The blots were incubated with a horseradish peroxidase-conjugated secondary antibody (1:1000, Thermo Scientific, IL, USA) for 1 h. Immunoreactive bands were visualized with the Pierce ECL Western blotting substrate (Thermo Scientific, IL, USA), using ChemiDoc (BioRad Laboratories, CA, USA).

2.6. Cell Culture

HaCaT cells were obtained from the Korean Cell Line Bank (Seoul, Korea). The cells were cultured in high-glucose Dulbecco's modified Eagle's medium supplemented with 10% fetal bovine serum (FBS, Gibco, NY, USA) and 1% penicillin–streptomycin (WelGENE, Daegu, Korea) in 5% CO_2 at 37 °C.

2.7. Cell Viability Assay

The cytotoxicity of UP extract was examined using the 3-(4, 5-dimethylthiazol-2-yl)-2,5-diphenyltetrazolium bromide (MTT, Sigma, MO, USA) assay. HaCaT cells were seeded into 96-well plates (4.0×10^4 cells/well) in 10% FBS-containing medium. The cells were treated with various concentrations of UP extract, diluted in serum-free media. After 24 h of incubation, 0.5 mg/mL MTT solution was added, and the cells were cultured for 1 h. The dark-blue formazan crystals were solubilized with dimethyl sulfoxide (DMSO, Sigma, MO, USA), and the absorbance at 570 nm was measured using a spectrophotometer (Molecular Devices, CA, USA).

2.8. Cell Migration Assay

HaCaT cells were seeded in 96-well plates (3.0×10^4 cells/well) for the scratching assay. Monolayers of cultured cells were subjected to scratch wounds with a Wound Maker tool (Essen Bioscience, MI, USA), and the media was removed by suction. The cells were then washed twice with PBS buffer and incubated for 12 h in the presence or absence of UP extract. IncuCyte ZOOM (Essen Bioscience, MI, USA) was used to inspect cultures every 2 h.

2.9. Statistical Analysis

Differences between groups were determined using a one-way analysis of variance (ANOVA). *p*-values of <0.05, <0.01, and <0.001 were considered statistically significant. Results are presented as the mean and the standard error of the mean (SEM).

3. Results

3.1. The Angle of Repose of Different Particle Sizes of the Root Bark Powder of *U. parvifolia*

The angle of repose indicates changes in the fluidity in the root bark of UP. The angle of repose for the different particle sizes of the root bark powder of UP is shown in Table 1. The root bark powder of UP with a particle size of 200 mesh (49.8 ± 1.1°) had a lower angle of repose than the others, followed by 100 mesh (51.9 ± 1.6°) and 50 mesh (52.9 ± 0.7°), with the highest being the 20 mesh (57.2 ± 0.8°). The angle of repose of the root bark powder decreased as the particle size decreased

Table 1. The angle of repose of *Ulmus parvifolia* (UP) root bark powder depending on particle size.

Mesh	Particle Size (μm)	Angle of Repose (θ)
20	355–850	57.2 ± 0.8
50	150	52.9 ± 0.7
100	75–150	51.9 ± 1.6
200	≤75	49.8 ± 1.1

3.2. Effect of the Particle Size of the Root Bark Powder of *U. parvifolia* on Wound Healing in Mice

We observed the regenerative effects of the root bark powder of UP using a SKH-1 hairless mouse model. To assess the efficacy of UP powder, wound closure was observed after treatment with UP powder (50, 100, and 200 mesh) for five days. Wounds treated with the 200 mesh powder showed a faster rate of wound closure and dermal regeneration compared with those treated with other sizes (Figure 1A). In the 200 mesh treatment group, wound sizes were significantly decreased on day 5, whereas those in the control group were not healed (Figure 1B). In addition, we investigated the tissue samples of skin wounds using H and E and MT staining. Treatment with 200 mesh UP powder resulted in increased granulation tissue formation, hair follicle, and glands, and decreasing of inflammatory cells in the epidermis was found compared with that in the untreated group (Figure 1C). Collagen formation was significantly increased in the 200 mesh treatment group (Figure 1D).

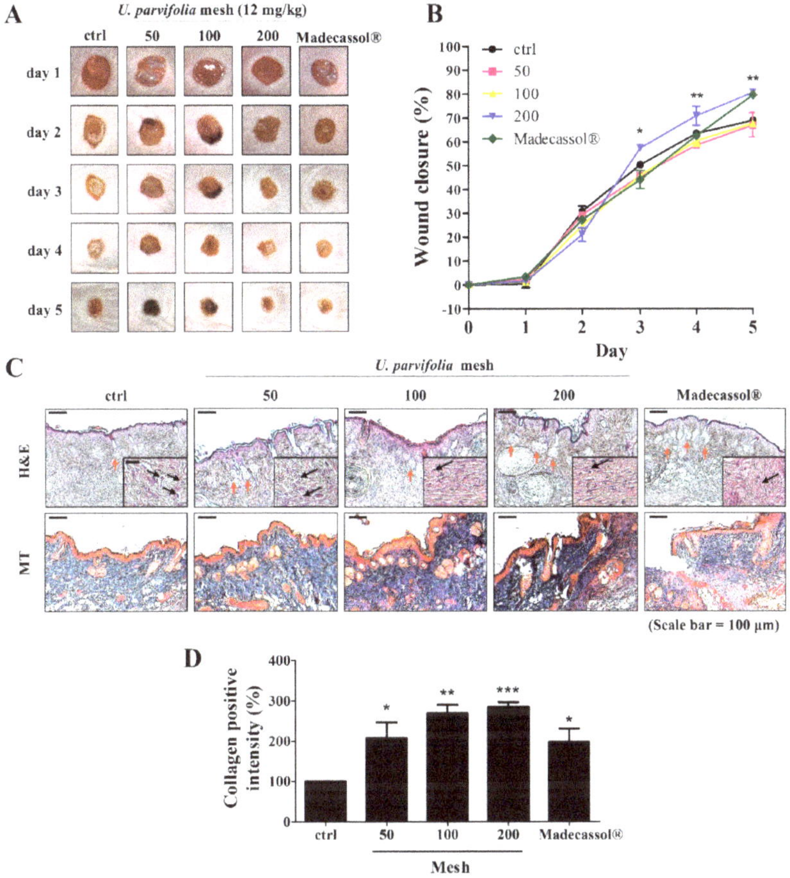

Figure 1. Effects of the root bark of *U. parvifolia* on wound healing in hairless mice. (**A**) Representative images of wounds from each group over a five-day period post-wounding. Madecassol® was used as positive control. (**B**) The graphical representation of the average wound closure in each group was measured using ImageJ software. (**C**) H and E-stained skin tissue sections and Masson's trichrome-stained sections on day 5. Scale bar = 200 µm. Black arrow indicates inflammatory cells and red arrow indicates the hair follicle and glands in the wound site. Insets of main figures represent granulation tissue (50 µm). (**D**) Graphical representation of expression of collagen formation in dorsal. The values are shown as mean ± SEM ($n = 7$). * $p < 0.05$, ** $p < 0.01$, and *** $p < 0.001$ vs. the control group.

3.3. Effects of Root Bark Extract of U. parvifolia on Migration in HaCaT Cells

To determine whether root bark extract of UP affected rejuvenation and wound repair, we induced wounds in skin keratinocyte (HaCaT cells) monolayer cultures and administered the root bark extract of UP. As shown in Figure 2A, no significant change in cell viability was noticed after treatment with root bark extract at 10 µg/mL. HaCaT cells grown in the presence of root bark extract of UP showed faster, dose-dependent growth rates compared with the untreated cells (Figure 2B,C).

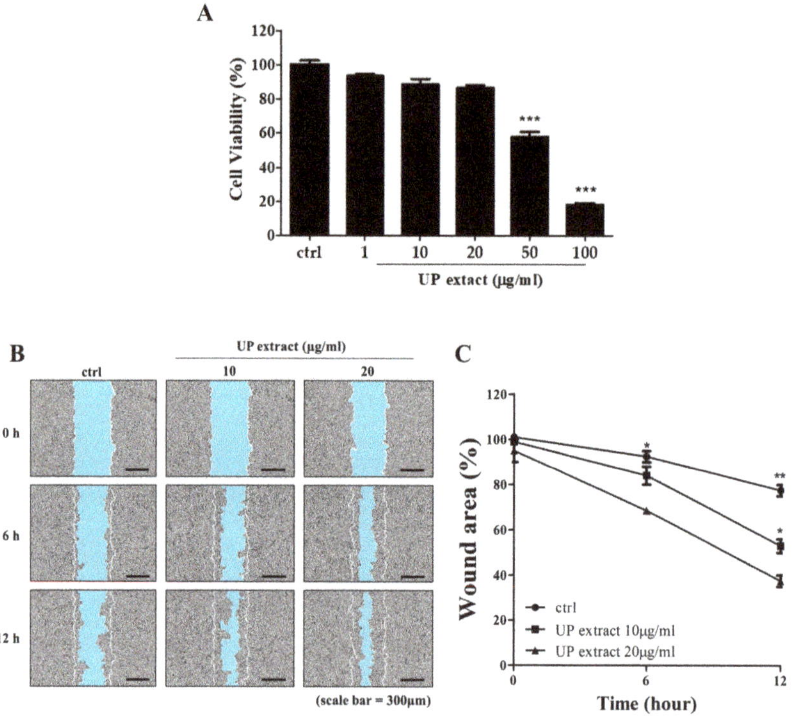

Figure 2. Effects of UP extract on migration in HaCaT cells. (**A**) Cells were cultured in 96-well plates and treated with UP extract (1, 10, 20, 50, and 100 μg/mL). After 24 h, cell viability was measured using the MTT assay. (**B**,**C**) Wound areas were recorded over time using the IncuCyte ZOOM™ live cell-imaging platform. HaCaT cells were cultured with or without UP extract. The red line indicates the initial scratch wound mask, created immediately after wound creation. The values are shown as mean ± SD ($n = 6$). * $p < 0.05$, ** $p < 0.01$, and *** $p < 0.001$ vs. the control group.

3.4. *Effect of the Root Bark Powder of U. parvifolia on Large-Scale Wound Healing in Mice*

To investigate the effect of the root bark powder (200 mesh) of UP in large-scale wound healing, we observed its regenerative effects using a 20 mm diameter wound created on SKH-1 mice. We also treated the wound with the root bark powders of UM to compare the effects of these with those of UP powder. Wounds treated with UP powder showed a faster rate of wound closure and dermal regeneration, similar to treatment with Madecassol® powder, 7 and 14 days post wound creation (Figure 3A). Seven and fourteen days post wound creation, the wound sizes in the UP-treated group were significantly decreased, whereas those in the control and UM-treated groups were not significantly different as they were not completely healed (Figure 3B,C). Masson's trichrome staining was done to investigate wound development in tissue samples of wounded skin. UP powder treatment resulted in more granulation tissue formation and collagen deposition than other treatments (Figure 3D). These results indicate that UP accelerates skin wound healing by enhancing collagen synthesis during the remodeling phase of the wound healing process.

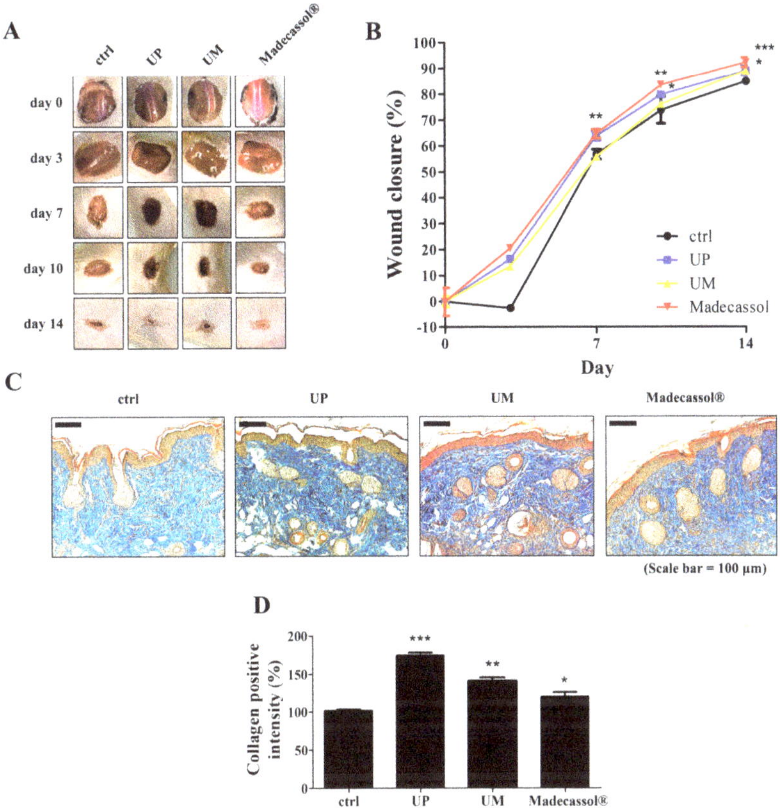

Figure 3. Effects of the root bark of *U. parvifolia* and *U. macrocarpa* on wound healing in hairless mice. (**A**) Two Ulmus root barks were applied to the wounds of SKH-1 mice for 14 days. Madecassol® was used as positive control. (**B**) The closure rates of 20 mm diameter wounds were measured. (**C**) Masson's trichrome-stained tissue sections on day 14. Scale bar = 100 μm. (**D**) Graphical representation of expression of collagen formation in dorsal. The values are shown as mean ± SEM ($n = 7$). * $p < 0.05$, ** $p < 0.01$, and *** $p < 0.001$ vs. the control group.

3.5. Effect of *U. parvifolia* on Skin Wound Healing in Hairless Mice by Regulating MMP and TGF-β1 Expression

We explored the expression levels of MMP-1, -2, -9, and TGF-β1 in the mice on day 14 of UP treatment (Figure 4A). As shown in Figure 4B–E, UP treatment significantly decreased the protein expression of MMP-1 (UP: 29.81%, UM: 22.56% Madecassol®: 43.51%). On the contrary, the expression of MMP-2 or -9 was significantly upregulated in the UP-treated group compared with the Madecassol®-treated group (MMP-2: UP; 65.90%, UM; 46.18% Madecassol®; −19.36%, MMP-9: UP; 101.12%, UM; 60.27% Madecassol®; 31.51%). TGF-β1 levels were also increased in the UP-treated groups (UP: 31.81%, UM: −37.90% Madecassol®: −8.02%). These results indicate that UP can accelerate wound healing by enhancing the expression of MMP-2 and -9 and increasing TGF-β1 levels.

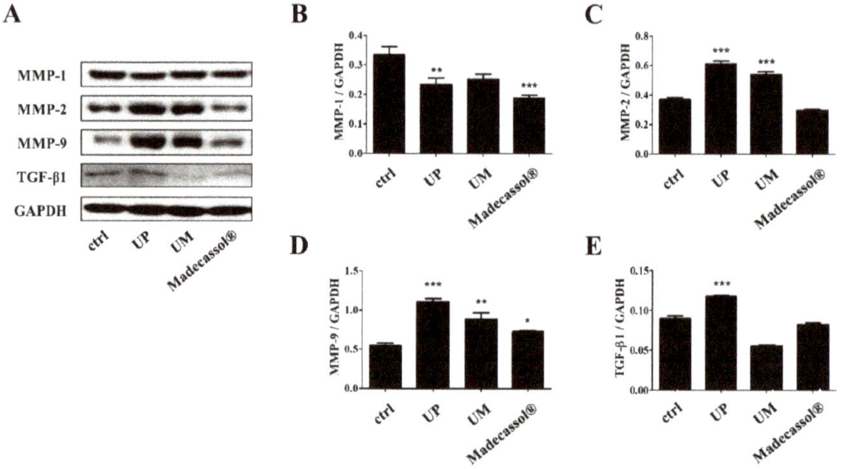

Figure 4. Effects of the root bark of *U. parvifolia* on the expression of MMPs and TGF-β1 in mouse dorsal skin tissue. (**A**) Western blot analyses of wounded skin showed the expression of (**B**) MMP-1, (**C**) MMP-2, (**D**) MMP-9, and (**E**) TGF-β1 on day 14 post-wounding. The values are shown as mean ± SEM (n = 7). * $p < 0.05$, ** $p < 0.01$, and *** $p < 0.001$ vs. the control group.

4. Discussion

Ulmus species have been widely used in Korean traditional medicine because of their anti-inflammatory and antimicrobial properties. Bioactive components, such as sesquiterpenoids, triterpenoids, flavonoids, coumarins, and lignans, are mainly present in this species [16]. It has been reported that UP has analgesic and anti-inflammatory effects [12,14]; however, its role in skin wound healing has not been reported. Therefore, in the present study, we demonstrated for the first time the skin wound healing effect of the root bark of UP in SKH-1 hairless mice.

As the population over 60 years of age grows, the burdens of nonhealing cutaneous wounds, such as pressure ulcers and diabetic foot ulcers, are increasing [17]. Cutaneous wounds are particularly hard to heal in aging, so it is necessary to develop effective treatments to heal wounds in aged skin.

For treatment of large-area wound injuries, such as pressure ulcers or rough or hard surfaces, a powder form of treatment is required and easy to apply. Treatment with powder in the wound area absorbs more wound exudate, forming a crust that prevents overdrying, and seals the wound from bacteria. It can modulate maintenance of moisture balance in the wound bed and also reduce the lingering of malodor compared to ointment application. [18]. In our study, it was observed that the wound closure and dermal regeneration effects of the 200 mesh root bark powder of UP were similar to those of Madecassol®, a commercially available wound healing ointment [19]. When the angle of repose and size of the particle were smaller, the solubility and water-retaining capacity of the powder were increased [20]. When the particle size of the UP powder was small, e.g., 200 mesh, it was able to hold more water than the UP powder with a larger size of particle (Figure S1). Interestingly, UP powder itself, instead of UP extract, has been used for many years in Korean traditional medicine. It is possible that the small particle size of UP powder itself may allow it to quickly absorb inflammatory exudate more than when presented in the form of a UP extract.

Maintaining hemostasis of collagen in the skin is a very important issue in skin rejuvenation and integrity for the wound matrix. It is also essential for re-epithelization and cell–cell and cell–matrix interactions. Deposition of collagen is important in wound healing and the development of wound strength [21]. The remodeling of collagenous proteins during wound healing can be influenced by proteolytic activities in the extracellular matrix by the MMPs. In our study, treatment of UP samples with different particle sizes showed that the finest UP powder (200 mesh) significantly decreased wound size in treated animals and also increased the collagen level in the dorsal skin.

During normal tissue remodeling and morphogenesis, MMPs play a crucial role in all stages of wound healing by modifying the wound matrix [22]. MMPs regulate cell–cell and cell–matrix signaling through the release of cytokines and growth factors sequestered in the ECM. Previously, it was shown that cytokines and hormones modulated MMP expression in skin tissues and could regulate inflammation and ECM on skin tissues [23]. In our study, expression of MMP-1 was downregulated by treatment of UP, similar to the positive control group. The loss of ECM may trigger MMP-1 expression in basal keratinocytes, thereby promoting migration, but keratinocytes downregulate the expression of MMP-1 in the final stage of tissue remodeling [24]. Furthermore, UP treatment upregulated MMP-2 and -9 expressions even more than those of Madecassol® treatment. Particularly, overexpressions of matrix metalloproteinases 2 and 9 impair the remodeling and re-epithelization phases in wound-damaged models. [25]. Downregulation of MMP-2 and -9 expressions in the wounds increased keratinocyte migration during wound closure. MMP-9 knockout mice delay wound re-epithelialization and inhibit cell proliferation through Smad2 signaling in delaying corneal wound healing [26,27]. Therefore, the potential of MMPs and their inhibitors could be as therapeutic agents in treating wounds during distinct phases of the wound healing.

Keratinocyte migration and fibroblast migration during the re-epithelization phase are important processes in mammalian skin healing. Keratinocytes are the predominant cell type in the epidermis and are responsible for the epithelialization phase of skin wound healing. During epithelialization, keratinocytes proliferate and migrate to the wound site. These processes help ameliorate the disruption of the skin barrier [28]. Impaired keratinocyte migration results in poor wound healing, leading to a chronic wound [29]. Therefore, regulation of keratinocyte migration by UP treatment may ameliorate wound lesions via regulating expression of MMPs.

TGF-β is a family of growth factors that play an essential role in wound healing by regulating the inflammatory response, keratinocyte proliferation and migration, angiogenesis, collagen synthesis, and ECM remodeling. Lower TGF-β expression was studied in skin of a human diabetic foot ulcer [30]. Our results suggest that the potential efficacy of wound healing by UP seems to be due to stimulation of keratinocyte migration directly or TGF-β expression in the wound lesion.

Previous investigations conducted with the leaves of UP have demonstrated that it contains flavonol glycosides in its leaves [31]. Phytochemical constituents in the barks of *U. parvifolia* have resulted in the isolation of sterols, sterol glucoside, and a catechin glycoside [13]. In particular, catechin derivatives are among the major components in UP root bark and have a regulating cell migration effect (data not shown). Nevertheless, the scope of these claims is limited to the effect of the powder only. A future study with a major compound in the UP root bark could be studied. However, our study is a step forward in adding ethnopharmacological validation to the use of UP powder in wound healing cases.

5. Conclusions

For the first time, we discovered that the root bark powder of *U. parvifolia* could accelerate wound healing and that the mechanism might involve the upregulation of the expression of MMPs and TGF-β. Therefore, root bark powder of *U. parvifolia* can be a potential candidate in treating cutaneous wound damages. A further, precise mechanism study on UP in skin cells and the effects of its main compound should be done.

Supplementary Materials: The following are available online at http://www.mdpi.com/2077-0383/9/1/59/s1, Figure S1: Effect of particle size and soaking time on the water-holding capacity of different sized UP particles.

Author Contributions: Conceptualization, S.Y.K. and M.-J.A.; methodology, M.C.K. and W.S.P.; data curation, M.C.K. and S.Y.; investigation, H.M.S.; writing—original draft preparation, M.C.K. and S.Y.; writing—review and editing, S.Y.K., K.H.K., and M.C.S.; visualization, M.C.K.; supervision, S.Y.K.; project administration, M.-J.A. All authors have read and agreed to the published version of the manuscript.

Funding: This work was supported by the R and D Program for Forest Science Technology (Project No. 2017036A00-1719-BA01) developed by the Korea Forest Service (Korea Forestry Promotion Institute).

Conflicts of Interest: The authors declare that they have no conflicts of interest.

References

1. Takeo, M.; Lee, W.; Ito, M. Wound healing and skin regeneration. *Cold Spring Harb. Perspect. Med.* **2015**, *5*, a023267. [CrossRef] [PubMed]
2. Martin, P. Wound healing—Aiming for perfect skin regeneration. *Science* **1997**, *276*, 75–81. [CrossRef] [PubMed]
3. Barrientos, S.; Stojadinovic, O.; Golinko, M.S.; Brem, H.; Tomic-Canic, M. Growth factors and cytokines in wound healing. *Wound Repair Regen.* **2008**, *16*, 585–601. [CrossRef] [PubMed]
4. Braiman-Wiksman, L.; Solomonik, I.; Spira, R.; Tennenbaum, T. Novel insights into wound healing sequence of events. *Toxicol. Pathol.* **2007**, *35*, 767–779. [CrossRef] [PubMed]
5. Olczyk, P.; Mencner, L.; Komosinska-Vassev, K. The role of the extracellular matrix components in cutaneous wound healing. *BioMed Res. Int.* **2014**, *2014*, 747584. [CrossRef] [PubMed]
6. Wathoni, N.; Motoyama, K.; Higashi, T.; Okajima, M.; Kaneko, T.; Arima, H. Enhancement of curcumin wound healing ability by complexation with 2-hydroxypropyl-gamma-cyclodextrin in sacran hydrogel film. *Int. J. Biol. Macromol.* **2017**, *98*, 268–276. [CrossRef] [PubMed]
7. Tasic-Kostov, M.; Arsic, I.; Pavlovic, D.; Stojanovic, S.; Najman, S.; Naumovic, S.; Tadic, V. Towards a modern approach to traditional use: In vitro and in vivo evaluation of Alchemilla vulgaris L. gel wound healing potential. *J. Ethnopharmacol.* **2019**, *238*, 111789. [CrossRef]
8. Jun, C.D.; Pae, H.O.; Kim, Y.C.; Jeong, S.J.; Yoo, J.C.; Lee, E.J.; Choi, B.M.; Chae, S.W.; Park, R.K.; Chung, H.T. Inhibition of nitric oxide synthesis by butanol fraction of the methanol extract of *Ulmus davidiana* in murine macrophages. *J. Ethnopharmacol.* **1998**, *62*, 129–135. [CrossRef]
9. Yang, H.J.; Ko, B.S.; Kwon, D.Y.; Lee, H.W.; Kim, M.J.; Ryuk, J.; Kang, S.; Kim, D.S.; Park, S. Asian Elm tree inner bark prevents articular cartilage deterioration in ovariectomized obese rats with monoiodoacetate-induced osteoarthritis. *Menopause* **2016**, *23*, 197–208. [CrossRef]
10. Gardiner, P.; Kemper, K.J. Herbs in pediatric and adolescent medicine. *Pediatr. Rev.* **2000**, *21*, 44–57. [CrossRef]
11. Lee, Y.; Park, H.; Ryu, H.S.; Chun, M.; Kang, S.; Kim, H.S. Effects of elm bark (*Ulmus davidiana* var. japonica) extracts on the modulation of immunocompetence in mice. *J. Med. Food* **2007**, *10*, 118–125. [CrossRef] [PubMed]
12. Mina, S.A.; Melek, F.R.; Adeeb, R.M.; Hagag, E.G. LC/ESI-MS/MS profiling of *Ulmus parvifolia* extracts and evaluation of its anti-inflammatory, cytotoxic, and antioxidant activities. *Z. Naturforschung* **2016**, *71*, 415–421. [CrossRef] [PubMed]
13. Moon, Y.H.; Rim, G.R. Studies on the constituents of *Ulmus parvifolia*. *Korean J. Pharmacogn.* **1995**, *26*, 1–7.
14. Kim, S.P.; Lee, S.J.; Nam, S.H.; Friedman, M. Elm Tree (*Ulmus parvifolia*) Bark Bioprocessed with Mycelia of Shiitake (*Lentinus edodes*) Mushrooms in Liquid Culture: Composition and Mechanism of Protection against Allergic Asthma in Mice. *J. Agric. Food Chem.* **2016**, *64*, 773–784. [CrossRef]
15. Cho, S.K.; Lee, S.G.; Kim, C.J. Anti-inflammatory and analgesic activities of water extract of root bark of *Ulmus parvifolia*. *Korean J. Pharmacogn.* **1996**, *27*, 274–281.
16. Kwon, J.H.; Kim, S.B.; Park, K.H.; Lee, M.W. Antioxidative and anti-inflammatory effects of phenolic compounds from the roots of Ulmus macrocarpa. *Arch. Pharm. Res.* **2011**, *34*, 1459–1466. [CrossRef]
17. Gould, L.; Abadir, P.; Brem, H.; Carter, M.; Conner-Kerr, T.; Davidson, J.; DiPietro, L.; Falanga, V.; Fife, C.; Gardner, S.; et al. Chronic wound repair and healing in older adults: Current status and future research. *J. Am. Geriatr. Soc.* **2015**, *63*, 427–438. [CrossRef]
18. Ghatnekar, A.V.; Elstrom, T.; Ghatnekar, G.S.; Kelechi, T. Novel wound healing powder formulation for the treatment of venous leg ulcers. *J. Am. Coll. Certif. Wound Spec.* **2011**, *3*, 33–41. [CrossRef]
19. Bylka, W.; Znajdek-Awizen, P.; Studzinska-Sroka, E.; Brzezinska, M. Centella asiatica in cosmetology. *Postep. Dermatol. Alergol.* **2013**, *30*, 46–49. [CrossRef]
20. Zhao, X.; Yang, Z.; Gai, G.; Yang, Y. Effect of superfine grinding on properties of ginger powder. *J. Food Eng.* **2009**, *91*, 217–222. [CrossRef]

21. Mehrtash, M.; Mohammadi, R.; Hobbenaghi, R. Effect of adipose derived nucleated cell fractions with chitosan biodegradable film on wound healing in rats. *Wound Med.* **2015**, *10*, 1–8. [CrossRef]
22. Fray, M.J.; Dickinson, R.P.; Huggins, J.P.; Occleston, N.L. A potent, selective inhibitor of matrix metalloproteinase-3 for the topical treatment of chronic dermal ulcers. *J. Med. Chem.* **2003**, *46*, 3514–3525. [CrossRef] [PubMed]
23. Koshikawa, N.; Giannelli, G.; Cirulli, V.; Miyazaki, K.; Quaranta, V. Role of cell surface metalloprotease MT1-MMP in epithelial cell migration over laminin-5. *J. Cell Biol.* **2000**, *148*, 615–624. [CrossRef] [PubMed]
24. Sudbeck, B.D.; Pilcher, B.K.; Welgus, H.G.; Parks, W.C. Induction and repression of collagenase-1 by keratinocytes is controlled by distinct components of different extracellular matrix compartments. *J. Biol. Chem.* **1997**, *272*, 22103–22110. [CrossRef]
25. Salo, T.; Makela, M.; Kylmaniemi, M.; Autio-Harmainen, H.; Larjava, H. Expression of matrix metalloproteinase-2 and -9 during early human wound healing. *Lab. Investig.* **1994**, *70*, 176–182.
26. Mulholland, B.; Tuft, S.J.; Khaw, P.T. Matrix metalloproteinase distribution during early corneal wound healing. *Eye* **2005**, *19*, 584–588. [CrossRef]
27. Hattori, N.; Mochizuki, S.; Kishi, K.; Nakajima, T.; Takaishi, H.; D'Armiento, J.; Okada, Y. MMP-13 plays a role in keratinocyte migration, angiogenesis, and contraction in mouse skin wound healing. *Am. J. Pathol.* **2009**, *175*, 533–546. [CrossRef]
28. Nardini, J.T.; Chapnick, D.A.; Liu, X.; Bortz, D.M. Modeling keratinocyte wound healing dynamics: Cell-cell adhesion promotes sustained collective migration. *J. Theor. Biol.* **2016**, *400*, 103–117. [CrossRef]
29. Eming, S.A.; Martin, P.; Tomic-Canic, M. Wound repair and regeneration: Mechanisms, signaling, and translation. *Sci. Transl. Med.* **2014**, *6*, 265sr266. [CrossRef]
30. Blakytny, R.; Jude, E. The molecular biology of chronic wounds and delayed healing in diabetes. *Diabet. Med.* **2006**, *23*, 594–608. [CrossRef]
31. Heimler, D.; Mittempergher, L.; Buzzini, P.; Boddi, V. Quantitative HPTLC separation of flavonoid glycosides in the taxonomy of elm (Ulmus spp.). *Chromatographia* **1990**, *29*, 16–20. [CrossRef]

Journal of
Clinical Medicine

MDPI

Article

Radioprotective and Antimutagenic Effects of *Pycnanthus angolensis* Warb Seed Extract against Damage Induced by X rays

Daniel Gyingiri Achel [1], Miguel Alcaraz-Saura [2], Julián Castillo [3], Amparo Olivares [2] and Miguel Alcaraz [2,*]

1 Applied Radiation Biology Centre, Radiological and Medical Sciences Research Institute, Ghana Atomic Energy Commission, Legon, Accra GE-257-046, Ghana; gachel@gmail.com
2 Radiology and Physical Medicine Department, School of Medicine, University of Murcia, 30100 Espinardo, Murcia, Spain; Miguel.Alcaraz@um.es (M.A.-S.); amparo.o.r@um.es (A.O.)
3 Nutrafur S. A., Camino Viejo de Pliego, Km.2, 30820 Alcantarilla, Murcia, Spain; j.castillo@Nutrafur.com
* Correspondence: mab@um.es; Tel.: +34-868-883-601; Fax: +34-868-884-150

Received: 8 November 2019; Accepted: 13 December 2019; Published: 18 December 2019

Abstract: Although different studies have demonstrated different applications of *Pycnanthus angolensis* extracts in traditional African and Asian medicine, its possible antimutagenic or genoprotective capacities have never been explored. We studied these capabilities of *Pycnanthus angolensis* seed extract (PASE) by means of the two micronucleus assays, determining the frequency of micronucleus (MN) yield in mouse bone marrow (in vivo) and in human lymphocytes blocked by cytochalasin B (in vitro). PASE exhibited a significant genoprotective capacity ($p < 0.001$) against X-rays with a protection factor of 35% in both in vivo and in vitro assays. Further, its radioprotective effects were determined by the 3-(4,5-dimethyl-2-thiazolyl)-2,5-diphenyl-tetrazolium bromide (MTT) cell viability test in two cell lines: one being radiosensitive (i.e., human prostate epithelium (PNT2) cells) and the other being radioresistant (i.e., B16F10 melanoma cells). In the radiosensitive cells, PASE showed a protection factor of 35.5%, thus eliminating 43.8% of X-ray-induced cell death ($p < 0.001$) and a dose reduction factor of 2.5. In the radioresistant cells, a protection factor of 29% ($p < 0.001$) with a dose reduction factor of 4 was realized. PASE elicited a greater radioprotective capacity than the substances currently used in radiation oncology and, thus, could be developed as a nutraceutical radioprotectant for workers and patients exposed to ionizing radiation.

Keywords: micronuclei; radioprotectors; radiation effects; melanoma; PNT2; B16F10 cells

1. Introduction

Numerous studies have portrayed the varied medical applications of different extracts of *Pycnanthus angolensis* in traditional African and Asian medicine [1–6]. Extracts of *P. angolensis* have been used as antibacterial [1,3] antiparasitic [4], anti-inflammatory and analgesic [1,3–5], and as antihemorrhagic agents [4]. There are also reports about its use as an antidote against poisons [4], for hyperglycemia [1,2], and even against female sterility [1]. References on its antimutagenic/antigenotoxic or radioprotective capacity is rare even though some authors suggest that its antioxidant potential could explain some of the applications described [2].

Our attention was drawn to *P. angolensis* because of the potential applications that may be derived from its suggested potent antioxidant and free radical scavenging capacities [2]. The ability of antioxidants to eliminate reactive oxygen species (ROS) produced by oxidative stress during exposure to ionizing radiation (IR) is considered a protection mechanism against cellular damage induced by IR both in vitro and in vivo [7–12].

Thus, in this study, we examined the radioprotective and antimutagenic potentials of *Pycnanthus angolensis* seed extract (PASE) both in vitro and in vivo and compared it with other compounds with known radioprotective properties. This aimed at assessing if the extract offers some level of protection to normal tissues and may uncover novel substances with protection for workers occupationally exposed to ionizing radiation and/or for patients undergoing diagnostic radiology.

2. Materials and Methods

2.1. Plant Material

Seeds of *P. angolensis* Warb were harvested from plants growing in the wild in cocoa farms in the eastern region of Ghana and authenticated by an established curator at the Ghana Herbarium, Department of Botany, University of Ghana, Accra. The seeds were picked during the maturity period in November 2015 and were initially dried under shade and finally under vacuum at ambient temperature to a moisture content of less than 5% measured as described in the European Pharmacopoeia version 7.0.

2.2. Seed Extraction

Dried seeds were chopped into small pieces, mixed with SiO_2 and diatomaceous earth (10:1:9 respectively), and ground in a laboratory mill to an average particle size of 1 μm. Two hundred grams of this ground material (equivalent to 100 g of seed) was extracted in 99% methanol at a ratio of 10% (w/v) at room temperature (range 22–24 °C) on a Heidolph mechanical stirrer (RZR 2020, Heidolph Instruments, Schwabach, Germany) for 1 h.

The extract was filtered by vacuum filtration through a Büchner funnel attached to a Kitasato flask fitted with a polypropylene filter cloth. The marc was squeezed to recover all the solvent, and the funnel was washed with fresh methanol (200 mL). The volume of extract recovered (1.924 mL) was concentrated under reduced pressure at 40–50 °C in a Heidolph rotary evaporator (Laborota 4000, Heidolph Instruments, Schwabach, Germany) to approximately 1/12th of its original volume, yielding 150–160 mL of a turbid, semiviscous, syrupy liquid. This syrup was mixed with 30 mL (5:1 ratio) of deionized water, prompting flocculation, that was clarified by filtration using a system comprising a Büchner-Kitasato filter system fitted with a one micron cellulose/silica filter membrane (filter plate AF100, Ref 2036-Filtrox, St. Gallen, Switzerland). The clarified extract was concentrated under vacuum at 40–45 °C using a Heidolph rotary evaporator (Laborota 4000) to yield 36 mL of a very dark brown viscous syrup.

This material was extracted in ether 1:7 (*v/v*) at room temperature (22–24 °C) for 3 h in a 500 mL Erlenmeyer flask with continual stirring on a Heidolph mechanical stirrer (model RZR 2020, Heidolph Instruments, Schwabach, Germany). The extraction process was repeated thrice, ensuring that the organic phase showed no taint of yellow-orange color. The resulting solutions were pooled and allowed for liquid–liquid partitioning in a 500 mL separatory funnel for one hour. This yielded a 737 mL ethereal layer that was evaporated to dryness at 30–35 °C on a Heidolph rotary evaporator, (Laborota 4000) affording 16.34 g of a dark brownish, oily, and viscous semisolid as final product (PASE).

2.3. Chemicals and Reagents

P. angolensis seed extract (PASE) was extracted from the seeds as described above. RPMI 1640, Ham's F10, phytohemagglutinin A (PHA), cytochalasin B, streptomycin, penicillin, phosphate-buffered saline (PBS), 3-(4,5-dimethyl-2-thiazolyl)-2,5-diphenyl-tetrazolium bromide (MTT), vitamin E (δ-tocopherol) (T), bovine serum albumin (BSA fraction V), and fetal bovine serum (FBS) were obtained from Gibco (USA). Glacial acetic acid and ethanol were obtained from Scharlao SL (Madrid, Spain). Methanol and methanol HPLC grade were obtained from Panreac (Madrid, Spain); 5% sodium heparin was obtained from Rovi Pharmaceutical Laboratories (Madrid, Spain).

Rosmarinic acid (RA), diosmin (D), and quercetin (Q) were obtained from Extrasynthese S.A. (Genay, France). Eriodictyol (E) and ascorbic acid (C) were obtained from Sigma-Aldrich Chemicals

SA (Madrid, Spain). Dimethyl sulfoxide (DMSO) was obtained from Merck (Darmstadt, Germany). Amifostine (AMF) (Ethyol®) was obtained from Schering-Plough S.A (Madrid, Spain). Green tea extract (Te), carnosic acid (CA), and apigenin (API), were supplied by Nutrafur S.A. (Alcantarilla, Murcia, Spain).

2.4. *Preparation of Plant and Plant Seed Extract (PASE) for Chromatographic Analysis*

Active compounds from different seeds of the plant (PASE) were extracted for analytical chromatography using HPLC-grade methanol in the ratio of 20 and 4 mg/mL, respectively. The extraction was done at 25 °C during 30 min in a stirred flask. All solutions were filtered through a 0.45 μm nylon filter membrane before undertaking HPLC analysis. The samples were aliquoted into small vials and stored at 4 °C until required.

2.4.1. HPLC Analysis of *P. angolensis* Seeds and *P. angolensis* Seed Extract (PASE)

Analyses were performed on an HP 1100 liquid chromatographic system (Hewlett- Packard, Waldbronn, Germany) series equipped with an LC-6A double pump (Shimadzu Corporation, Kyoto, Japan). The chromatograms were monitored by a UV–vis diode array detector at a wavelength of 250 nm. The stationary phase was a 250 × 4 mm id., 5 μm, C_{18} reversed-phase HPLC column (Shimadzu Shim-Pack CLC (M)) thermostated at 30 °C. The flowrate was 1 mL/min.

Analysis was made using a gradient between mobile phase A (1% acetic acid) and phase B (methanol) at a flow rate of 1 mL/min as follows: 0–5 min, 50% of A and B; 5–25 min, 50% A and B; 25–35 min, 100% B. The column was finally re-equilibrated with the initial solvent for 5 min (total time 40 min). The main compounds were identified by comparison of their retention times and UV spectra obtained with the diode-array detector with standard compounds. Three experiments were conducted on each sample, while solvent blanks were intermittently injected into columns (column washing) to eliminate peak splitting or tailing during the analysis.

2.4.2. Identification of Extracted Compounds

Further analysis was performed on an Agilent 1100 series HPLC (Agilent Technologies, Germany) coupled to an ion trap VL mass spectrometer detector (Agilent Technologies, Germany) to confirm the identities of the compounds present in the raw seed material and the PASE extract.

The separation was executed on a Waters SunFire® C_{18} column (5 μm particle size and column dimensions of 120 μm, 150 mm × 4.6 mm i.d.). The mobile phase was an isocratic system composed of 20:80 water/methanol and 1% acetic acid, at a flow rate of 0.8 mL/min, thermostated at 30 °C and a total run time of 20 min.

Two signals were acquired, one with a diode array detector at a wavelength of 280 nm and one in the range of 190–380 nm. The mass spectrometer was operated in a scan mode with the electrospray (ESI) source in the positive ion mode (ESI +), a mass detection range of 100–800 amu, and a target mass of 400 m/z. The optimized conditions were nebulizer pressure of 60 psi, a drying gas flow rate of 9 mL/min, and a gas temperature of 350 °C.

2.4.3. Chromatographic Analysis of Used Flavonoids and Polyphenols

HPLC analyses were conducted to confirm the concentrations of active compounds in all flavonoids, polyphenols, and plant extracts used in this structural comparative study (D, Q, Te, and API served as flavonoids; CA and RA as diterpenic caffeoyl compounds respectively). All compounds were dissolved in DMSO at a concentration of 1 mg/mL. All solutions were filtered through a 0.45 μm nylon filter membrane before undertaking HPLC analysis.

Analyses were performed in an HP 1100 liquid chromatographic system (Hewlett- Packard, Waldbronn, Germany) series equipped with an LC-6A double pump (Shimadzu Corporation, Kyoto, Japan). The chromatograms were monitored simultaneously by a UV–vis diode array detector at 280 and 340 nm. The stationary phase was a 250 × 4 mm id., 5 μm, C_{18} reversed-phase HPLC column (Shimadzu Shim-Pack CLC (M)) thermostated at 30 °C. The flow-rate was 1 mL/min.

The following mobile phases were used for chromatographic analysis: (A) acetic acid/water (2.5:97.5) and (B) acetonitrile. A linear gradient was run from 95% (A) and 5% (B) to 75% (A) and 25% (B) during 20 min; changed to 50% (A) and (B) for 20 min (40 min total run time); and changed to 20% (A) and 80% (B) for 10 min (50 min total run time). The column was re-equilibrated for 10 min in the initial solvent (60 min run time).

2.5. Genoprotective Studies

2.5.1. Micronucleus Test (CBMN)

Venous blood was obtained by venipuncture from the arm veins of three supposedly healthy young female donors into heparinized tubes. Twenty microliters (20 μL) of a 20 μM concentration of the test substances was added to 2 mL of the heparinized human blood samples at two different times: immediately before exposure to X-rays (treatment before irradiation) or immediately after exposure to the X-rays (post irradiation treatment). Immediately after irradiation with X-rays, the cytokinesis-block micronucleus (CBMN) assay, as described by Fenech and Morley [13] and adapted by the International Atomic Energy Agency [14], was used to access damage in the cultured irradiated human lymphocytes. The number of micronuclei in at least 3000 CB cells for each treatment was determined by three specialists who analyzed the slides using optical microscopes in a double-blind study.

2.5.2. Micronucleus Assay in Mouse Bone Marrow (PCEs)

In the in vivo experiments, male Swiss mice 12 weeks old, distributed in groups of 6 for each of the substances tested, with weights ranging from 27 to 35 g were used. All solutions were prepared daily, and the test substances were dissolved to a concentration of 0.2% in their drinking water. This treatment commenced one week prior to X-ray exposure.

The animals were housed in the Animal Service Laboratory of the University of Murcia (REGAES300305440012), and the procedures used were approved by the Ethical Committee of the Autonomous Community of the Region of Murcia (Spain) (CECA:510/2018).

An in vivo micronucleus assay was performed on the bone marrow of the mice, as described by Schmid [15]. Twenty-four hours after X-ray exposure, the numbers of micronucleated polychromatic erythrocytes (MNPCEs) among 1000 PCEs per mouse were determined by three specialists in a double-blind study. To ensure that the substances tested were nontoxic, the number of normochromatic erythrocytes and of total erythrocytes in each animal were also determined.

2.6. Radioprotective Effects: Cell Lines and Culture Conditions

In this study, two cell types selected based on their radiosensitivity status were used: cells traditionally considered radiosensitive (PNT2) and B16F10 cells, which are traditionally considered to be very radioresistant [16]. The normal epithelium prostatic cell line (PNT 2) was obtained from the European Collection of Cell Cultures (ECACC, Salisbury, UK), Health Protection Agency, Culture Collection (catalogue no.:95012613, Salisbury, UK). The PNT2 cells were cultivated in RPMI 1640 (Sigma-Aldrich, Madrid, Spain) supplemented with 10% FBS, 2 mM glutamine, and streptomycin and penicillin (100 μg/mL and 100 IU/mL respectively). The mouse metastatic melanoma cell (B16F10) line was kindly provided by Dr. V. Hearning (NIH, Bethesda, MA, USA) and cultured in Dulbecco's modified Eagle´s medium (DMEM)/F12K (1:1) (Sigma-Aldrich, St. Louis, MI, USA) supplemented with 10% FBS (Gibco, BRL, Louisville, KY, USA), 4 mM L-glutamine, penicillin (100 IU/mL), and streptomycin (100 μg/mL).The cultures were maintained at 37 °C, a relative humidity of 90%–95%, and an atmosphere of 7.5% CO_2. Tests were carried out to confirm the absence of *Mycoplasma* spp. throughout the study.

Radioprotective Effects: (MTT) Test

To analyze the radioprotective effects of the substances on PNT2 and B16F10 cell lines, two MTT assay types, as previously described [17,18], were carried out. One of these tests lasting 24 h was used to assess cytotoxicity, and the other lasting 48 h was to evaluate cell proliferation after treatment with test substances with and without exposure to X-ray. Briefly, the cultures were incubated in 200 μL growth medium and allowed to adhere for 24 h after cell seeding in both types of assays so cells could adapt to the culture conditions and adhere to the bottom of the wells. For the PNT2 cells 3200 cells/wells and for B10F16 2500 cells/well were established as optimal cell seeding concentrations. Different concentrations of the test substances to be assayed were put into each well (at least 6 wells per test substance), and the plates were exposed to different doses of X-rays (0, 4, 6, 8, and 10 Gy), 15 min post substance addition. After the requisite incubation period (i.e., 24 or 48 h), cell survival was determined by the MTT test as previously described [17,18].

2.7. Irradiation

An Andrex SMART 200E (Yxlon International, Hamburg, Germany) X-ray producing equipment with the following characteristics was used: 200 kV, 4.5 mA, filtration of 2.5 mm of Al, and dose rate of 1.3 cGy/s at a focus object distance (FOD) of 35 cm. The experiments were performed at room temperature. For the determination of in vitro genotoxicity, whole human blood samples were exposed to 2 Gy X-rays at an FOD of 35 cm; while for the in vivo study, conscious and immobilized animals were whole body irradiated to a dose of 500 mGy at an FOD of 74 cm. For the determination of the radioprotective capacity, cell cultures grown in microplates were irradiated to different doses of X-rays (0, 4, 6, 8, and 10 Gy) at an FOD of 35 cm. At all times, the doses of radiation administered were continuously monitored inside the X-ray cabin by means of UNIDOS® Universal Dosimeter with PTW Farme® ionization chambers TW30010 (PTW-Freiburg, Freiburg, Germany), and the final radiation dose was confirmed by means of thermoluminescent dosimeters (TLDs) (GR-200®; Conqueror Electronics Technology Co Ltd., Beijing, China).

2.8. Statistical Analysis

Two different analysis were performed in this study. In the genoprotective study, analysis of variance complemented by a contrast of means to determine the degree of dependence and correlation between the variables was performed and further complemented with regression and linear correlation analysis amongst the quantitative variables. In the radioprotective study, the percentages of the surviving cells in the presence of the different substances were compared using analysis of variance (ANOVA) of repeated means, complemented by a least significant differences analysis to contrast pairs and means. p values of less than 0.01 ($p < 0.01$) were deemed significant.

In addition, in the genotoxicity analysis, we used the formula described by Sarma and Kesavan [19] to evaluate the protection factor (PF) regarding the reduction of the frequency of occurrence of MN:PF (%) = (Fcontrol − Ftreated/Fcontrol) × 100, where Fcontrol is the frequency of micronuclei in the irradiated control samples, and Ftreated is the frequency of micronuclei in the treated and irradiated samples. In the radioprotection analysis we modified this formula to adapt it to the cell survival cultures exposed to 10 Gy and incubated over a period of 48 h: PF (%) = (Mcontrol − Mtreated/Mcontrol) × 100, where Mcontrol is the mortality of the irradiated control cells, and Mtreated is the mortality of the cells treated with each substance and irradiated.

Finally, the dose reduction factor (DRF) was calculated as a ratio of radiation dose required to produce the same biological effect in the presence and absence of the radioprotector as described by Hall [16].

3. Results

3.1. Identification and Quantification of the Main Active Compounds in P. angolensis Seeds

The chromatogram produced according to HPLC analytical assay of *P. angolensis* seeds pointed to the presence of some plastoquinones/ubiquinones. Figure 1 shows the chromatogram of material obtained from *P. angolensis* seeds. The composition of the extracts in the chromatograms was assessed by comparing their relative retention times and UV spectra, which are a function of their molecular structures, and subsequently confirmed by mass spectrometry (HPLC-MS). The proposed compounds were the plastoquinones/ubiquinones sargahydroquinoic acid, (peak 1), sargaquinoic (peak 2), and sargachromenol (peak 3).

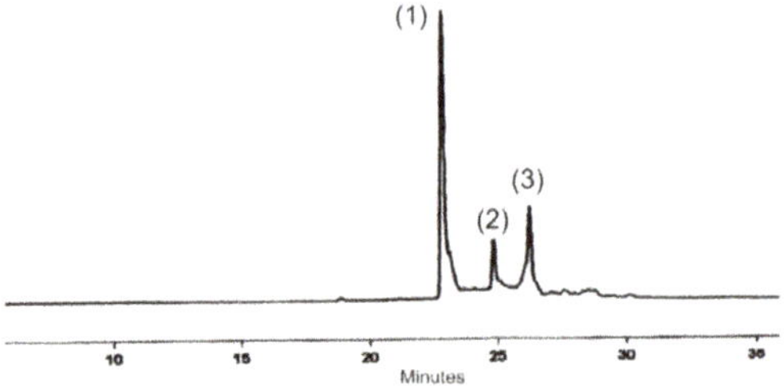

Figure 1. Characteristic chromatogram (Materials and Methods 2.4.1) of *Pycnanthus angolensis* seed extract (PASE), monitored at 250 nm. Peaks: (1) Rt 22.7 min, sargahydroquinoic acid; (2) Rt 24.8 min, sargaquinoic acid; (3) Rt 26.4 min, sargachromenol.

To confirm the structure of the above-mentioned compounds, the HPLC mass spectra data (Materials and Methods 2.4.2) of the three main peaks present in *Pycnanthus angolensis* seed extract were evaluated (Table 1).

Table 1. Experimental results (Materials and Methods 2.4.2) versus theoretical structural data of proposed compounds present in *Pycnanthus angolensis* seeds, monitored at 280 nm (HPLC-MS).

Parameter	Peak 1	Peak 2	Peak 3
Proposed structure	Sargahydroquinoic acid	Sargaquinoic acid	Sargachromenol
Molecular weight of proposed compound	426	424	424
Molecular formula of proposed compound	$C_{27}H_{38}O_4$	$C_{27}H_{36}O_4$	$C_{27}H_{36}O_4$
Retention time in HPLC-MS analysis	27.4 min	29.3 min	31.6 min
$M + H^+$	449	447	447
M + Na	471	469	469
Molecular weight obtained from HPLC-MS	448	446	446
Theoretical and experimental mass difference	+ 22	+ 22	+ 22

Based on the results obtained, we propose that the peaks obtained in the HPLC-MS correspond to the potential generation of two adducts, one of which probably is due to Na+ binding $[M + Na^+]$ to the primary carboxyl group in the plastoquinone/ubiquinone molecule/skeleton and the other on the sterically less hindered hydroxyl group on the phenol ring of the type $[M + 2Na\text{-}H]^+$. Thus, the case of sargahydroquinoic acid specifically has

426 (theoretical molecular weight) + (1 × 23) = 449 (signal shown);

426 (theoretical molecular weight) + (2 × 23 -1H) + = 471 (signal appearing).

Based on the deductions made from these results, it may be reasonable and consistent to imagine that the molecular structure of the main actives (peaks 1, 2 and 3) present in the plant material used in the study are compatible with sargahydroquinoic acid, (peak 1), sargaquinoic (peak 2), and sargachromenol (peak 3). Figure 2 shows the chemical structures of these compounds. Quantitative analysis of these compounds shows the following amounts (% weight) in the crushed seeds: sargahydroquinoic acid, 7.48%; sargaquinoic, 0.41% (peak 2); and sargachromenol, 1.42%.

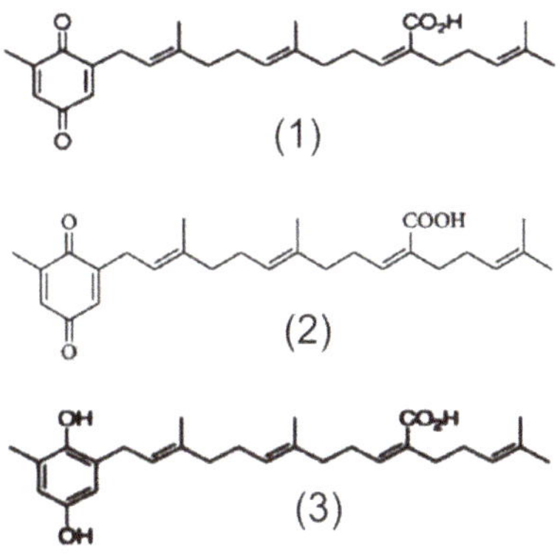

Figure 2. Possible chemical structures related to the results obtained from the PASE.

3.2. *Quantification of the Main Active Compounds in P. angolensis Seeds Extract (PASE)*

Figure 3 shows the characteristic chromatogram of PASE. This HPLC chromatogram was characterized by a selective and significant increase in the sargahydroquinoic acid level. The contents (%weight) of the three main identified compounds in the ether extract of the crushed seeds were: sargahydroquinoic acid, 40.14% (peak 1); sargaquinoic, 0.35% (peak 2); and sargachromenol, 0.56% (peak 3). This extract was used in all the assays.

3.3. *HPLC Analysis of Used Flavonoids, Polyphenols, and Plant Extracts*

HPLC analysis of polyphenol distribution in the different extracts used in this study is as shown in Table 2. Diosmin is a very well-known flavonoid, specifically a flavone compound (C2=C3 double bond on flavonoid skeleton), widely used in the pharmaceutical field as peripheral vasoprotective agent. Quercetin is another flavonoid from the flavonol family (C2=C3 double bond and 3-OH radical), also widely used as reference compound in flavonoid research and a pharmaceutical raw material. Eriodictyol is a flavanone aglycone with the same substitution pattern as quercetin but without a C2=C3 double bond and 3-OH radical group. Apigenin is also a flavone compound with very significant anti-inflammatory properties. Green tea extract is one of the most popular extracts used as nutritional supplement for several health applications, with flavan-3-ol family of compounds (also named "catechins") being the main flavonoid compounds present. Carnosic acid is the main diterpene from rosemary leaf extract, widely used as lipid antioxidant in food applications. Rosmarinic acid, a polyphenol with the "caffeoyl" structure, is widely present in the plant kingdom with interesting antioxidant and photoprotective properties. The chemical structures of the main flavonoids and polyphenols in the different extracts used in this study and the chemical structures of sulfur-containing compounds (amifostin and DMSO) are shown in Figure 3.

Table 2. Distribution of chemical structures by HPLC analysis in the different extracts used in this study.

Used Compound Extracts	Chemical Structure	Main Compounds	Content (%) [1]
Diosmin	Flavone	Diosmin	93.44
	Flavanone	Hesperidin	1.78
	Flavone	Isorhoifolin	0.23
	Flavone	Diosmetin	0.18
		Other flavonoids	0.43
Quercetin	Flavonol	Quercetin	94.37
	Flavonol	Isoquercitrin	1.12
	Flavonol	Rutin	0.75
		Other flavonoids	0.56
Apigenin	Flavone	Apigenin	95.72
	Flavone	Rhoifolin	1.38
	Flavanone	Naringenin	0.64
		Other flavonoids	0.67
Eriodictyol	Flavanone	Eriodictyol	93.12
	Flavanone	Eriocitrin	2.56
	Flavanone	Hesperidin	0.52
		Other flavonoids	0.71
Green Tea Extract	Flavan-3-ol	Epigallocatechin 3-O-gallate	57.89
	Flavan-3-ol	Epigallocatechin	14.65
	Flavan-3-ol	Epicatechin 3-O-gallate	6.71
	Flavan-3-ol	Epicatechin	6.11
Carnosic acid	Diterpene	Carnosic acid	76.44
	Diterpene	Carnosol	4.68
	Diterpene	12-methyl-carnosic acid	3.70
		Other diterpenes	1.23
Rosmarinic acid	Di-caffeoyl compound	Rosmarinic acid	94.22
	Caffeoyl co.	Di-hydroxy-cinnamic acid	0.65
		Other polyphenols	1.78

[1] Absolute value as is.

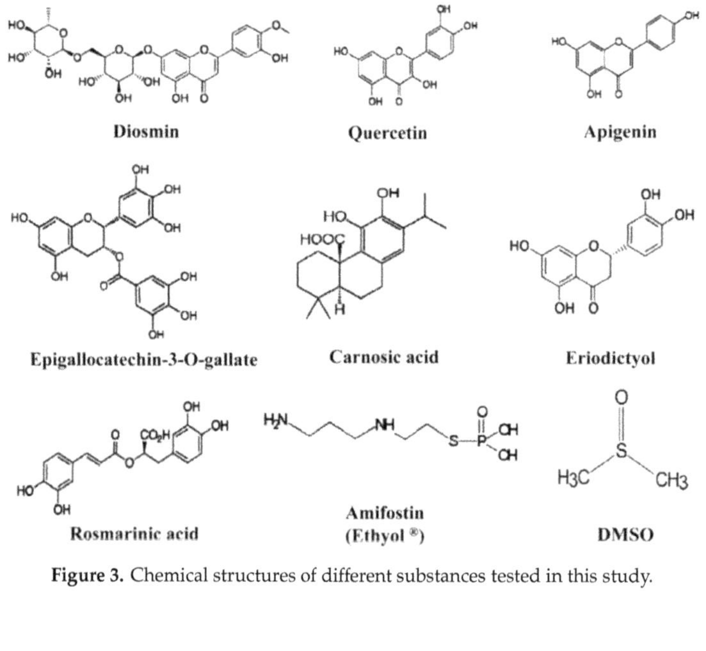

Figure 3. Chemical structures of different substances tested in this study.

3.4. X-ray Genoprotective Effects: Antimutagenic Activity

No significant differences were determined between the frequency of occurrence of MN in human lymphocytes treated with the different substances tested and control lymphocytes, indicating the absence of genotoxicity effects of these substances. X-ray exposure produced a significant increase in MN frequencies in irradiated human peripheral blood lymphocytes (26 ± 2.1 MN/500 CB) when compared to the baseline micronuclei frequency portrayed in nonirradiated blood samples (10 ± 1.1 MN/500 BC) ($p < 0.001$), showing a genotoxic capacity of the 2 Gy of X-rays administered. Figure 4a shows the influence of timing of sample treatment (i.e., addition before and after X-ray exposure) on the frequency of MN in irradiated human lymphocytes. There was an observed decrease in the frequency of MN produced when the different test substances were administered, revealing the individual antigenotoxic capacity of each substance tested. It was further observed that the induced MN frequency was strongly influenced by the sequence and timing of the two treatment modalities. When human lymphocytes were treated with test substances before exposure to X-rays, the frequency of MN showed the following order with respect to irradiated control samples: RA < CA = API = T < D < AMF = C < PASE < Te ($p < 0.001$), where CA, API, and T did not show statistically significant differences between them (CA = API = T), and AMF and C also showed no significant differences between them (AMF = C). Finally, DMSO also showed a smaller reduction with respect to the frequency of occurrence of MN in the irradiated control samples ($p < 0.01$). However, unlike all previous substances, E and Q showed an increase in the frequency of MN with respect to irradiated controls ($p < 0.001$) that could be interpreted as an increase in the radiosensitivity of the samples treated with these substances.

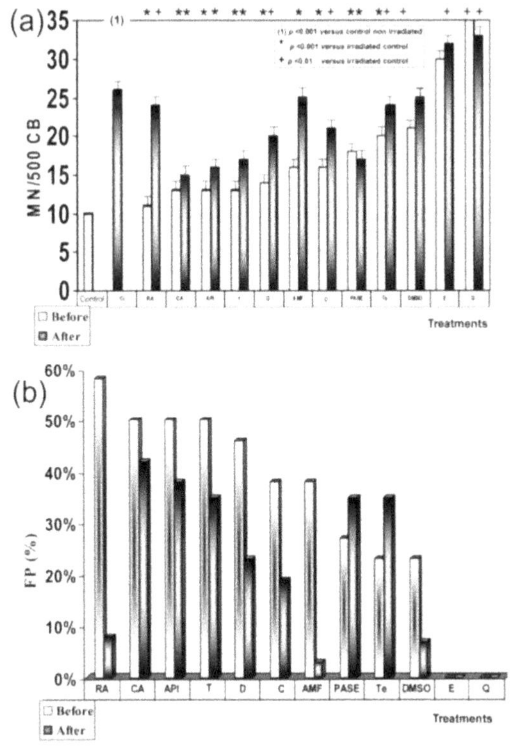

Figure 4. "In vitro" genoprotective effects against X-rays: (**a**) frequency of MN/500 CB in irradiated human lymphocytes blocked with cytochalasin B; (**b**) protection factor of PASE and of the other substances tested.

However, when the different substances were administered after X-ray exposure, the MN frequencies were higher than what was observed in the pre X-ray treatments. It is clear that while CA showed significant antimutagenic activity, RA demonstrated a low degree of genoprotective activity, and DMSO along with AMF (sulfur-containing compounds) lost their genoprotective capacities against X-rays. The order of genoprotection from lowest to highest level of radiation induced MN frequency was CA < API < PASE = T < D < C < Te = RA < AM = DMSO < E < Q ($p < 0.001$). Figure 4b shows the protection factors of each treatment and how they varied according to the time of administration (before and after exposure to ionizing radiation).

Significant differences were not established between the frequency of MNPCEs/1000 PCEs in the animals treated with the different substances and the control animals, and no significant changes in the P/N and P/E ratios in any of the exposed animals compared with the control groups were observed, indicating the absence of genotoxicity of these substances. Exposure to X-rays produced a significant increase in MNPCEs/1000 PCEs (18.7 ± 1.1 MNPCEs/1000 PC) with respect to the baseline frequency presented by control animals (3.1 ± 1.1 MNPCEs/1000 PC) ($p < 0.001$), showing a genotoxic capacity of the 500 mGy of X-rays administered. Figure 5a shows the influence of timing of treatments before and after exposure to X-rays on in vivo MN frequency induced in polychromatic erythrocytes (PCEs) of mouse bone marrow in vivo, which also permits a comparison of the potential genotoxicity of X-rays irradiated control, versus the antimutagenic capacities of the different substances assayed. The frequency of induced micronuclei varied with the time of administration of the test substances and exposure to radiation. When the test substances were administered prior to irradiation, the radiation-induced MN frequencies (MNPCEs) ordered from lowest to highest was RA < CA < API < PASE = D < AMF = Te = DMSO ($p < 0.001$). However, when the different substances were administered after X-ray irradiation, the induced MN frequencies (MNPCEs) were higher than that observed in the groups that received treatment before X-ray. It is clear that while CA showed significant antimutagenic activity, RA demonstrated a low degree of genoprotective activity, while DMSO and AMF (sulfur-containing compounds) lost their genoprotective capacities against X-rays. The genoprotective capacity of these substances were as follows: CA < API < PASE < D = Te < RA < AMF < DMSO ($p < 0.001$).

Figure 5b shows the protection capacities of the substances tested, the order of efficacies being RA > CA > API > PASE = D > AMF = Te = DMSO for treatments before X-ray exposure and CA > AP > PASE > D = Te > RA > AMF > DMSO for treatments after X-irradiation. Differences in effects between CA, RA, and PASE in relation to the timing of substance administration (i.e., before or after exposure to radiation) can also be appreciated.

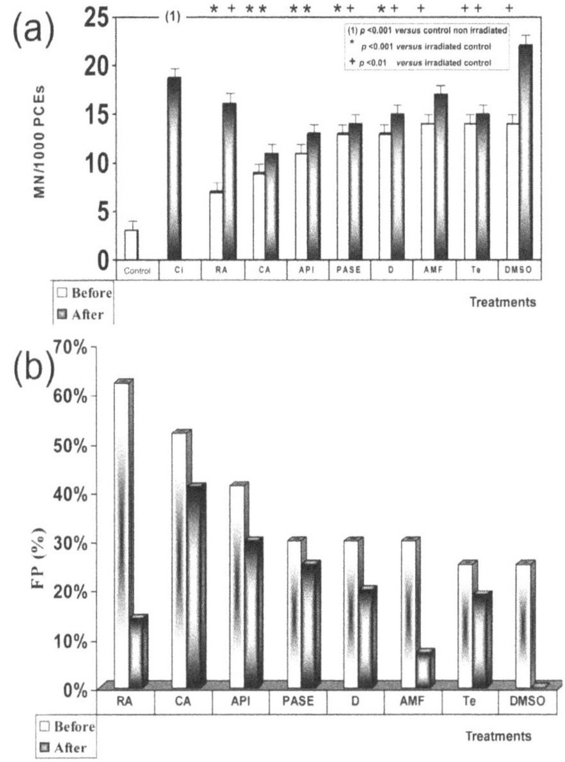

Figure 5. "In vivo" genoprotective effects against X-rays: (**a**) frequency of MN/1000 PCEs in mouse bone marrow; (**b**) protection factor of PASE and of the other substances tested. Radioprotective effects against X-rays. Protection capacities of the substances tested.

3.5. Radioprotective Effects against X-rays: Growth Inhibition

The concentrations of the tested substances that we selected for this study had no effect on cell survival. All cultures treated with the test substances but not exposed to irradiation were found to have cell survivals within 100% ± 5% for the different incubation periods. Moreover, no significant differences in cell survival induced by the treatments were established, demonstrating the absence of toxic effects of the substances administered. Figure 6 shows the percentage cell survival (%) of PNT2 and B16F10 melanoma cells assessed by the MTT cell viability test after administration of PASE during 24 and 48 h post irradiation incubation periods. In the irradiated PNT2 cells, PASE elicited an increase in cell survival at the highest radiation dose of 10 Gy used, which expressed the radioprotective capability of PASE for the two cell lines and at the two incubation periods studied (24 and 48 h) ($p < 0.001$). In the PNT2 cells, we established a protection factor of 35.5% and a dose reduction factor of 2.5 ± 0.2, respectively, after 48 h of incubation and exposure to 10 Gy of radiation, whereas in the B16F10 melanoma cells, a protection factor of 41.2% and DRF of 4 ± 0.2 were observed for the same incubation period (48 h).

Figure 7 shows an increase in the survival (%) of PNT2 cells after 24 and 48 h of incubation when treated with different substances (CA, API, RA, and PASE) and irradiated compared with cells that received only irradiation (irradiated controls), indicating the radioprotective capacities of these substances ($p < 0.001$).

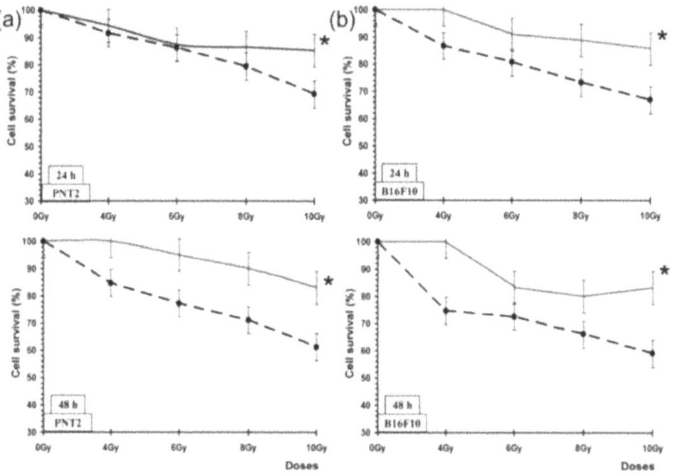

Figure 6. Cell survival (%) of PNT2 and B16F10 melanoma cells assessed by the MTT cell viability test after administration of PASE: (**a**) PNT2 cells after 24 h and 48 h incubation periods; (**b**) B16F10 melanoma cells after 24 h and 48 h incubation periods. * $p < 0.001$ versus control irradiated. Data are the mean ± standard error of eight independent experiments.

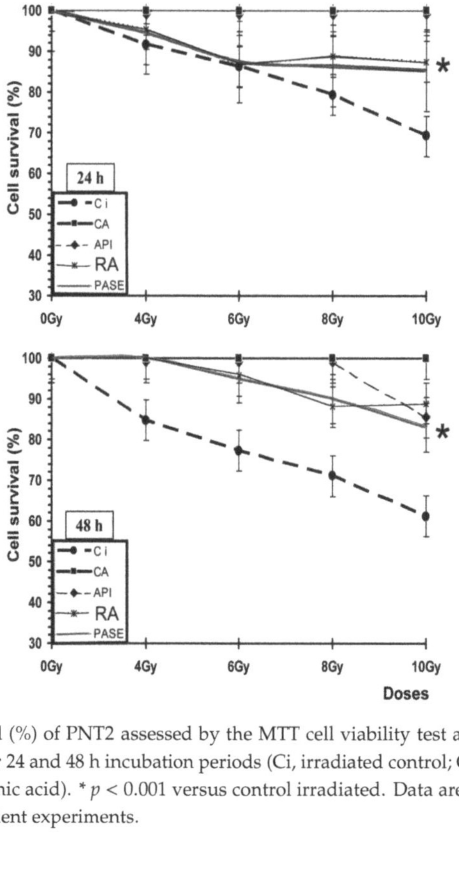

Figure 7. Cell survival (%) of PNT2 assessed by the MTT cell viability test after administration of different substances for 24 and 48 h incubation periods (Ci, irradiated control; CA, carnosic acid; API, apigenin; RA, rosmarinic acid). * $p < 0.001$ versus control irradiated. Data are the mean ± standard error of eight independent experiments.

4. Discussion

X-ray exposure produces a massive generation of reactive oxygen species (ROS)/free radicals in vivo. These ROS are formed by a sequential mechanism of electron transfer, through which molecular oxygen successively gives rise to a superoxide radical, hydrogen peroxide, and hydroxyl radical [12,20–22]. In general, ionizing radiation produces in the vicinity of DNA and its environs a large number of different radicals such as •OH, e^{-}_{aq}, and H• [7], which are mostly produced by the radiolysis water even in the absence of molecular oxygen. Its high reactivity produces an immediate reaction in the vicinity of its generation. However, when its generation is massive as a result of exposure to X-rays, the cytotoxic effect is no longer only local but can spread through reactive species and other radicals within the intracellular and even extracellular environment, increasing interaction with cellular phospholipids structures and inducing lipid peroxidation processes that increase the oxidative damage of DNA [20,21].

It is generally accepted that endogenously generated ROS and ROS that arise after exposure to X-rays are similar, but not necessarily identical. Both can be perpetuated through side reactions, for example, they can react with polyunsaturated fatty acids, which can cause tertiary biochemical reactions. However, the particular difference between metabolic ROS and those induced by ionizing radiation are based on their compartmentalization and their rate of appearance. In mammalian cells, ROS occur steadily and abundantly at frequent and changing time intervals, partly the result of metabolic reactions. An antioxidant enzyme system maintains an intracellular ROS concentration within a physiological range. In X-ray exposure, the generation of these ROSs is massive and can exceed any intracellular protection mechanism, affecting any place in the cell, and with an intensity that depends on the dose rate of absorbed radiation and the linear transfer of energy of the ionizing radiation administered [23].

Several authors have shown that under conditions of intense oxidative stress, such as during exposure to X-rays, when the endogenous antioxidant systems may be insufficient or defective, exogenous supplements or agents with the ability react with and eliminate free radicals could be used, as long as they contribute with a high degree of stability of the new intermediate neoformed radicals [21]. However, although the genoprotective effects are mentioned as being scavenging of •OH radicals [10–14,19,23–27], new DNA protection mechanisms have been described in recent years: the displacement of water in the extended hydration shell of DNA, the energy loss of low-energy electrons due to the scattering at vibrational water modes [28,29], the resulting decrease in secondary structure, and the ability to protect cells from stress conditions and to prevent cell damage by maintaining an elevated level of the Hsp70 [30]. To quantify the relative contributions of these different protective mechanisms, further work is needed.

This study attempted to obtain an extract from a suitable part of African nutmeg *Pycnanthus angolensis* (PASE) as well as quantify its radioprotective capacity when administered before (pre) and immediately after (post) exposure to ionizing radiation in line with results of our previous studies. In those studies, different test substances were evaluated for radioprotection, some of which expressed higher degrees of protection against harmful damage induced by ionizing radiation when compared with reference radioprotective compounds. In order to achieve these objectives and to enable effective comparisons, the same experimental protocols used in those previous studies were adapted for this study [8,9,17,18] but used a different ionizing agent, X-rays, which also conditioned new exposure times and dose rate.

We have previously described the antimutagenic capacity of some of the substances used in this study as comparative controls (RA, CA, API, D) against genotoxic damage induced by gamma radiation [8,10,11,27]. In this study, when these substances are administered before or after exposure to X-rays, they have lower anitmutagenic capacities that show no statistically significant differences. According to previous authors, our results show that when ionizing radiation has similar linear energy transfers, it conditions a similar relative biological effectiveness; therefore, the intensity of the radio-induced damage is similar [7,16]. This would explain that the genoprotective capacity of some substances tested in this study are similar to X-rays as well as gamma radiation [8].

We have not found specific information on the cellular uptake of the different compounds in relation to the micronucleus or MTT assays. We have previously shown that the reduction of micronuclei induced by ionizing radiation in biological systems cannot be directly ascribed to one single compound with a peculiar chemical structure, although the observed genoprotective effects induced by the presence of some compounds seem to be related to their antioxidant capacities and bioavailability in the cellular milieu [8]. Consequently, we observed that flavan-3-ols showed the greatest protective capacity of all polyphenols evaluated in our previous study [12], while other flavonoids known to have high antineoplastic and antiproliferative capacities showed lower antimutagenic capacities [31,32]. This may explain the increase in micronuclei formation obtained after treatments with Q and E since both present a flavonoid structure with a catechol group in the B ring that gives them pro-oxidant capacities, even at the low concentrations used in this study. When reacted with the superoxide radical, this can lead to the generation of hydrogen peroxide, thus increasing its cytotoxic capacity [33–36].

In addition, this genoprotective capacity was also found to depend on the degree of polymerization and solubility of the substances assessed, since both modify their bioavailability [8,10,11]. We believe that all of the above are equally relevant to PASE, which we used as a genoprotective substance against IR-induced damage in this study.

We have not found references on antigenotoxic activity of *Pycnanthus angolensis*. However, its genoprotective capacity is greater than that shown by the AMF, the only radioprotector used in radiation oncology. In this sense, when an extract of PASE is administered before exposure to IR, it is observed to have a medium radioprotective capacity similar to that of AMF; however, it is found to be superior to AMF when administered after exposure to X-rays, an observation which could be explained by the increased activity in the lipid peroxidation process [8,9].

We have not found references on the radioprotective activity of *Pycnanthus angolensis*. Our results on cell survival, protection factor (PF), and dose reduction factor (DRL) also confirm the radioprotective effect of PASE against cytotoxic damage induced by IR on normal prostate (traditionally considered as radiosensitive cells) and melanoma tumor cells (considered as radioresistant cells). This radioprotective effect is less intense than determined for RA and CA for PNT2 cells, but it did not portray the paradoxical radiosensitizing effect of these substances that we previously described in melanoma cells treated with RA and CA. In B16F10 melanoma cells irradiated with X-rays, both substances (RA and CA) are shown as potent radiosensitizing agents to reduce cell survival, suggesting a mechanism of activation of pheomelanin production that would consume intracellular glutathione causing the decrease of endogenous protection mechanisms [17,18].

Regardless of its applications in traditional medicine, components of PASE are habitually consumed in human diets and have been included in dietary supplements for decades within certain concentration ranges without reported toxicity. With the exception of AMF, which is known to have a high degree of toxicity, the substances analyzed in this study are also common components of human diets [22,25]. Evidently, before administering any compounds to humans in an ionizing radiation exposure scenario, studies should be performed on a wider range of cell lines, especially since different types of tissues can act quite diversely to the same compound with/without radiation exposure. Further, the effects of antioxidant supplements in oncology may be harmful. Although some studies have suggested that antioxidants can protect normal tissues from chemotherapy- or radiation-induced damage, others have claimed that supplementary antioxidants during chemotherapy and radiation therapy should be discouraged because they may actually protect the tumor cells and so reduce survival of the patient [8].

In this regard, it is worth pointing out two scenarios in which a dietary supplement containing these substances, specifically AR and PASE, may have utility in the reduction of the stochastic effects induced by ionizing radiation: the protection of workers professionally exposed to ionizing radiation and patients undergoing medical radiodiagnostic examinations. In this way, it offers a possibility of increasing the levels of endogenous protection against damage induced by ionizing radiation in professionally exposed workers by scavenging the free radicals produced and reducing the harmful effects of accidental exposures; while patients who consume these substances prior to performing radiological examinations would be endowed with the capacity to reduce or eliminate a possible stochastic effect induced by IR. PASE offers an improved protective capability over RA as it offers the possibility of protecting cells against damage even after exposure to ionizing radiation, a property which could be exploited to mitigate the harmful effects of ionizing radiation during accidental or emergency situations in which workers are exposed to radiation without prior knowledge. In conclusion, given the possibility of stochastic effects, the use of innocuous substances, such as PASE, may offer protection against biological damage induced by ionizing radiation by augmenting the endogenous antioxidant protection mechanisms of the individual.

Author Contributions: Conceptualization, M.A., A.O., J.C., D.G.A., and M.A.-S.; Methodology, M.A., J.C., and A.O.; Software, J.C. and M.A.; Validation, J.C., D.G.A., M.A.S., A.O., and M.A.; Formal Analysis, J.C.; Investigation, D.G.A.; M.A.-S., and A.O.; Writing—Original Draft Preparation, D.G.A. and M.A.; Resources, M.A.-S. and A.O.; Writing—Review & Editing, D.G.A. and M.A.; Visualization, M.A., A.O., J.C., and M.A.S.; Supervision, M.A.; Project Administration, D.G.A.; A.O. and M.A.; Funding Acquisition: D.G.A.; A.O.; M.A. All authors have read and agreed to the published version of the manuscript.

Funding: This study was supported by a grant from the National Spanish R&D Programme CENIT of the Spanish Ministry of Science and Technology named "Industrial Research and Experimental Development of Intelligent Foods (Acronym: SMARTFOODS); D.G.A. was able to take part in this study because of a sponsored fellowship (GHA/0021) from the International Atomic Energy Agency (IAEA) in the project "Biological Dosimetry for radiation workers and the evaluation of extracts from African Nutmeg (Pycnanthus angolensis) for their radioprotective potential".

Conflicts of Interest: The authors declare no conflicts of interest.

Abbreviations

AMF: amifostine; API: apigenin; C: ascorbic acid; CA: carnosic acid; CB: cells blocked; CBMN: cytokinesis-blocked micronucleus; D: diosmin; DMSO: dimethyl sulfoxide; DRF: dose reduction factor; E: eriodictyol; FBS: fetal bovine serum; PF: protection factor; IR: ionizing radiation; MC: mortality of the irradiated control cells; MN: micronucleus; MNPCEs: micronucleus in polychromatic erythrocytes; MT: mortality of the cells irradiated and treated; MTT: 3-(4,5-dimethyl-2-thiazolyl)-2,5-diphenyl-tetrazolium bromide; PASE: *Pycnanthus angolensis* Warb seed extract; PBS: phosphate-buffered saline; PCEs: polychromatic erythrocytes; PHA: phytohemagglutinin A; Q: quercetin; RA: rosmarinic acid; ROS: reactive oxygen species; Te: green tea extract; T: δ-tocopherol; TLDs: thermoluminescent dosimeters.

References

1. Fort, D.M.; Ubillas, R.P.; Mendez, C.D.; Jolad, S.D.; Inman, W.D.; Carney, J.R.; Chen, J.L.; Ianiro, T.T.; Hasbun, C.; Bruening, R.C.; et al. Novel Antihyperglycemic Terpenoid-Quinones from Pycnanthus angolensis. *J. Org. Chem.* **2000**, *65*, 6534–6539. [CrossRef] [PubMed]
2. Achel, D.G.; Alcaraz, M.; Kingsford-Adaboh, R.; Nyarko, A.K.; Gomda, Y. A review of the medicinal properties and applications of Pycnanthus angolensis (Welw) Warb. *Pharmacologyonline* **2012**, *2*, 1–22.
3. Tsaassi, V.B.; Hussain, H.; Tamboue, H.; Dongo, E.; Kouam, S.F.; Krohn, K. Pycnangloside: A new cerebroside from bark of Pycnanthus angolensis. *Nat. Prod. Commun.* **2010**, *5*, 1795–1798. [CrossRef] [PubMed]
4. Onocha, P.A.; Ajaiyeoba, E.O.; Ali, M.S. In vitro antileishmaniasis, phyto and cytotoxicity of Pycnanthus angolensis methanolic extracts. *Res. J. Med. Sci.* **2008**, *2*, 178–181.
5. Gbolade, A.A.; Adeyemi, A.A. Investigation of in vitro anthelmintic activities of Pycnanthus angolensis and Sphenocentrum jollyanum. *Fitoterapia* **2008**, *79*, 220–222. [CrossRef]
6. Govindasamy, R.; Simon, J.; Puduri, V.S.; Juliani, H.R.; Asante-Dartey, J.; Arthur, H.; Diawuo, B.; Acquaye, D.; Hitimana, N. Retailers and wholesalers of African herbal and natural products: Case studies from Ghana and Rwanda. In *New Crops and New Uses*; ASHP Press: Seattle, VA, USA, 2007; pp. 332–337.
7. Von Sonntag, C. *Free-Radical-Induced DNA Damage and Its Repair. A Chemical Perspective*; Springer: Berlin, Germany, 2016; pp. 1–45.
8. Alcaraz, M.; Acevedo, C.; Castillo, J.; Benavente-Garcia, O.; Armero, D.; Vicente, V.; Canteras, M. Liposoluble antioxidants provide an effective radioprotective barrier. *Br. J. Radiol.* **2009**, *82*, 605–609. [CrossRef]

9. Alcaraz, M.; Armero, D.; Martínez-Beneyto, Y.; Castillo, J.; Benavente-García, O.; Fernandez, H.; Alcaraz-Saura, M.; Canteras, M. Chemical genoprotection: Reducing biological damage to as low as reasonably achievable levels. *Dentomaxillofac. Radiol.* **2011**, *40*, 310–314. [CrossRef]
10. Castillo, J.; Benavente-García, O.; Lorente, J.; Alcaraz, M.; Redondo, A.; Ortuño, A.; Del Rio, J.A. Antioxidant Activity and Radioprotective Effects against Chromosomal Damage Induced in Vivo by X-rays of Flavan-3-ols (Procyanidins) from Grape Seeds (Vitis vinifera): Comparative Study versus Other Phenolic and Organic Compounds. *J. Agric. Food Chem.* **2000**, *48*, 1738–1745. [CrossRef]
11. Castillo, J.; Benavente-García, O.; del Baño, M.J.; Lorente, J.; Alcaraz, M.; Dato, M.J. Radioprotective Effects Against Chromosomal Damage Induced in Human Lymphocytes by γ-Rays as a Function of Polymerization Grade of Grape Seed Extracts. *J. Med. Food* **2001**, *4*, 117–123. [CrossRef]
12. Benavente-García, O.; Castillo, J.; Lorente, J.; Alcaraz, M. Radioprotective Effects in Vivo of Phenolics Extracted from Olea europaea L. Leaves Against X-Ray-Induced Chromosomal Damage: Comparative Study Versus Several Flavonoids and Sulfur-Containing Compounds. *J. Med. Food* **2002**, *5*, 125–135. [CrossRef]
13. Fenech, M.; Morley, A.A. Measurement of micronuclei in lymphocytes. *Mutat. Res. Mutagenes. Relat. Subj.* **1985**, *147*, 29–36. [CrossRef]
14. International Atomic Energy Agency. *Cytogenetic Dosimetry: Applications in Preparedness for and Response to Radiation Emergencies*; IAEA: Vienna, Austria, 2011; pp. 1–247.
15. Schmid, W. The micronucleus test. *Mutat. Res. Mutagenes. Relat. Subj.* **1975**, *31*, 9–15. [CrossRef]
16. Hall, E.J. *Radiobiology for the Radiologist*, 2nd ed.; Harper & Row: Philadelphia, PA, USA, 1978; pp. 93–110.
17. Alcaraz, M.; Achel, D.G.; Olivares, A.; Olmos, E.; Alcaraz-Saura, M.; Castillo, J. Carnosol, radiation and melanoma: A translational possibility. *Clin. Transl. Oncol.* **2013**, *15*, 712–719. [CrossRef] [PubMed]
18. Alcaraz, M.; Alcaraz-Saura, M.; Achel, D.G.; Olivares, A.; López-Morata, J.A.; Castillo, J. Radiosensitizing effect of rosmarinic acid in metastatic melanoma B16F10 cells. *Anticancer Res.* **2014**, *34*, 1913–1921. [PubMed]
19. Sarma, L.; Kesavan, P.C. Protective Effects of Vitamins C and E Against γ-ray-induced Chromosomal Damage in Mouse. *Int. J. Radiat. Biol.* **1993**, *63*, 759–764. [CrossRef] [PubMed]
20. Sáez-Tormo, G.; Oliva, M.R.; Muñoz, P.; Valls, V.; Irandi, A.; Ramos, M.; Climent, J. Oxidative stress and genetic damage, in: Health and Orange. In *Fundación Valenciana de Estudios Avanzados*; FVEA: Valencia, Spain, 1994; pp. 51–60.
21. Benavente-García, O.; Castillo, J.; Marin, F.R.; Ortuño, A.; Del Río, J.A. Uses and Properties of Citrus Flavonoids. *J. Agric. Food Chem.* **1997**, *45*, 4505–4515. [CrossRef]
22. Prasad, K.N. Rationale for using multiple antioxidants in protecting humans against low doses of ionizing radiation. *Br. J. Radiol.* **2005**, *78*, 485–492. [CrossRef]
23. Prasad, K.N.; Cole, W.C.; Haase, G.M. Radiation protection in humans: Extending the concept of as low as reasonably achievable (ALARA) from dose to biological damage. *Br. J. Radiol.* **2004**, *77*, 97–99. [CrossRef]
24. Baliga, M.S.; Jagetia, G.C.; Venkatesh, P.; Reddy, R.; Ulloor, J.N. Radiprotective effect of abana, a polyherbal drug following total body irradiation. *Br. J. Radiol.* **2004**, *77*, 1027–1035. [CrossRef]
25. Feinendegen, L.E. Significance of basic and clinical research in radiation medicine: Challenges for the future. *Br. J. Radiol.* **2005**, *78*, 185–195. [CrossRef]
26. Abraham, S.K.; Sarma, L.; Kesavan, P.C. Protective effects of chlorogenic acid, curcumin and β-carotene against γ-radiation-induced in vivo chromosomal damage. *Mutat. Res. Lett.* **1993**, *303*, 109–112. [CrossRef]
27. Del Baño, M.J.; Castillo, J.; Benavente-García, O.; Lorente, J.; Martín-Gil, R.; Acevedo, C.; Alcaraz, M. Radioprotective−Antimutagenic Effects of Rosemary Phenolics against Chromosomal Damage Induced in Human Lymphocytes by γ-rays. *J. Agric. Food Chem.* **2006**, *54*, 2064–2068. [CrossRef] [PubMed]
28. Hahn, M.B.; Meyer, S.; Schroter, M.; Kunte, H.; Solomun, T.; Sturn, H. DNA protection by Ectoine from ionizing radiation: Molecular Mechanisms. *Phys. Chem. Phys. Chem.* **2017**, *19*, 25717–277122. [CrossRef] [PubMed]
29. Rieckmann, T.; Gatzemeier, F.; Christiansen, S.; Rothkamm, K.; Münscher, A. The inflamation-reducing compatible solute ectoine does not impair the cytotoxic effect of ionizing radiation on head and neck cancer cells. *Sci. Rep.* **2019**, *9*, 6594–6601. [CrossRef] [PubMed]
30. Buomino, E.; Schiraldi, C.; Baroni, A.; Paoletti, M.; De Rosa, M.; Tufano, M.A. Ectoine from halophilic microorganisms induces the expression of hsp70 and hsp70B′ in human keratinocytes modulating the proinflammatory response. *Cell Stress Chaperones* **2005**, *10*, 197–203. [CrossRef] [PubMed]

31. Martínez Conesa, C.; Vicente Ortega, V.; Yáñez Gascón, M.J.; Alcaraz Baños, M.; Canteras Jordana, M.; Benavente-García, O.; Castillo, J. Treatment of Metastatic Melanoma B16F10 by the Flavonoids Tangeretin, Rutin, and Diosmin. *J. Agric. Food Chem.* **2005**, *53*, 6791–6797. [CrossRef] [PubMed]
32. Yanez, J.; Vicente, V.; Alcaraz, M.; Castillo, J.; Benavente-Garcia, O.; Canteras, M.; Teruel, J.A.L. Cytotoxicity and Antiproliferative Activities of Several Phenolic Compounds Against Three Melanocytes Cell Lines: Relationship Between Structure and Activity. *Nutr. Cancer* **2004**, *49*, 191–199. [CrossRef]
33. Zhou, L.; Elias, R.J. Factors influencing the antioxidant and pro-oxidant activity of polyphenols in oil-in-water emulsions. *J. Agric. Food Chem.* **2012**, *60*, 2906–2915. [CrossRef]
34. Miura, T.; Muraoka, S.; Fujimoto, Y. Inactivation of creatine kinase induced by quercetin with horseradish peroxidase and hydrogen peroxide. pro-oxidative and anti-oxidative actions of quercetin. *Food Chem. Toxicol.* **2003**, *41*, 759–765. [CrossRef]
35. Raja, S.B.; Rajendiran, V.; Kasinathan, N.K.; Amrithalakshmi, P.; Venkatabalasubramanian, S.; Murali, M.R.; Devaraj, H.; Devaraj, S.N. Differential cytotoxic activity of Quercetin on colonic cancer cells depends on ROS generation through COX-2 expression. *Food Chem. Toxicol.* **2017**, *106*, 92–106. [CrossRef]
36. Dajas, F.; Abin-Carriquiry, J.A.; Arredondo, F.; Blasina, F.; Echeverry, C.; Martínez, M.; Rivera, F.; Vaamonde, L. Quercetin in brain diseases: Potential and limits. *Neurochem. Int.* **2015**, *89*, 140–148. [CrossRef] [PubMed]

Journal of
Clinical Medicine

MDPI

Review

Role of Vacha (*Acorus calamus* Linn.) in Neurological and Metabolic Disorders: Evidence from Ethnopharmacology, Phytochemistry, Pharmacology and Clinical Study

Vineet Sharma [1], Rohit Sharma [1,*], DevNath Singh Gautam [1], Kamil Kuca [2,*], Eugenie Nepovimova [2] and Natália Martins [3,4,*]

1 Department of Rasa Shastra and Bhaishajya Kalpana, Faculty of Ayurveda, Institute of Medical Sciences, BHU, Varanasi, Uttar Pradesh 221005, India; vinitbhu93@gmail.com (V.S.); drdnsgautam@gmail.com (D.S.G.)
2 Department of Chemistry, Faculty of Science, University of Hradec Králové, Rokitanskeho 62, 50003 Hradec Králové, Czech Republic; eugenie.nepovimova@uhk.cz
3 Faculty of Medicine, University of Porto, Alameda Prof. Hernani Monteiro, 4200-319 Porto, Portugal
4 Institute for research and Innovation in Heath (i3S), University of Porto, Rua Alfredo Allen, 4200-135 Porto, Portugal
* Correspondence: rohitsharma@bhu.ac.in or dhanvantari86@gmail.com (R.S.); kamil.kuca@uhk.cz (K.K.); ncmartins@med.up.pt (N.M.)

Received: 23 March 2020; Accepted: 14 April 2020; Published: 19 April 2020

Abstract: Vacha (*Acorus calamus* Linn. (Acoraceae)) is a traditional Indian medicinal herb, which is practiced to treat a wide range of health ailments, including neurological, gastrointestinal, respiratory, metabolic, kidney, and liver disorders. The purpose of this paper is to provide a comprehensive up-to-date report on its ethnomedicinal use, phytochemistry, and pharmacotherapeutic potential, while identifying potential areas for further research. To date, 145 constituents have been isolated from this herb and identified, including phenylpropanoids, sesquiterpenoids, and monoterpenes. Compelling evidence is suggestive of the biopotential of its various extracts and active constituents in several metabolic and neurological disorders, such as anticonvulsant, antidepressant, antihypertensive, anti-inflammatory, immunomodulatory, neuroprotective, cardioprotective, and anti-obesity effects. The present extensive literature survey is expected to provide insights into the involvement of several signaling pathways and oxidative mechanisms that can mitigate oxidative stress, and other indirect mechanisms modulated by active biomolecules of *A. calamus* to improve neurological and metabolic disorders.

Keywords: *Acorus calamus*; ethnomedicinal; phytochemistry; toxicity; pharmacological action; clinical trial; neuroprotective; neurological; metabolic application

1. Introduction

Globally, an estimated 450 million people are suffering from mental disorders and about 425 million are known diabetics [1,2]. In 2016, 650 million adults were obese and about 23.6 million people were estimated to die of cardiovascular diseases (CVDs) by the year 2030 [3]. Metabolic disorders are characterized by hypertension, hyperglycemia, abdominal obesity, and hyperlipidemia, which may worsen the neurological disease risk. Improper diet (high calorie intake), lifestyle (e.g., smoking, chronic alcohol consumption, sedentary habits), and/or low level of nitrosamines (through processed food, tobacco smoke, and nitrate-containing fertilizers) affect the liver and can further lead to fatty liver disease [4,5]. In this condition, fatty changes may be due to increased production or decreased use of fatty acids, which may lead to inflammatory injury of hepatocytes, where inflammatory mediators, such as cytokines and interleukins, are released, which, along with lower adipokines, may eventually develop hepatic insulin resistance [6]. The same pathology also mediates diabetes, obesity, and peripheral insulin resistance. Insulin resistance also promotes the release of ceramides and other toxic lipids which enter the circulation and cross the blood–brain barrier leading to brain insulin resistance, inflammatory changes, and further progression to neurodegeneration and neurological disorders (Figure 1) [7].

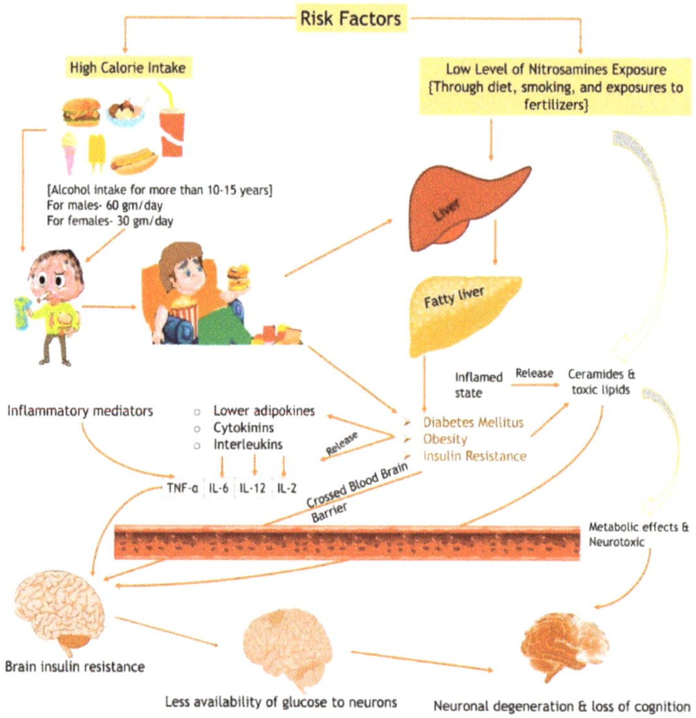

Figure 1. Pathophysiology of insulin resistance, metabolic malfunction, and progression to a neurological disorder. TNF, tumor necrosis factor; IL, interleukin.

Acorus calamus Linn. (Acoraceae), also known as Vacha in Sanskrit, is a mid-term, perennial, fragrant herb which is practiced in the Ayurvedic (Indian traditional) and the Chinese system of medicine. The plant's rhizomes are brown in color, twisted, cylindrical, curved, and shortly nodded. The leaves are radiant green, with a sword-like structure, which is thicker in the middle and has curvy margins (Figure 2) [8]. Several reports ascertained a wide range of biological activities involving its myriad of active phytoconstituents. In this sense, the intent of this review is to assemble and summarize the geographical distribution, ethnopharmacology, phytochemistry, mechanism of action of *A. calamus* along with preclinical and clinical claims that are relevant to manage neurological and metabolic disorders. To the best of our knowledge, so far, none of the published reviews has described all the characteristics of this medicinal plant [9–11]. The present report is expected to produce a better understanding of the characteristics, bioactivities, and mechanistic aspects of this plant and to provide new leads for future research.

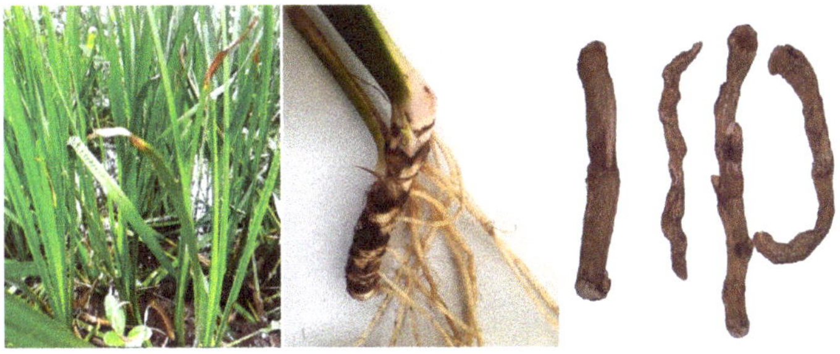

(A) (B) (C)

Figure 2. Photographs of *Acorus calamus*: (**A**) Natural habitat; (**B**) Fresh rhizome; (**C**) Dried rhizome.

2. Methodology

The literature available in the Ayurvedic classical texts, technical reports, online scientific records such as SciFinder, Google Scholar, MEDLINE, EMBASE, Scopus directory were explored for ethnomedicinal uses, geographical distribution, phytochemistry, pharmacology, and biomedicine by applying the following keywords: "*Acorus calamus*", "Vacha", "Medhya", "neuroprotective", "phytochemistry", "obesity", "oxidative stress", "anticonvulsant", "antidepressant", "antihypertensive", "anti-inflammatory", "immunomodulator", "antioxidant", "diabetes", "mechanism of action" with their corresponding medical subject headings (MeSH) terms using conjunctions OR/AND. The search was focused on identifying Ayurvedic claims in the available ethnomedicinal, phytochemical, preclinical, clinical, and toxicity reports to understand the role of *A. calamus* in neurological and metabolic disorders. This search was undertaken between January 2018 and January 2020. Searches were restricted to the English language. The search methodology as per the Preferred Reporting Items for Systematic Reviews and Meta-Analysis (PRISMA) is stipulated in the flowchart in Figure 3.

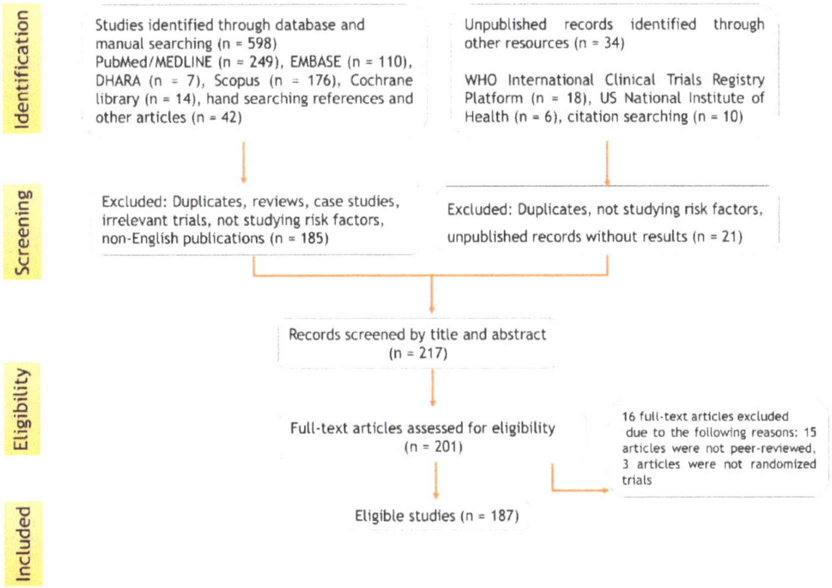

Figure 3. Flowchart of the selection process.

3. Geographical Distribution

A. calamus grows in high (1800 m) and low (900 m) altitudes and it is found to be geographically available in 42 countries [8]. Furthermore, as per the Global Biodiversity Information Facility records [12], the distribution of this plant in several parts of the world, as well as in India, is highlighted in Figure 4.

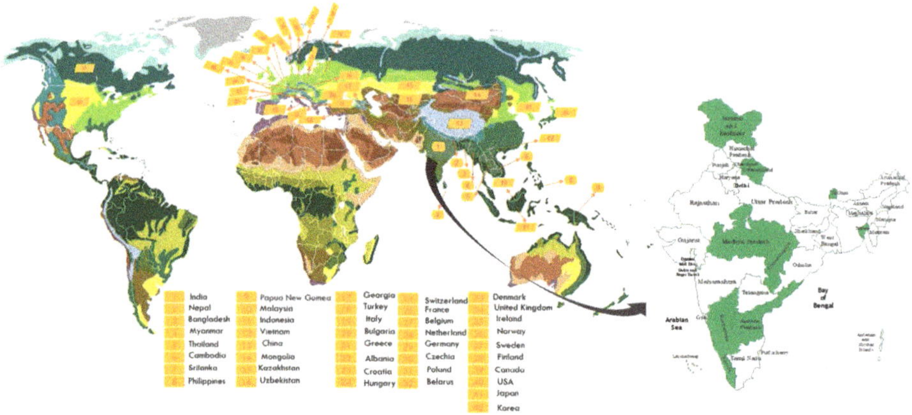

Figure 4. Distribution of *A. calamus* worldwide and in India.

4. Ethnomedicinal Use

This plant is being practiced traditionally in the Indian Ayurvedic tradition, as well as in the Chinese system of medicine for analgesic, antipyretic, tonic, anti-obesity, and healing purposes; it is highly effective for skin diseases, along with neurological, gastrointestinal, respiratory, and several other health disorders. Rhizomes and leaves are found to be profusely practiced in the form of infusion, powder, paste, or decoction [13–72]. The ethnomedicinal uses of the *A. calamus* are detailed in Table 1.

A. calamus rhizomes and leaves are also used as an active pharmaceutical ingredient in various Ayurvedic formulations (Table 2).

Table 1. Ethnomedicinal use of *A. calamus* in various countries.

Country	Ailment/Use	Part Used/ Dosage Form	Route of Administration	References
India	Eczema	The paste of *A. calamus* rhizomes are given with the paste of *Curcuma aromatica* rhizomes and *Azadirachta indica* leaves	Oral	[13]
	Skin diseases	Rhizomes paste *A. calamus* and *C. aromatica* are applied with the seed paste of *Argemone Mexicana*		
	Cough, stuttering, ulcer, fever, dermatitis, scab, sores	Rhizomes		[14]
	Cold, cough, and fever	Rhizomes paste of *A. calamus* is given to children with mother's milk, *Myristica fragrance*, and *Calunarejan spinosa* fruits		[15]
		Two teaspoonfuls of herbal powder containing *A. calamus* rhizomes, *Boerhaavia diffusa* roots, *Calonyction muricutum* flower pedicles, *Ipomoea muricate* seeds, *Senna* leaves, *Cassia fistula* fruits pulp, *Curcuma longa* rhizomes, *Helicteres isora* fruits, and *Mentha arvensis* leaves, black pepper is taken with lukewarm water		[16]
	Gastric disorders	*A. calamus* rhizomes paste is given with cow milk		[17]
	Carminative, flavoring, tonic, and head lice infestation	Infusion of a dried rhizomes (collected and stored in the autumn season)		[17–19]
	Epilepsy, dysentery, mental illnesses, diarrhea, kidney and liver disorders	*A. calamus* rhizomes paste is given with honey		[20]
	Wounds, fever, body pain	Rhizomes		[21,22]
	Dysentery	Fresh ground rhizomes is mixed with hot water and given for 3 days		[23]
	Stimulant	Dry powder of *A. calamus* is given with honey		[24]
	Injuries	External application of the *A. calamus* rhizomes paste	Dermal	[25]
	Stomachache	Ash of the *A. calamus* rhizomes paste		[26]
	Otitis externa	*A. calamus* roots paste is given with coconut husk juice		[27]
	Lotion	Fresh leaves of *A. calamus*		[28]
	Cough, cancer, and fever	*A. calamus* roots juice is given with honey and *MyristicaDactyloides*		[29]

Table 1. *Cont.*

Country	Ailment/Use	Part Used/ Dosage Form	Route of Administration	References
	Analgesic	*A. calamus* rhizomes are given with cinchona bark		[30]
	Gastrointestinal, respiratory, emmenagogue, antihelmintic	Rhizomes		
	Prolonged labor	Rhizomes is applied with saffron and horse milk		
	Paralysis, arthritis	Rhizomes ash is applied with castor oil		
	Neurological disorder, gastrointestinal, respiratory, increases menstrual flow, analgesic, contraceptive	Rhizomes		[31–33]
	Herpangina, analgesic, neurological disorder, gastrointestinal, respiratory			[34]
Pakistan	Colic and diarrhea	Whole plant	Oral	[35]
Nepal	Blood pressure	Roots infusion of *A. calamus*		[36]
	Cough, headache, snake bite, sore throat, and pain	Rhizomes		[37]
	Dysentery	Rhizomes juice is given with hot water		
	Neurological, respiratory	Rhizomes		[38]
Malaysia	Rheumatism, diarrhea, dyspepsia, and hair loss	Whole plant		[39]
Tibet	Fever, gastrointestinal	Dried rhizomes is given with *Saussurea lappa*, *Ferula foetida*, *Terminalia chebula*, *Cuminum cyminum*, *Inula racemosa*, and *Zingiber officinale*		[40]
	Cancer	Rhizomes		[41]

Table 1. *Cont.*

Country	Ailment/Use	Part Used/ Dosage Form	Route of Administration	References
China	Gastrointestinal, respiratory, neuroprotective, analgesic, contraceptive, cancer	Rhizomes		[42–44]
	Antipyretic and ear-related disease	Rhizomes given with squeezed *Coccinia cordifolia* stems along with water		[45]
	Detoxification	Rhizomes with vinegar, *Alpinia galanga*, *Zingiber purpureum*		
	Analgesic	Herbal baths of the rhizome	External	
	Hemorrhage	Rhizomes paste		[46]
	Aphrodisiac	Rhizomes	Oral	[47]
	Hallucination	Rhizomesare mixed with Indian hemp and *Podophyllum pleianthum*		[48]
	Fair skin	Leaves of *A. calamus* are given with *Artemisia vulgaris*	Dermal	[49]
Indonesia	Gastrointestinal	Rhizomes	Oral	[50]
England		Rhizomes blended with chalk and magnesium oxide		[51]
	Gastrointestinal, antibacterial, analgesic	Rhizomes		[52]
	Neurological, dysentery, and chronic catarrh	Rhizomesare given with *Gentiana campestris* L.		
	Malaria	Rhizomes		[53]
Europe	Obesity, influenza, gastrointestinal, respiratory			[54,55]
Republic of South Africa	Tooth powder, gastrointestinal, tonic, aphrodisiac			[56]
Sweden	Liquor			[57]
Germany	Increases menstrual flow, gastrointestinal			[58,59]
Java	Lactation			[60]

Table 1. *Cont.*

Country	Ailment/Use	Part Used/ Dosage Form	Route of Administration	References
Lithuania	Chest pain, diarrhea	Rhizomes and leaves are taken with sugar		[52]
	Relieves pain, gout, rheumatism	Leaves decoction	External	[61]
New Guinea	Miscarriage	Rhizomes	Oral	[62]
Philippines	Gastrointestinal, rheumatism			[56]
Russia	Typhoid, syphilis, baldness, fever, cholera			[63]
Thailand	Blood purifier, fever			[64]
Turkey	Wound healing, cough, tuberculosis		External and oral	[61]
	Gastrointestinal		Oral	[65,66]
Arab countries	Gastrointestinal, tuberculosis			[67,68]
Brazil	Destroys parasitic worms			[68]
Argentina	Dysmenorrhea			[69]
United States	Gastrointestinal, abortifacient, stimulant, tonic, respiratory disorder	Rhizomes		[70]
Korea	Improves memory and life span			[71]
Sri Lanka	Cough, worm infestation	Rhizomes paste are given with milk		[72]

Table 2. Pharmaceutical products of *A. calamus* available in the market.

Medicine/Formulations	Indications/Use	Manufacturers
Pilochek tablets	Hemorrhoids	Dabur India Limited
Brahm Rasayan	Nervine tonic	
Mahasudarsan Churna	Malaria	
Janma Ghunti Honey	Babies growth, Constipation, Diarrhea	
Brahmi Pearls capsules	Brain Nourisher	Kerala Ayurveda
GT capsules	Osteoarthritis, osteoporosis, hyperlipidemia	
Histantin tablets	Anti-allergic	
Santhwanam oil	Antioxidant, rejuvenate	
Mahathikthaka Ghrita capsules	Skin disease, malabsorption syndrome	
Calamus root tincture	Stimulates the digestive system	Florida Herbal Pharmacy
Vacha capsules	Food supplements	DR Wakde's Natural Health Care, London
Mentat tablets and syrup	Nervine tonic	Himalaya Herbal Healthcare
Abana	Cardiovascular disorders, hyperlipidemia, dyslipidemia	
Mentat tablets and Syrup	Anxiety, depression, insomnia	
Muscle & Joint Rub	Backaches, muscular sprains, pain	
Anxocare	Anxiety	
Erina-EP	Ectoparasites	
Himpyrin, Himpyrin Vet	Analgesic and anti-inflammatory	
Scavon Vet	Anti-bacterial, anti-fungal	
Vacha powder	Brain tonic, improves digestion, and prevents nausea	Bixa Botanical
Amalth	Herbal supplements	Mcnow Biocare Private Limited
Sunarin capsules	Anal fissures, piles, rectal inflammation, congestion	SG Phyto Pharma

Table 2. *Cont.*

Medicine/Formulations	Indications/Use	Manufacturers
Dr Willmar Schwabe India *Acorus calamus* mother tincture	Intestinal worms and stomach disorders, fever, nausea	Dr Willmar Schwabe India Pvt Ltd.
Himalayan calamus root essential oil	Pain relief and calm mind	Naturalis Essence of Nature
Calamus oil	Body, skin care, hair growth	Kazima Perfumers
Calamus root powder	Mental health problems	Heilen Biopharm
Winton tablets and syrup	Reduce tension, stress, and anxiety	Scortis Healthcare
Chesol syrup	Muscular aches and pains, chest colds, and bronchitis	J & J Dechane Laboratories Private Limited
Enzo Fast	Acidity, gastritis, flatulence, indigestion	Naturava
Dark Forest Vekhand powder	Abdomen pain, worms (infants)	Simandhar Herbal Pvt. Ltd.
Nervocare	Insomnia	Deep Ayurveda
Antress tablets	Anxiety and stress disorders	Ayursun Pharma
Grapzone syrup	Mental wellness	Alna Biotech Pvt Ltd.
Memoctive syrup	Improves memory power	Aayursh Herbal India
Smrutihills capsules	Stress, anxiety, adaptogenic	Ayush Arogyam
Gastrin capsules	Gastritis, dyspepsia	Sarvana Marundhagam
Pigmento tablets	Leukoderma or vitiligo	Charak Pharma
Paedritone drops	Digestive functions	
Vacha Churna	Brain tonic, digestion, nausea	Sadvaidyasala
Alert capsules	Immunomodulator, anxiety	Vasu Healthcare
Brento tablets	Increasing cognitive functions	Zandu Realty Limited
Livotrit Forte	Hepatitis, jaundice	
Zanduzyme	Indigestion and dyspepsia	

Table 2. *Cont.*

Medicine/Formulations	Indications/Use	Manufacturers
Vedic Slim	Anti-obesity	Vedic Bio-Labs Pvt. Ltd.
Hinguvachaadi Gulika	Anorexia, indigestion, appetite loss	Nagarajuna Pvt. Ltd.
Nilsin capsules	Sinusitis and allergic rhinitis	Phytomarketing
Norbeepee tablet	Hypertension	AVN Formulations
Sooktyn tablet	Antacid, antispasmodic	Alarsin Pharma Pvt. Ltd.
Deonac oil	Pain reliving oil	Doux Healthcare Pvt. Ltd.
Smrutisagar Rasa	Memory enhancer	Shree Dhootpapeshwar Limited
Yogaraj Guggul	Vitiligo, anorexia, indigestion, loss of appetite	
Kankayan Bati	Gastritis, flatulence, dyspepsia	Baidyanath Pvt. Ltd.
Brahmi Ghrita	Insanity and memory issues	
Fat Go	Controls high cholesterol level	Jolly Healthcare
Divya Medha Vati	Improves memory power	Patanjali Ayurveda
Divya Mukta Vati	High blood pressure	

5. Phytochemistry

The phytochemical investigation of this plant has been ongoing since the year 1957 [73,74]. To date, about 145 compounds were isolated from *A. calamus* rhizomes and leaves, viz. phenylpropanoids, sterols, triterpene glycosides, triterpenoid saponins, sesquiterpenoids, monoterpenes, and alkaloids (Table 3). Amongst those, phenylpropanoids (chiefly, asarone and eugenol) and sesquiterpenoids have been considered the principal effective compounds of *A. calamus*. Chemical structures of isolated compounds from *A. calamus* are illustrated in Figure 5.

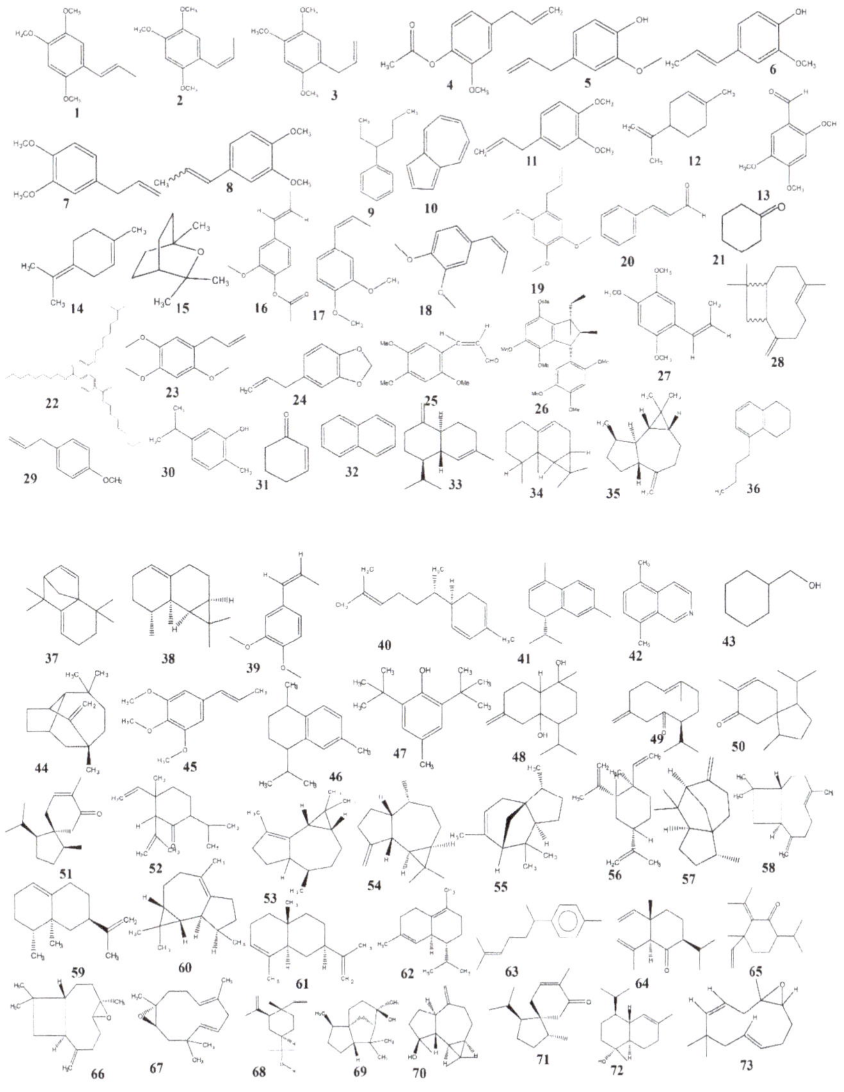

Figure 5. *Cont.*

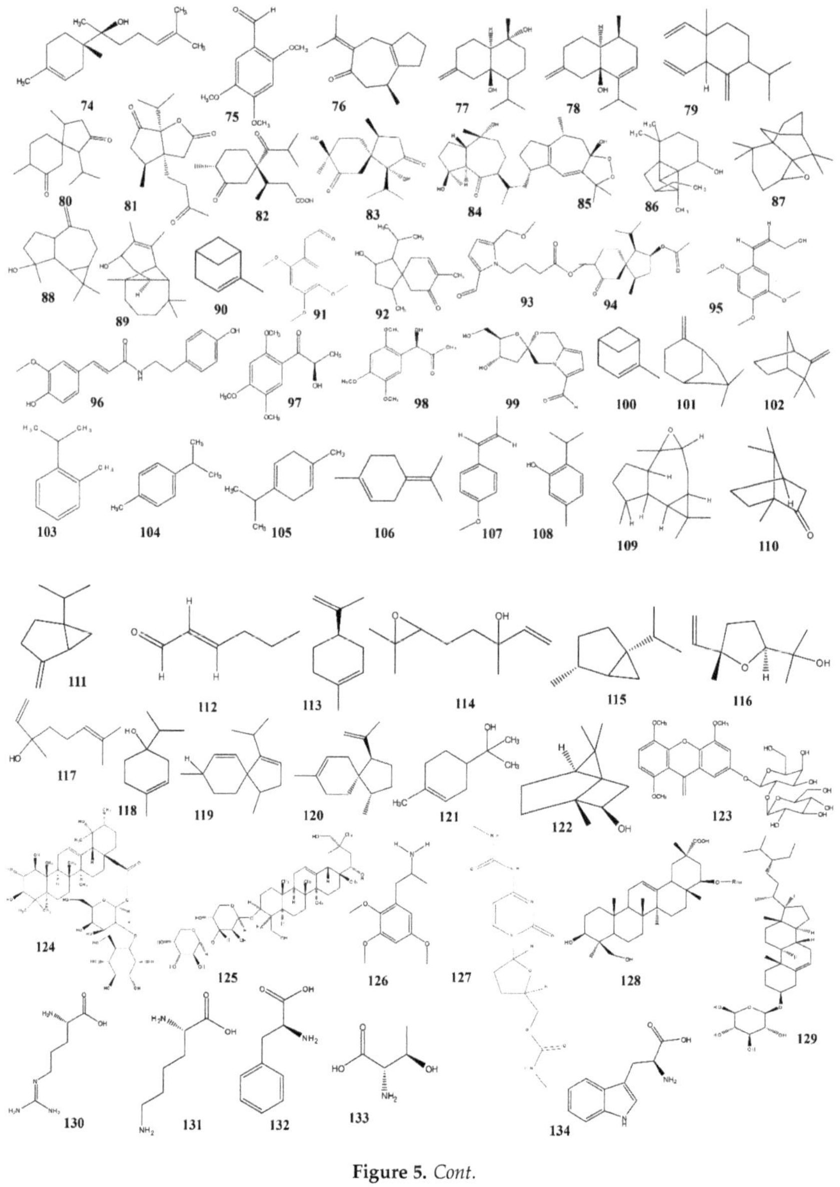

Figure 5. *Cont.*

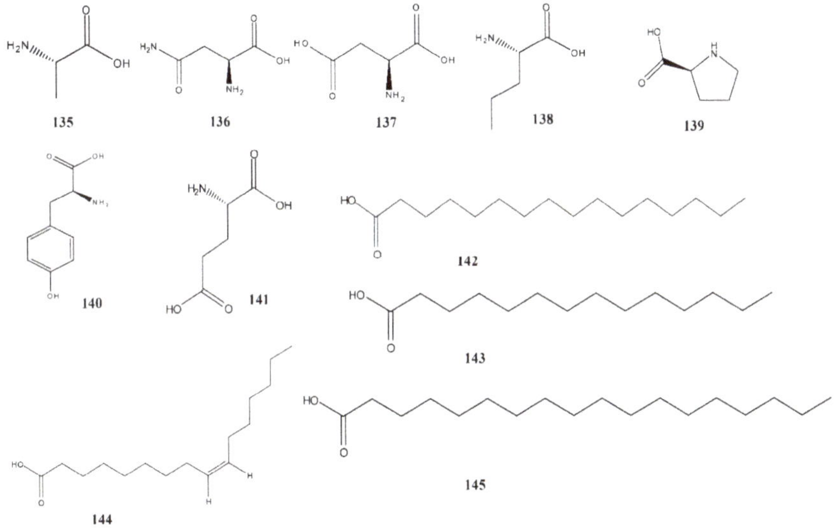

Figure 5. Chemical structures of isolated compounds from *A. calamus*.

5.1. Phenylpropanoids

Phenylpropanoids have an aromatic ring with a structurally diverse group of phenylalanine-derived secondary plant metabolites (C_6–C_3), like α-asarone, β-asarone, eugenol, isoeugenol, etc. [75]. A number of phenylpropanoids have been identified from *A. calamus* rhizome and leaves **(1-45)**. α and β-asarone isolated from the rhizome are the predominant compounds present in this plant. A series of aromatic oils from the rhizome with diverse structures are also reported [74–98].

Table 3. Chemical compounds isolated from different botanical parts of *A. calamus*.

Classification	Compound No.	Chemical Ingredient	Methods of Characterization	Parts/Extract	References
Phenylpropanoids	**1**	α-Asarone			
	2	β-Asarone	GC-FID, GC-MS	Rhizomes/n-hexane, aqueous, methanol, ethanol	[74,78,84,89–91]
	3	γ-Asarone			
	4	Eugenyl acetate			
	5	Eugenol		Rhizomes/aqueous extract	[74,78,91]
	6	Isoeugenol			
	7	Methyl eugenol		Rhizomes/n-hexane, ethyl acetate	[92]
	8	Methyl isoeugenol		Rhizomes/hexane	[74,78,91,94]
	9	Calamol	GC-MS		
	10	Azulene			
	11	Eugenol methyl ether			
	12	Dipentene			[74,78,91]
	13	Asaronaldehyde		Rhizomes/aqueous extract	
	14	Terpinolene			
	15	1,8-cineole			
	16	(*E*)-isoeugenol acetate			
	17	(*E*)-methyl isoeugenol			[89]
	18	Cis-methyl isoeugenol	GC-FID, GC-MS		
	19	Euasarone		Rhizomes/n-hexane, ethyl acetate	[92]
	20	Cinnamaldehyde			
	21	Cyclohexanone	GC-MS	Rhizomes/hexane	[94]
	22	Acorin			
	23	Isoasarone	NMR	Rhizomes/chloroform	[95]
	24	Safrole			

Table 3. *Cont.*

Classification	Compound No.	Chemical Ingredient	Methods of Characterization	Parts/Extract	References
Phenylpropanoids	24	Safrole			
	25	Z-3-(2,4,5-trimethoxyphenyl)-2-propenal	FTIR, NMR	Rhizomes/ethanol	[96]
	26	2,3-dihydro-4,5,7-trimethoxy-1-ethyl-2-methyl-3 (2,4,5-trimethoxyphenyl) indene			
	27	(Z)-asarone	GC-MS	Leaves/n-hexane	[97]
	28	(E)-caryophyllene			
	29	Estragole		Rhizomes/aqueous	[98]
	30	Carvacrol			
	31	2-cyclohexane-1-one			
	32	Naphthalene			
	33	γ-Cadinene			
	34	Aristolene			
	35	1(5),3-aromadenedradiene			
	36	5-n-butyltetraline			
	37	4,5-dehydro-isolongifolene			
	38	Calarene			
	39	Isohomogenol			
	40	Zingiberene			
	41	α-Calacorene			
	42	5,8-dimethyl isoquinoline			
	43	Cyclohexane methanol			
	44	Longifolene			
	45	Isoelemicin			

Table 3. *Cont.*

Classification	Compound No.	Chemical Ingredient	Methods of Characterization	Parts/Extract	References
Sesquiterpenoids	**46**	Calamene		Rhizomes/aqueous	[74,78,91]
	47	Calamenenol			
	48	Calameone			
	49	Preisocalamendiol			
	50	1,4-(trans)1,7(trans)-acorenone			[93]
	51	1,4-(cis)-1,7-(trans)-acorenone			
	52	2,6 diepishyobunone			
	53	α-Gurjunene			
	54	β-Gurjunene			
	55	α-Cedrene			[98]
	56	β-Elemene			
	57	β-Cedrene			[93]
	58	β-Caryophyllene			
	59	Valencene			
	60	Viridiflorene			
	61	α-Selinene	GC-FID, GC-MS		[89,93]
	62	δ-Cadinene	GC-MS		[93]
	63	α-Curcumene			
	64	Shyobunone			[84,93,99,100]
	65	Isoshyobunone			[93,99,101]
	66	Caryophyllene oxide			[93]
	67	Humulene oxide II	GC-FID, GC-MS		[89,93]
	68	Elemol	GC-MS		[93]
	69	Cedrol			
	70	Spathulenol			
	71	Acorenone			
	72	α-Cadinol			
	73	Humulene epoxide II	GC-FID, GC-MS		[89]
	74	α-Bisabolol			

Table 3. *Cont.*

Classification	Compound No.	Chemical Ingredient	Methods of Characterization	Parts/Extract	References
Sesquiterpenoids	75	Asaronaldehyde	NMR	Rhizomes/chloroform	[95]
	76	Calamusenone	GLC, IR, NMR	Rhizomes/petroleum ether	[99]
	77	Isocalamendiol			
	78	Dehydroxyiso-calamendiol			
	79	Epishyobunone			
	80	Acorone	NMR	Rhizomes/hydro alcoholic	[100]
	81	Neo-acorane A		Rhizomes/ethanol	[102]
	82	Acoric acid			
	83	Calamusin D			
	84	$1\beta,5\alpha$-Guaiane-$4\beta,10\alpha$-diol-6-one			[103]
	85	Dioxosarcoguaiacol	HPLC	Rhizomes/petroleum ether	[101]
	86	7-tetracycloundecanol,4,4,11,11-tetramethyl	GC-MS	Rhizomes/ethanol	[84]
	87	4α,7-Methano-4α-naphth[1,8a-b] oxirene,			
	88	Spathulenol		Rhizomes/aqueous	[98]
	89	Vulgarol B			
	90	Tatanan A	HPLC, NMR	Rhizomes/95% ethanol	[104]
	91	Acoramone			
	92	2-hydroxyacorenone			
	93	4-(2-formyl-5-methoxymethyl pyrrol-1-yl) butyric acid methyl ester			
	94	2-acetoxyacorenone			
	95	Acoramol			
	96	N-transferuloyl tyramine			
	97	Tatarinoid A			
	98	Tatarinoid B			
	99	Acortatarin A			

Table 3. *Cont.*

Classification	Compound No.	Chemical Ingredient	Methods of Characterization	Parts/Extract	References
Monoterpenes	**100**	α-Pinene	GC-MS	Rhizomes, roots/aqueous	[74,78,91,93]
	101	β-Pinene			
	102	Camphene			[74,78,91,93,98]
	103	o-Cymol			[98]
	104	p-Cymene	GC-FID, GC-MS		[89,93,98]
	105	γ-Terpinene	GC-MS		[98]
	106	α-Terpinolene			
	107	Anethole			
	108	Thymol			
	109	Isoaromadendrene epoxide			
	110	Camphor		Rhizome, leaves, roots/aqueous, hexane	[93,97]
	111	Sabinene		Roots/aqueous	[93]
	112	2-hexenal			
	113	Limonene			[93,98]
	114	Cis-linaloloxide			[93]
	115	Cis-sabinene hydrate			
	116	Trans-linalol oxide			
	117	Linalool			[93,97]
	118	Terpinen-4-ol			[93]
	119	α-Acoradiene			
	120	β-Acoradiene			
	121	α-Terpineol			
	122	Isoborneol		Leaves/hexane	[97]

Table 3. *Cont.*

Classification	Compound No.	Chemical Ingredient	Methods of Characterization	Parts/Extract	References
Xanthone glycosides	**123**	4,5,8-trimethoxy-xanthone-2-O-β-D-glucopyranosyl (1-2)-O-β-D-galactopyranoside	NMR	Rhizome/ethanol	[83]
Triterpenoid saponins	**124**	1β,2α,3β, 19α-Tetrahydroxyurs-12-en-28-oic acid-28-O- {(β-D-glucopyranosyl (1-2)}-β-D galactopyranoside			[82]
	125	3-β, 22-α-24,29-Tetrahydroxyolean-12-en-3-O-(β-Darabinosyl (1,3)}-β-D-arabinopyranoside			
Alkaloids	**126**	Trimethoxyamphetamine,2,3,5	GC-MS		[84]
	127	Pyrimidin-2-one,4-[N-methylureido]-1-[4methyl amino carbonloxy methy]			
Triterpene glycoside	**128**	22-[(6-deoxy-α-L-rhamnopyranosyl) oxy]-3,23-dihydroxy-, methyl ester, (3β,4β,20α,22β)	NMR	Root, Rhizomes/ethyl acetate	[85]
Steroids/Sterols	**129**	β-daucosterol			
Amino acids	**130**	Arginine	HPLC	Roots/ethanol	[86,87]
	131	Lysine			
	132	Phenylalanine			
	133	Threonine			
	134	Tryptophan			
	135	α-alanine			
	136	Asparagine			
	137	Aspartic acid			
	138	Norvaline			
	139	Proline			
	140	Tyrosine			
	141	Glutamic acid			
Fatty acids	**142**	Palmitic acid	GLC	Rhizome/petroleum ether	[88]
	143	Myristic acid			
	144	Palmitoleic acid			
	145	Stearic acid			

GC-FID, gas chromatography – flame ionization detector; GC-MS, gas chromatography – mass spectrometry; NMR, nuclear magnetic resonance; FTIR, Fourier-transform infrared spectroscopy; GLC, gas liquid chromatography; IR, infrared spectroscopy; HPLC, high-performance liquid chromatography.

5.2. Sesquiterpenoids

About 44 sesquiterpenes, including lactones, were characterized and identified in *A. calamus* rhizomes. Sesquiterpene lactones are produced of 3 isoprene units and composed of lactone rings. α–β unsaturated γ-lactonic ring in sesquiterpene lactones is believed to be responsible for pharmacological activity (46-99) [74,78,89,91,93,98–104].

5.3. Monoterpenes

Monoterpenes (C-10) are the simplest class of the terpene series that belongs to two isoprene units (tricyclic, bicyclic, monocyclic, etc.). Monoterpenes can have different functional groups, like aldehydes, ketones, esters, ethers, phenols, and alcohols [80]. These organic compounds emit the characteristic flavor and fragrance of *A. calamus* leaves and rhizomes (100-122) [74,78,89,91,93,97,98].

5.4. Triterpenoid Saponins

Triterpenoid saponins are made up of a pentacyclic C-30 terpene skeleton as a pillar. Limited reports studying triterpenoid saponins in *A. calamus* are available, and only two triterpenoid saponins (124, 125) have been isolated from *A. calamus* rhizomes (Table 3) [85].

5.5. Other Compounds

To date, one xanthone glycoside (123) [82,83], two alkaloids (126-127) [84], one triterpene glycoside (128), one steroid (129) [85], 12 amino acids (130-141) [86,87], and 4 fatty acids (142-145) [88] have been identified in *A. calamus* rhizomes [83–88].

6. Pharmacological Properties

Diverse bioactivities of *A. calamus* extracts are evident from preclinical (in vitro and in vivo) and clinical reports, such as antidiabetic, anti-obesity, antihypertensive, antioxidant, anti-inflammatory, immunomodulatory, anticonvulsant, and neuroprotective [105–173]. The summarized information on *A. calamus* botanical parts, extract type, and their bioactivities in neurological and metabolic disorders is stipulated in Table 4.

Table 4. Preclinical claims of *A. calamus* in neurological and metabolic disorders.

Action	Parts of Plant	Extract/Compound	Animal Model	Dosage	Results	References
Antidiabetic effects	Rhizomes	Methanol	STZ-induced	50, 100, and 200 mg/kg, p.o. to rats	↓ Lipid profile and blood glucose, while ↑ levels of plasma insulin, tissue glycogen, and G6PD	[105]
			Alloxan-induced	150 and 200 mg/kg, p.o. to rat	↓ Blood glucose level	[106]
		Ethyl acetate	Genetically obese diabetic C57BL/Ks db/db mice	100 mg/kg, p.o.	↓ Levels of triglycerides and serum glucose	[107]
			GLP-1 expression and secretion with STZ-induced	100 mg/kg, i.g.	↑ Secretion of GLP-1 and ↓ blood glucose levels	[108]
			In vitro HIT-T15 cell line and alpha-glucosidase enzyme	6.25, 12.5, and 25 μg/mL	↑ Insulin secretion in HIT-T15 cells	[109]
			Glucose tolerance	400 and 800 mg/kg, p.o. to mice	↓ Serum glucose, and abolished the ↑ level of blood glucose	
Anti-obesity effects		Ethanol and aqueous	HFD-induced	100 and 200 mg/kg to rats	↓ Levels of serum cholesterol and triglycerides, ↑ lipoprotein fraction	[110]
		Diethyl ether	HFD-induced	20 and 40 mg/kg, p.o. to rats	↓ Total cholesterol and low-density lipoprotein levels, ↑ plasma fibrinogen levels	[111]
		Methanol	Triton-X-100-induced hyperlipidemic	250 and 500 mg/kg to rats	Dose-dependent anti-hyperlipidemic effect	[112]
			HFD-induced	250 and 500 mg/kg, p.o. to rats	↓ Level of total cholesterol, triglycerides, and LDL, ↑ HDL cholesterol	[113]
		Aqueous	HFD-induced	100, 200, and 300 mg/kg, p.o. to rats	↓ Levels of serum glucose, leptin, and insulin along with ↓ triglyceride, low-density lipoprotein, very LDL cholesterol, total cholesterol, phospholipids, and free fatty acid increased levels	[114]
Antihypertensive effects		Ethyl acetate	Clamping the left kidney artery for 4 h	250 mg/kg, p.o. to rats	↓SBP and DBP, blood urea nitrogen, creatinine and LPO, ↑ level of nitric oxide, SOD, CAT, GPX	[115]
		Crude extract, ethyl acetate and n-hexane	Blood pressure lowering effect in normotensive	10, 30, and 50 mg/kg to anesthetized rats	Relaxant effects mediated through Ca^{+2} antagonism and NO pathways	[116]
		Ethanol and α-asarone	Dimethyl sulfoxide-induced noise stress to rats	100 and 9 mg/kg, p.o. to rats	↓ Destructive effect of stress enlightening the morphological changes of hippocampus	[117]
Anti-inflammatory effects	Leaves	Ethanol	Carrageenan-induced paw edema	100 and 200 mg/kg to rats	↓ Histamine, 5-HT, and kinins	[118]
Antioxidant effects	Rhizomes	α-asarone	Noise stress induced to rats	3, 6, and 9 mg/kg, i.p. to rats	↑ SOD and LPO, decreased ↓ CAT, GPX, GSH, vitamins C and E, and protein thiol levels	[119]
	Leaves and rhizomes	Ethyl acetate and methanol	DPPH radical scavenging chelating ferrous ions, FRAP	200, 100, 80, 60, 40, 20, 10, and 5 μg/mL	Prominent DPPH scavenging activity, chelating ferrous ions, and reducingpower	[120,121]
	Rhizomes	Ethanol	Acetaminophen-induced	250, 500 mg/kg, p.o. to rats	↓ MDA and ↑ SOD, CAT, GPX, GSH levels	[122]

Table 4. *Cont.*

Action	Parts of Plant	Extract/Compound	Animal Model	Dosage	Results	References
Anticonvulsant effects	Roots	Ethanol and β-asarone	Kainic acid-induced convulsion	35 and 20 mg/kg	↓ Epileptic seizure, neuroprotective, and regenerative ability	[123]
		Methanol	PTZ-induced convulsion	100 and 200 mg/kg, p.o. to mice	↑ Latency period and ↓ PTZ-induced seizure time	[124]
	Rhizomes	Calamus oil	MES, PTZ, and MCS model	30, 100, and 300 mg/kg, p.o. to mice	Calamus oil is found stable	[125]
		Ethanol	MES and PTZ-induced convulsion	250, 500 mg/kg, p.o. to mice	↓ Hind limb extension and tonic flexion of forelimbs	[126]
		Methanol	MES and PTZ-induced	250 and 150 mg/kg, p.o. to rats	↓ Immobility time at 250 mg/kg; however, ineffective at 150 mg/kg	[127]
Antidepressant effects			TST and FST	50 and 100 mg/kg, i.p. to mice	↓ Immobility time in a dose-dependent manner	[128]
	Leaves		TST and FST	50 and 100 mg/kg	↓ Immobility time	[129]
	Roots	Aqueous	TST and FST	100, 150, 200 mg/kg, p.o. to mice	↓ Immobility time	[130]
		Hydro-alcoholic extract	TST and FST	75 and 150 mg/kg, p.o. to mice	↓ Corticosteroid levels	[131]
	Rhizomes	Ethanol	OFB and HPM test	72 mg/kg, p.o.	No stimulation of postsynaptic 5-HT1A receptors	[132]
		Methanol and acetone	Behavioral despair test	5, 20, and 50 mg/kg, p.o.	↓ Spontaneous locomotor activity	[133]
		β-asarone	EPM and FST	25, 50, and 100 mg/kg, p.o.	↓ Immobility time	[134]
Neuroprotective effects		Hydro-alcoholic	CCI of sciatic nerve-induced neuropathic pain	10 mg/kg to rats	Significantly ameliorated CCI-induced nociceptive pain	[135]
			CCI of sciatic nerve-induced peripheral neuropathy	100 and 200 mg/kg to rats	Prevented CCI-induced neuropathy through ↓ oxidation and inflammation	[136]
	Leaves	Methanol and acetone	Apomorphine-induced stereotypy and haloperidol-induced catalepsy	20 and 50 mg/kg to mice	Reversed stereotypy induced by apomorphine and significantly potentiated catalepsy induced by haloperidol	[137]
	Rhizomes	Ethanol	Spontaneous electrical activity and monoamine levels of the brain	200 and 300 mg/ kg to rats	Depressive response by altering electrical activity, including changing brain monoamine levels	[138]
		Hydro-alcoholic	MCAo-produced brain ischemia	25 mg/kg to rats	Improvement in neurobehavioral performance, ↓ levels of GSH, SOD, and ↑ LPO level	[139]
		Ethanol	Methotrexate-induced stress	5, 10, 15, 20, 25 ppm concentration to fruit flies	↓ Elevated ROS, SOD, CAT, and GPX levels	[140]
Cardioprotective effects	Whole plant		DOX-induced myocardial toxicity	100 and 200 mg/kg to rats	↓ Serum enzyme levels and protected the myocardium from the toxic effect of DOX	[141]
	Rhizomes	Crude, n-hexane, ethyl acetate	Guinea pig tracheal segments	0.01 mg/mL	↓ Force and rate of contractions at higher concentrations	[142]

CAT, catalase; CCI, chronic constriction injury; COX, cyclooxygenase; DBP, diastolic blood pressure; DOX, doxorubicin; DPPH, 2,2-diphenyl-1-picrylhydrazyl radical; EPM, elevated plus maze; FRAP, ferric reducing antioxidant power; FST, forced swim test; GLP-1, glucagon-like peptide-1; GPX, glutathione peroxidase; GR, glutathione reductase; GSH, reduced glutathione; HDL, high-density lipoproteins; HFD, high-fat diet; HPM, high plus maze; i.g., intragastric; i.p., intraperitoneal; LDL, low-density lipoprotein; LPO, lipid peroxides; MCAo, middle cerebral artery occlusion; MCS, minimal clonic seizure; MDA, malondialdehyde; MES, maximal electroshock; NO, nitric oxide; OFB, open field behavior; p.o., per oral; PTZ, pentylenetetrazol; ROS, reactive oxygen species; SBP, systolic blood pressure; SOD, superoxide dismutase; STZ, streptozotocin; TST, tail suspension test.

6.1. Antidiabetic Effect

The antidiabetic effect of *A. calamus* ethyl acetate fraction was evaluated in streptozotocin (STZ)-induced and diabetic (db/db) mice. Glucagon-like peptide-1 (GLP-1) levels, plasma insulin, "and related gene expression were evaluated. The fraction (100 mg/kg, intragastric (i.g.)) indicated a significant reduction in blood glucose levels. For in vitro, at the concentration of 12.5 μg/mL, a significant increment in GLP-1 levels was found in the insulin-secreting L-cell culture medium [108]. The ethyl acetate radix fraction exhibited a significant effect on the HIT-T15 cell line and α-glucosidase enzyme. The ethyl acetate fraction also enhanced insulin secretion in HIT-T15 cells and blocked the α-glucosidase in vitro activity with 0.41 μg/mL of inhibitory concentration (IC_{50}) [109]."

6.2. Anti-Obesity Effect

The β-asarone compound isolated from the rhizome was investigated against high-fat diet (HFD)-induced obesity in animals. β-Asarone-treated adipose rats showed weight loss, but also inhibited metabolic transformations, as well as glucose intolerance, elevated cholesterol, and adipokine variance [143]. The in vitro investigation on the *A. calamus* aqueous extract showed lipid-lowering activity through inhibition of the pancreatic lipase percentage (28.73%) [144].

6.3. Antihypertensive Effect

The antihypertensive effects of *A. calamus* were studied on their own, in isolation, and in combination with *Gymnema sylvestre* in the HFD-induced hypertension in rats. The HFD was given for 4 weeks, which significantly increased the average systolic blood pressure (SBP). At a 200 mg/kg dose, *A. calamus* in combination with *G. sylvestre* reduced the SBP and heart rate significantly. *A. calamus* with *G. sylvestre* exhibited synergistic effect as compared with individual herbs [145].

6.4. Anti-Inflammatory and Immunomodulatory Effect

The methanolic *A. calamus* rhizome extract (12.5 μg/mL) prevented the VCAP-1 and intercellular expression on the surface of mouse myeloid leukemia cells and murine endothelial cells, respectively [146]. In an in vitro anti-inflammatory study (Red blood cell membrane stabilization method), the *A. calamus* aqueous rhizome extract at the highest concentration of 10 mg/mL showed insignificant activity against hemolysis inhibition and the RBC membrane stabilization percentage [144]. Aqueous *A. calamus* leave extract was studied on HaCaT cells and restricted the characteristics of interleukin (IL)-8, IL-6 RNA protein levels alongside interferon regulatory factor 3 (IRF3) and nuclear factor kB (NF-κB) activation [147]. N-hexane, butanolic, and aqueous fractions of *A. calamus* were evaluated against cyclooxygenase (COX) and lipoxygenase (LOX)-mediated eicosanoid production by arachidonic acid. The butanolic fraction inhibited the COX-mediated production of thromboxane B2 (TXB2) and lipoxygenase product 1 (LP1). Investigation of the underlying signaling pathways revealed that the butanolic fraction inhibited phospholipase C (PLC) pathway in platelets, presumably acting on protein kinase C (PKC) [148]. The essential oil isolated from *A. calamus* was evaluated by protein denaturation assay, where at the concentration level of 300 μg/mL, 69.56% of the inhibition level was observed [149].

6.5. Antioxidant Effect

The in vitro antioxidant activity of acetone, acetonitrile, alcoholic, and aqueous extracts of *A. calamus* rhizomes exhibited free radical scavenging activity on the [2,2′-azinobis (3-ethylbenzothiazoline-6-sulphonic acid)] free radical scavenging activity assay (ABTS), the (1, 1-diphenyl-2-picrylhydrazyl) free radical scavenging activity assay (DPPH), and the ferric ion reducing antioxidant power assay (FRAP). Strong antioxidant effect was noticed in the acetone extract, followed by acetonitrile and methanol, while in the aqueous extract, poor antioxidant activity was found [150]. The aqueous extract exhibited superior antioxidant effects in metal ion chelation, lipid peroxidation (LPO), and DPPH assays [144,151]. The in vitro antioxidant activity of ethanol, hydro-ethanol, and aqueous whole plant extracts of

A. calamus was investigated using FRAP, DPPH, nitric oxide, hydroxyl radical, reductive ability, and superoxide radical scavenging activity. The existence of phenolics and flavonoids in *A. calamus* are believed to contribute to the promising antioxidant effect. IC_{50} values of the ethanol extract were found to be 54.82, 109.85, 38.3, 118.802 μg/mL for the scavenging activities of DPPH, hydroxyl radical, superoxide radical, and nitric oxide, respectively. The irreversible potential of the above results and the FRAP values of the extracts were found to augment in a concentration-dependent manner [152]. "Ethanol and hydro-alcoholic extracts of *A. calamus* roots and rhizomes were studied for antioxidant potential against DPPH compared with butylated hydroxyanisole (BHA) and silymarin. Ethanol and hydro-alcoholic extracts showed free radical scavenging activity of 59.13 ± 18.95 and 56.71 ± 19.54, respectively [153–155]. The essential oil isolated from *A. calamus* showed strong antioxidant efficacy against the β-carotene/linoleic acid bleaching test and DPPH free radicals [156]. The methanol extract of the *A. calamus* rhizome was evaluated against the free radical scavenging activity, and the reported IC_{50} value was 704 μg/mL [157]. The IC_{50} of the essential oil was 1.68 μg/mL, which showed virtuous free radical scavenging activity in the DPPH test [149]."

6.6. Anticonvulsant Effect

The methanol extract shows anticonvulsant effects feasibly through potentiating the action of gamma-aminobutyric acid (GABA) pathway in the central nervous system [124]. When it comes to the purification of *A. calamus* rhizome in cow urine, it is advocated in the Ayurvedic pharmacopoeia of India (API) before its therapeutic use. The purified rhizome was investigated in a maximal electroshock (MES) seizure model, and phenytoin was used as the standard drug. The raw and processed rhizome (11 mg/kg, p.o.) exhibited notable anticonvulsant activity by minimizing the span of the tonic extensor period in rats, whereas the processed rhizome showed better therapeutic activity than when it was raw [158]. The calamus oil isolated from the *A. calamus* rhizome was evaluated at varying dose levels of 30, 100, and 300 mg/kg, p.o., body weight (b.w.), against MES, pentylenetetrazol (PTZ), and minimal clonic seizure (MCS) models. The calamus oil was found to be neurotoxic at 300 mg/kg, though it was effective in the MCS test at 6 Hz. The protective index value of calamus oil was found to be 4.65 [125].

6.7. Antidepressant Effect

Interaction of the methanolic *A. calamus* rhizome extract with the adrenergic, dopaminergic, serotonergic, and GABAergic system was found responsible for the expression of antidepressant activity [128]. In another study, the methanolic *A. calamus* leave extract showed significant activity through a reduction in the immobility period in the TST and FST [129]. Through interaction with the adrenergic and dopaminergic system, the hydro-alcoholic extract was normalized to the over-activity of the hypothalamic pituitary adrenal (HPA) axis [131]. Sobers capsules (a herbo-mineral formulation containing *A. calamus*) were evaluated by tail suspension and forced swimming tests in mice. At the oral dose of 50 mg/kg for 14 days, capsules exhibited insignificant impact on locomotor activity, and caused antidepressant effects in experimental animals [159]. Tensarin (the traditional medicine of Nepal containing *A. calamus*) was evaluated for the anxiolytic effect in mice using the open field test (OFT), activity monitoring along with the passive avoidance test. At all three dose levels (50, 100, 200 mg/kg), Tensarin produced an anxiolytic effect in a dose-dependent way by an improvement in rearing, number of passages, and duration of the period employed by mice [160].

6.8. Neuroprotective Effect

The ethanolic extract was studied (25, 50, and 100 mg/kg doses, oral and intraperitoneal routes) for learning and memory-enhancing activity. The subjects used consisted of male rates, through Y maze and shuttle box tests models. The findings showed an increase in acquisition–recalling and spatial recognition data [161]. The ethanolic *A. calamus* rhizome extract (0.5 mL/kg, i.p.) potentiated pentobarbitone-created sleep periods, which caused significant inhibition of conditioned avoidance response in rats and marked (40–60%) protection against PTZ-induced convulsions, although it did not show any spontaneous motor activity and impact the aggressive or fighting behavior response in male rat pairs [162].

6.9. Cardioprotective Effect

The alcoholic *A. calamus* rhizome extract (100 and 200 mg/kg) considerably attenuated isoproterenol-led cardiomyopathy in rats and showed a significant reduction in the heart/body weight ratio, level of serum calcineurin, serum nitric oxide, serum lactate dehydrogenase (LDH), and thiobarbituric acid reactive substances (TBARS) level. However, the level of the antioxidant enzyme was found increased at the 100 mg/kg extract dose level [163]. The crude extract and its fractions (0.01–10 mg/mL) were investigated in an isolated rabbit heart, which showed mild reduction in the force of forced vital capacity (FVC), hazard ratio (HR), and cystic fibrosis (CF), while the ethyl acetate extract exhibited complete suppression, and the n-hexane fraction showed the same effect on FVC and HR, but enhanced CF. The extract and its fractions exhibited controlled coronary vasodilator effect, interceded maybe by an endothelial-derived hyperpolarizing factor [164]. The cardioprotective potential of the whole plant's ethanolic extract (100 and 200 mg/kg) reduced serum enzyme levels and shielded the myocardium from the lethal effect of DOX [141].

6.10. Cytochrome Inhibitory Activities

Cytochromes P450 (CYPs) are the prime enzymes that catalyze the oxidative metabolism of a wide variety of xenobiotics. It is known that 2,4,5-trimethoxycinnamic acid is the main metabolite of α- or β- asarone [165]. The metabolism rate of α- and β-asarone was shown to be directly proportional to the CYPs concentration in rat hepatocytes and liver microsomes [166,167]. CYP3A4 (CYP isoforms) has been reported for bioactivation of α-asarone [168]. The hydro-alcoholic *A. calamus* extract and α-asarone were evaluated by the CYPs-carbon monoxide complex method. The extract exhibited moderate potential interaction in CYP3A4 (IC_{50} = 46.84 μg/mL) and CYP2D6 (IC_{50} = 36.81 μg/mL), while α-asarone showed higher interaction in CYP3A4 (IC_{50} = 65.16 μg/mL) and CYP2D6 (IC_{50} = 55.17 μg/mL) [169]. These outcomes indicated that both extracts and α-asarone interacted quite well in drug metabolism and also had an inhibitory effect on CYP3A4 and CYP2D6. The drug-drug interaction effect of the *A. calamus* extract and its main chemical constituent (α and β-asarone) needs to be studied in more CYPs isomers, like CYP2C9 and CYP2E1.

6.11. Toxicity and Safety Concerns

In acute and sub-acute toxicity of the hydro-alcoholic extract of *A. calamus* in rats, at the highest dose level of 10 gm/kg, no severe changes were observed, and the lethal dose (LD_{50}) was found to be 5 g/kg [170]. The petroleum ether extracts (obtained by cold rolling, water distillation, and Soxhlet extraction methods) of the *A. calamus* rhizome showed mild toxicity in two-day-old oriental fruit flies [171]. The ethanolic extract of the *A. calamus* rhizome at oral dosage of 175, 550, 1750, and 5000 mg/kg b.w. was given for 14 days within an acute toxicity study, while at the dose level of 0, 200, 400, and 600 mg/kg, p.o., the extract was given for 90 days within a chronic toxicity study. At the doses of 1750 and 5000 mg/kg, piloerection, tremors, and abdominal breathing were found for 30 min [172]. In that study, *A. calamus* was purified for 3 h in cow urine, decoction of *Sphaeranthus indicus*, and decoction of leaves of *Mangifera indica*, *Eugenia jambolana*, *Feronia limonia*, *Citrus medica*, and *Aegle marmelos*, followed by fomentation with Gandhodaka (decoction of six aromatic herbs) for 1 h. The acute oral toxicity test of raw and purified *A. calamus* was performed in albino rats at 2000 mg/kg for 2 weeks. At the 2000 mg/kg dose, *A. calamus* did not produce any toxic symptoms within 14 days [173].

The β-asarone compound isolated from *A. calamus* was found to be carcinogenic and toxic [174]. The LD_{50} value of β-asarone by oral and intraperitoneal route was found to be 1010 and 184 mg/kg, respectively, in mice and rats [175]. The LD_{50} of calamus oil was found to be 8.88 gm/kg b.w. [176], while in the calamus oil obtained from Jammu, India, the LD_{50} was 777 mg/kg b.w. [177]. Overall, several investigations have been carried out on *A. calamus* regarding its toxicity; however, no noticeable data on toxicity have been found so far.

7. Clinical Reports

A. calamus has also been clinically investigated as a monotherapy as well as in combination with other medicinal herbs in healthy subjects and sufferers of various metabolic and neurological ailments. Most clinical research has looked at the *A. calamus* effect on obesity, depression, neuroprotection, and cardiovascular disease [178–191]. The data obtained so far can be found in Table 5. Furthermore, a systematic review reveals that *A. calamus* (alone or in combination therapy) exhibits anti-obesity, antidepressant, and cardioprotective effects, as well as helps physical and mental performance.

Table 5. Clinical claims of *A. calamus* in neurological and metabolic disorders.

Formulations/Dosage forms *A. calamus*	Subjects	Study Design	Intervention	Primary Endpoint	Outcome	Evidence Quality	Reference
A. calamus rhizome powder	24 patients of both sexes with hyperlipidemia	Randomized single-blind controlled study	500 mg twice daily after meal for 1 month	BMI, body perimeter, skinfold depth	Significant reduction in skinfold depth, fatigue, and excessive hunger	III	[178]
Davaie Loban capsules (*A. calamus*, nut grass, incense, ginger, and black pepper)	24 patients of both sexes with Alzheimer's disease	Double-blind randomized clinical study	500 mg capsule thrice daily for 3 months	ADAS-cog and CDR-SOB scores	At 4 weeks and 12 weeks: significant reduction in the ADAS-cog and CDR-SOB scores	III	[179]
70% hydro-alcoholic extract of *A. calamus*	33 patients of both sexes (20 male and 13 female) with anxiety disorder	Non-randomized, open-label, single-arm study	500 mg extract of one capsule twice daily after meal for 2 months	BPRS score	Significant reduction of anxiety and stress-related disorder	III	[180]
Vachadi Churna (*A. calamus*, *Cyperus rotundus*, *Cedrus deodara*, ginger, *Aconitum Heterophyllum*, *T. chebula*)	30 obese patients of both sexes aged 14–50 years	Non-randomized, open-label, single-arm study	3 g powder twice daily with lukewarm water before meal for 1 month	BMI, girth measurements of mid-thigh, abdomen, hip, chest	Significant improvement in extreme sleep, body heaviness, fatigue, and excessive hunger	III	[181]
Guduchyadi Medhya Rasayana, (*A. calamus*, *Tinospora cordifolia*, *Achyranthes aspera*, *Embelia ribes*, *Convolvulus pluricaulis*, *T. chebula*, *S. lappa*, *Asparagus racemosus*, cow ghee, and sugar)	138 patients of both sexes aged 55–75 years with senile memory impairment	Randomized, two-parallel-group study	3 g granule thrice daily after meal for 3 months	Mini–Mental State Examination, BPRS score, and estimation of serum acetylcholinesterase	Significant improvement in terms of recall memory, cognitive impairment, amnesia, concentration ability, depression, and stress	III	[182]
Dried aqueous extract of *A. calamus*	40 healthy volunteers, both sexes aged 18–50 years with a premedicant for anesthesia	Open-label randomized, two- parallel-group study	90 min before anesthesia; In the control group: 0.2 mg intramuscular (IM) glycopyrrolate and a 0.2 mg IM 50 mg tablet of promethazine hydrochloride with water; In the second group: 0.2 mg IM glycopyrrolate and 100 mg *A. calamus* extract	Pulse rate, blood pressure, respiratory rate, body temperature	The dried aqueous extract exhibited anti-hyperthermic and sedative effect without producing any respiratory depression	III	[183]
Shankhapushpyadi Ghana Vati (*A. calamus*, *C. pluricaulis*, *Bacopa monnieri*, *T. cordifolia*, *C. fistula*, *A. indica*, *S. lappa*, *Tribulus terrestris*)	20 hypertensive patients of both sexes	Randomized single-blind controlled study	1 g twice daily after meal for 2 months	SBP and DBP	Significant relief in raised SBP and DBP	III	[184]
Brahmyadiyoga (*A. calamus*, *Centella asiatica*, *Rauvolfia serpentina*, *Saussurea lappa*, *Nardostachys jatamansi*)	10 schizophrenia patients of both sexes aged 18–40 years	Non-randomized, open-label, single-arm study	4 tablets thrice daily for three months after meal	Symptoms rating scale	Significant effect as a brain tonic, tranquillizer, hypnotic, and sedative	III	[185]
Bala compound (*A. calamus*, *Emblica officinalis*, *E. ribes*, *T. cordifolia*, *Piper longum*, *Glycyrrhiza glabra*, *C. rotundus*, *A. heterophyllum*)	24 neonates, both sexes, 2.5–3 kg body weight	Randomized single-blind controlled study	5 oral drops twice daily for 6 months	Change in serum immunoglobulins (IgG, IgM, and IgA) levels	Significant improvement in immunoglobulin levels after 6 months	Ib	[186]
Vachadi Ghrita (*A. calamus*, *T. cordifolia*, *Hedychium spicatum*, *C. pluricaulis*, *E. ribes*, ginger, *A. aspera*, *T. chebula*, and cow ghee)	90 healthy individuals of both sexes aged 40–50 years for assessment of cognition	Non-randomized positive-controlled study	10 g twice daily for 1 month with lukewarm water	Post Graduate Institute Memory Scale (PGIMS) test	Significant change in the mental balance score, holding of like and different pairs, late-immediate memory, and also improved digestion	III	[187]

Table 5. *Cont.*

Formulations/Dosage forms *A. calamus*	Subjects	Study Design	Intervention	Primary Endpoint	Outcome	Evidence Quality	Reference
Bramhi Vati (*A. calamus*, *B. monnieri*, *C. pluricaulis*, *Onosma bracteatum*, copper pyrite, iron pyrite, mercuric sulphide, *Piper nigrum*, *N. jatamansi*)	68 essential hypertension patients of both sexes aged 20–70 years	Randomized, double-blind, parallel-group comparative study	500 mg tablets twice daily for 1 month	Hamilton anxiety rating scale, SBP and DBP, and MAP	Significant improvement in the Hamilton anxiety rating scale, SBP and DBP, and MAP	III	[188]
Tagaradi Yoga (*A. calamus*, *Valeriana wallichii*, *N. jatamansi*)	24 insomnia patients of both sexes aged 18–75 years	Non-randomized positive-controlled study	500 mg hydro-alcoholic extract capsule twice daily after meal for 15 days	Sleep duration, initiating time of sleep, quality of sleep	Significant improvement in sleep duration, in the initiating time of sleep, and in quality of sleep	III	[189]
Acorus calamus rhizome powder	20 obese patients of both sexes	Randomized single-blind study	250 mg rhizome powder twice daily for 1 month	Body weight, height according to age, waist-hip ratio, and BMI	Significant improvement in extreme sleep, body heaviness, fatigue, and excessive hunger	III	[190]
Acorus calamus rhizome powder	45 ischemic heart disease patients	Non-randomized positive-controlled study	3 gm rhizome powder twice daily for 3 months	ECG, serum cholesterol level	Improvement of chest pain, dyspnea on effort, reduction of the body mass index, improved ECG: reduced serum cholesterol, reduced serum LDL, and increased serum HDL	Ib	[191]

ADAS-cog, alzheimer's disease assessment scale–cognitive subscale; BMI, body mass index; BPRS, brief psychiatric rating scale; CDR-SOB, clinical dementia rating scale sum of boxes; DBP, diastolic blood pressure; ECG, electrocardiogram; Ib, evidence from at least one randomized study with control; HDL, high-density lipoprotein; Ig, immunoglobulin; III, evidence from well-performed nonexperimental descriptive studies, as well as from comparative studies, correlation studies, and case studies; LDL, low-density lipoprotein; MAP, mean arterial pressure; SBP, systolic blood pressure.

8. Mechanistic Role

The proposed mechanism of action of *A. calamus* in neurological and metabolic disorders includes a synergic integration of antioxidant defense, GABAergic transmission, brain stress hormones modulation, pro-inflammatory cytokines, leptin and resistin levels, adipocytes inhibition, calcium channel blocker effect, protein synthesis, oxidative stress, acetylcholinesterase (AChE) inhibition, and anti-dopaminergic properties. A compendium of mechanisms of action of *A. calamus* in neurological and metabolic protection is illustrated in Figure 6 and Table 6. *A. calamus* significantly affects fasting blood sugar, insulin resistance, HbA1c, and the adipogenic transcription expression factor through various mechanisms, viz. antioxidant, anti-inflammatory, β-cells regeneration, improving insulin sensitivity, gluconeogenesis, nicotinamide adenine dinucleotide phosphate (NADPH) oxidase, and glucose transporter type 4 (GLUT-4)-mediated transport inhibition.

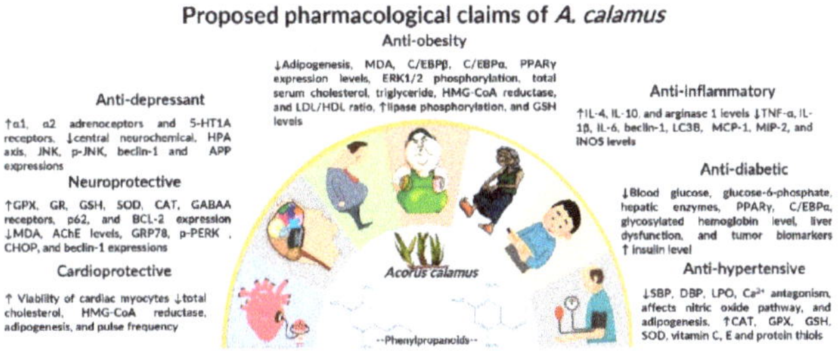

Figure 6. Illustration of role of *A. calamus* mechanisms in the treatment of neurological and metabolic disorders. AChE, acetylcholinesterase; APP, amyloid precursor protein; Bcl-2, B-cell lymphoma 2; CHOP, C/EBP homologous protein; CCAAT (cytosine-cytosine-adenosine-adenosine-thymidine)-enhancer-binding protein homologous protein; C/EBP, CCAAT enhancer-binding protein; GABAA, γ-Aminobutyric acid type A; GRP78, 78-kDa glucose-regulated protein; HMG-CoA, 3-hydroxy-3-methylglutaryl coenzyme A; iNOS, inducible nitric oxide synthase; JNK, c-Jun NH2-terminal kinase; LC3b, microtubule-associated proteins 1A/1B light chain 3B; MCP, modified citrus pectin; MDA, malondialdehyde; MIP, macrophage inflammatory protein; p-PERK, phospho-protein kinase RNA-like ER kinase; PPARγ, peroxisome proliferator-activated receptor gamma; ERK1/2, extracellular signal-regulated protein kinase.

Table 6. Mechanistic role of phytochemicals of *A. calamus* in the treatment of neurological and metabolic disorders.

Study	Compound	Model	Increased Level	Decreased Level	References
Anti-Parkinson	β-Asarone	6-OHDA parkinsonian	Bcl-2 expression	GRP78, p-PERK, CHOP, and Beclin-1 expression	[192]
		6-OHDA parkinsonian	-	mRNA levels of GRP78 and CHOP and p-IRE1and XBP1	[193]
		Dopamine in the striatum	TH plasma concentrations	Striatal COMT levels	[194]
		6-OHDA parkinsonian	L-DOPA, DA, DOPAC, and HVA levels	P-gp, ZO-1, occludin, actin, and claudin-5	[195]
Alzheimer's		Aβ25-35-induced inflammation	Bcl-2 level	TNF-α, IL-1β, IL-6, Beclin-1, and LC3B level	[196]
		NG108 cells	-	Upregulated SYP and GluR1 expression	[197]
		PC12 cells	-	Aβ-induced JNK activation, Bcl-w and Bcl-xL levels, cytochrome c release, and caspase-3 activation	[198]
		Aβ-induced cytotoxicity	Cell viability, p-Akt and p-mTOR	NSE levels, Beclin-1 expression	[199]
Neuroprotective		Pb-induced impairments	NR2B protein expression along with Arc/Arg3.1 and Wnt7a mRNA levels	-	[200]
	β-Asarone, eugenol	Scopolamine-induced	Improvement of neuron organelles and synaptic structure	APP expression	[201]
	Neotatarine	MTT reduction assay	-	Aβ25-35–induced PC12 cell death	[202]
	β-asarone, paeonol	MCAo model	Cholecystokinin and NF-κB signaling	TNF-α, IL-1β, IL-6 production	[203]

Table 6. *Cont.*

Study	Compound	Model	Increased Level	Decreased Level	References
Neuroprotective	β-Asarone	Cultured rat astrocytes	NGF, BDNF, and GDNF expression	-	[204]
		SN4741 cells	p62, Bcl-2 expression	JNK, p-JNK and Beclin-1 expressions	[205]
	Tatarinolactone	hSERT-HEK293 cell line	-	SERTs activity	[206]
	β-Asarone	RSC96 Schwann cells	GDNF, BDNF, and CNTF expression	-	[207]
		Aβ-induced	p-mTOR and p62 expression	AChE and $A\beta_{42}$ levels, p-Akt, Beclin-1, and LC3B expression, APP mRNA and Beclin-1 mRNA levels	[208]
		Aβ1–42-induced injury	-	GFAP, AQP_4, IL-1β, and TNF-α expression	[209]
Anti-depression		Chronic unpredictable mild stress	BDNF expression	Blocked ERK1/2-CREB signaling	[210]
	α-Asarone	Noradrenergic and serotonergic neuromodulators in TST	α_1 and α_2 adrenoceptors and 5-HT_{1A} receptors	-	[211]
Anticonvulsant and sedative	Eudesmin	MES and PTZ	GABA contents, expressions of GAD65, GABAA, and Bcl-2	Glu contents and ratio of Glu/GABA, caspase-3	[212]
Anti-anxiety	α-Asarone	BLA or CFA-induced	Down-regulation of $GABA_A$ receptors	Up-regulation of GluR1-containing AMPA, NMDA receptors	[213]
Anti-epilepsy		Temporal lobe epilepsy	Levels of GABA, GAD67, and GABAAR-mRNA expression	GABA-T	[214]
		Mitral cells	Down-regulation of $GABA_A$ receptors	Na^+ channel blockade	[215]
	β-Asarone	KA-induced	GABA	Glu	[216]

Table 6. *Cont.*

Study	Compound	Model	Increased Level	Decreased Level	References
Anti-inflammatory	α-Asarone	Spinal cord injury	IL-4, IL-10, and arginase 1 levels	TNF-α, IL-1β, IL-6, MCP-1, MIP-2, iNOS levels	[217]
Cytoprotective	β-Asarone	tBHP-induced astrocyte injury	GST, GCLM, GCLC, NQO1, Akt phosphorylation	-	[218]
Cardioprotective		Cultured neonate rat cardiac myocytes	Viability of cardiac myocytes	Pulse frequency	[219]
Arteriosclerosis		ECV304 cell strain	Apoptotic rate of ECV304 cells	Apoptotic rate of MMP, stabilized MMP and VSMC proliferation	[220]
Anti-adipogenic		3T3-L1 preadipocytes	-	C/EBPβ, C/EBPα, and PPARγ expression levels, ERK1/2 phosphorylation	[89]
Antioxidant		Cerebral artery occlusion	Antioxidant activity	Focal cerebral ischemic/ reperfusion injury	[221]
Anti-diabetic	α-Asarone + β-asarone + metformin HCl	STZ-induced	Insulin level	Glucose, glycosylated hemoglobin level, liver dysfunction, and tumor biomarkers	[222]
	Asarone	3T3-L1 preadipocytes	Hormone-sensitive lipase phosphorylation	Intracellular triglyceride levels, down-regulation of PPARγ and C/EBPα	[223]

6-OHDA, 6-hydroxydopamine; Ox-LDL, oxidized low-density lipoprotein; BDNF, brain-derived neurotrophic factor; NGF, nerve growth factor; GDNF, glial derived neurotrophic factor; SERTs, serotonin transporters; MCAo, middle cerebral artery occlusion; Aβ, β-amyloid; NSE, neuron specific enolase; AMPA, α-amino-3-hydroxy-5-methyl-4-isoxazolepropionic acid; NMDA, NR2A-containing N-methyl-D-aspartate; $GABA_A$, γ-aminobutyric acid A; BLA, basolateral amygdala; CFA, complete Freund's adjuvant; CNTF, ciliary neurotrophic factor; COMT, catechol-O-methyltransferase; TH, tyrosine hydroxylase; DA, dopamine; DOPAC, 3,4-dihydroxyphenylacetic acid; HVA, homovanillic acid; P-gp, P-glycoprotein; ZO-1, zonula occludens-1; SYP, synaptophysin; GluR1, glutamatergic receptor 1; GABA-T, GABA transaminase; TST, tail suspension test; KA, kainic acid; MCP-1, monocyte chemoattractant protein 1; MIP-2, macrophage inflammatory protein 2; iNOS, inducible nitric oxide synthase; GST, glutathione S-transferase; GCLM, glutamate-cysteine ligase modulatory subunit; GCLC, glutamate-cysteine ligase catalytic subunit; NQO1, NAD(P)H quinone oxidoreductase; GFAP, glial fibrillary acidic protein; AQP, aquaporin; VSMC, vascular smooth muscle cells; MMP, mitochondrial membrane potential; C/EBP, CCAAT enhancer-binding protein; PPARγ, peroxisome proliferator-activated receptor gamma; ERK1/2, extracellular signal-regulated protein kinase; XBP1, x-box binding protein; IRE1, inositol-requiring enzyme 1; Aβ1-42, amyloid β peptide; mTOR, mammalian target of rapamycin; MTT, 3-(4,5-dimethythiazol-. 2-yl)-2,5-diphenyl tetrazolium bromide; CREB, cAMP response element-binding protein; GABAAR, gamma-aminobutyric acid type-A receptor, tBHP, t-butyl hydroperoxide.

The antihypertensive effect of *A. calamus* may be explained by Ca^{2+} antagonists that affect the nitric oxide pathway. The chemical constituents of *A. calamus* upregulate the antioxidant effect, suppress pro-inflammatory cytokines, and act as detoxifying enzymes through the NF-κB and nuclear factor erythroid 2-related factor 2 (Nrf2) signaling pathways. The Nrf2 pathway may be activated by phenylpropanoids, sesquiterpenoids, and monoterpenes by interaction of active phytoconstituents with nitric oxide derivatives react with thiol groups between KEAP1 and Nrf2, along with Nrf2 phosphorylation. "When Nrf2 is released from the Kelch-like erythroid-derived CNC (cap'n'collar) homology protein (ECH)-associated protein 1 (KEAP1), it transfers into the nucleus, where it induces the genes encoding protein expression impenetrable in glutathione (GSH) synthesis, antioxidant, and detoxifying phase 2 enzymes. Oxidative stress and ligands for tumor necrosis factor receptors (TNFRs) and toll-like receptors (TLRs) activate upstream Ik-B kinases (IKKs), ensuing phosphorylation of IkB that is generally bound to the inactive NF-kB dimer in the cytoplasm. After that, IkB is targeted for proteasomal degradation and NF-kB, then it moves into the nucleus where it induces inflammatory cytokine expression in addition to the genes encoding proteins like superoxide dismutase (SOD) 2 and B cell chronic lymphocytic leukemia (CLL)/lymphoma 2 (Bcl2) involved in adaptive stress response (Figure 7). The bioactive molecules of *A. calamus* can inhibit NF-kB in inflammatory immune cells, while other phytoconstituents may activate NF-kB in neuronal cells to improve stress resistance." *A. calamus* phytoconstituents regulate NF-kB, LOX, and COX-2 activity. These compounds dose-dependently suppress the production of inflammatory factors like NO, TNF-α, IL-6, IL-1β, and JNK signaling, acting as anti-inflammatory agents. In addition, it was also noted that the inflammation induced by various chemicals was inhibited by bioactive constituents through suppression of IkB/NF-kB and JNK/AP-1 signaling pathways. Thus, over several studies, it has been reported that asarone compounds have a potential against neurodegenerative diseases.

PPAR gene and C/EBP are involved in the differentiation process. PPAR-δ and PPAR-γ promote adipogenesis. In the same way, amino acids and glucose react with C/EBP- δ and C/EBP-β. If low levels of glucose induce gadd153, the inactive dimer is formed, with C/EBP-β inhibiting the progress of adipocyte development. C/EBP delta activates C/EBP-α. This is mainly involved in the formation of mature adipocytes and lipid accumulation in adipose tissue. In 3T3-L1 preadipocytes, α-asarone and β-asarone inhibited adipocyte differentiation and reduced the intracellular lipid accumulation, and also decreased the expression levels of adipogenic transcription factors (PPARγ and C/EBPα). These phytochemicals significantly promoted adenosine monophosphate-activated protein kinase (AMPK), which is known to suppress adipogenesis. It was also found that pretreatment with α-asarone and β-asarone, a typical inhibitor of AMPK, attenuated the inhibitory effect of asarone on AMPK phosphorylation. The asarone-induced AMPK activation leads to a decrease in adipogenic transcription factor expression, and suppresses adipogenesis.

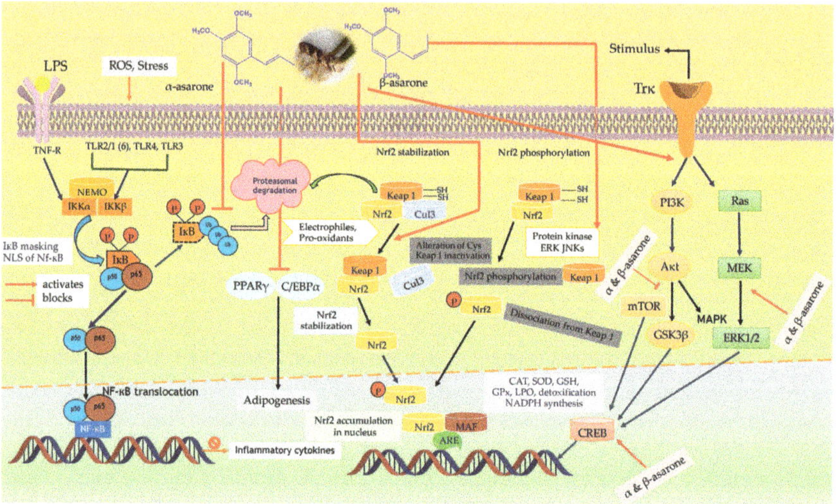

Figure 7. The role of the Nrf-2, NF-κB, PI3K/AKT, Ras/MAPK, and PPARγ signaling pathways as affected by phytoconstituents of *Acorus calamus* to upregulate antioxidant, neuroprotective, detoxifying enzymes and suppress inflammation. Ub, ubiquitin; NEMO, NF-kB essential modulator; ARE, antioxidant response element; Maf, musculoaponeurotic fibrosarcoma oncogene homolog; NLS, nuclear localization signal; CAT, catalase; GPX, glutathione peroxidase; Trk, tyrosine kinase receptor; LPS, lipopolysaccharide; TLRs, toll-like receptors; PI3K, phosphatidylinsoitol-3-kinase; MAPK, mitogen-activated protein kinase; mTOR, mammalian target of rapamycin; ERK, extracellular signal-regulated kinases; Nrf2, nuclear factor e2-related factor 2; Keap-1, kelch-like ECH-associated protein-1; MEK, mitogen-activated protein kinase; JNK, c-Jun N-terminal kinase;NADPH, nicotinamide adenine dinucleotide phosphate; NF-κB, nuclear factor-kappa B; IkB, inhibitor of kB; IKK, inhibitor of kB kinases.

9. Perspectives and Future Directions

The present review provides a plethora of information apropos ethnomedicinal uses, marketed formulations, geographical distribution, chemical constituents, pharmacological activities of crude, n-hexane, ethyl acetate, methanolic, ethanolic, hydro-alcoholic, aqueous extracts along with pure compounds, and clinical trials related to *A. calamus*.

Investigations on extracts and compounds of *A. calamus* suggested antidiabetic, anti-obesity, antihypertensive, anti-inflammatory, antioxidant, anticonvulsant, antidepressant, neuroprotective, and cardioprotective potentials with distinct underlying signaling pathways. The biological potential and mechanisms of action of some of the chemical constituents (α-asarone, β-asarone, eugenol) are known. However, other compounds need to be scientifically explored for their bioactivities and molecular modes of action, which could provide a lead for further development into therapeutics. More systematic, well-designed, and multi-center clinical studies are warranted to evaluate standardized extracts of *A. calamus* therapeutically and to identify the pharmacokinetic-dynamic roles of pharmacologically active biomolecules. There is scarce data from experimental and clinical reports on hypertension, diabetes, and atherosclerosis, and less supporting evidence is available on the use of *A. calamus* to treat hypertension and diabetes. Based on the available data, it is suggested that this plant could be used as an adjuvant to the established targeted drugs for neurological and metabolic disorders.

In 1974, United States food & drug administration (USFDA) banned *A. calamus* due to its carcinogenic effects following animal studies. They reported β-asarone as a carcinogenic agent, but the study was conducted on the calamus oil which consists of β-asarone in about 80%, while its different genotype in Europe and India contains β-asarone in lower concentrations. *A. calamus* cultivated in various geographical regions may have different chemical compositions along with therapeutic properties challenging quality control, toxicity, and safety concerns of *A. calamus*. In addition, the heavy metal, mycotoxin, and pesticide concentrations are required to be addressed in all toxicity studies.

10. Conclusions

Compelling in vitro, in vivo and clinical evidence suggests that the potential role of *A. calamus* rhizomes for modulating metabolic and neurological disorders could be due to their richness in several classes of active phytoconstituents. The predominant compounds present in rhizomes and leaves responsible for expression of potent bioactivities include α-asarone, β-asarone, eugenol, and calamine. The present report is expected to fill the gaps in the existing knowledge and could provide a lead for researchers working in the areas of phytomedicine, ethnopharmacology, and clinical research.

Author Contributions: R.S. and V.S. conceived the idea and wrote the manuscript. D.S.G., K.K., E.N., and N.M. edited and proofread the document. The entire team approved the submission of the final manuscript. All authors have read and agreed to the published version of the manuscript.

Funding: This paper was supported by the UHK Excellence project.

Acknowledgments: The authors express their sincere gratitude to Bharat Ratna Mahamana Pandit Madan Mohan Malviya, the founder of the Banaras Hindu University, Varanasi, for his services to humanity, great vision, and blessings. This work was also supported by University of Hradec Kralove (Faculty of Science, VT2019-2021) [KK, EN].

Conflicts of Interest: The authors declare no conflict of interest.

References

1. World Health Report. Available online: https://www.who.int/whr/2001/media_centre/press_release/en/ (accessed on 4 October 2019).
2. Toniolo, A.; Cassani, G.; Puggioni, A.; Rossi, A.; Colombo, A.; Onodera, T.; Ferrannini, E. The diabetes pandemic and associated infections: Suggestions for clinical microbiology. *Rev. Med. Microbiol.* **2019**, *30*, 1–17. [CrossRef]
3. Younossi, Z.M. Non-alcoholic fatty liver disease-A global public health perspective. *J. Hepatol.* **2019**, *70*, 531–544. [CrossRef]
4. Després, J.P. Is visceral obesity the cause of the metabolic syndrome. *Ann. Med.* **2006**, *38*, 52–63. [CrossRef]
5. Farooqui, A.A.; Farooqui, T.; Panza, F.; Frisardi, V. Metabolic syndrome as a risk factor for neurological disorders. *Cell. Mol. Life Sci.* **2012**, *69*, 741–762. [CrossRef]
6. Tilg, H.; Hotamisligil, G.S. Nonalcoholic fatty liver disease: Cytokine-adipokine interplay and regulation of insulin resistance. *Gastroenterology* **2006**, *131*, 934–945. [CrossRef] [PubMed]
7. Suzanne, M.; Tong, M. Brain metabolic dysfunction at the core of Alzheimer's disease. *Biochem. Pharmacol.* **2014**, *88*, 548–559.
8. Quraishi, A.; Mehar, S.; Sahu, D.; Jadhav, S.K. In vitro mid-term conservation of *Acorus calamus* L. via cold storage of encapsulated microrhizome. *Braz. Arch. Biol. Technol.* **2017**, *60*, 1–9. [CrossRef]
9. Balakumbahan, R.; Rajamani, K.; Kumanan, K. *Acorus calamus*: An overview. *J. Med. Plant Res.* **2010**, *4*, 2740–2745.
10. Sharma, V.; Singh, I.; Chaudhary, P. *Acorus calamus* (The Healing Plant): A review on its medicinal potential, micropropagation and conservation. *Nat. Prod. Res.* **2014**, *28*, 1454–1466. [CrossRef]
11. Singh, R.; Sharma, P.K.; Malviya, R. Pharmacological properties and ayurvedic value of Indian buch plant (*Acorus calamus*): A short review. *Adv. Biol. Res.* **2011**, *5*, 145–154.
12. Global Biodiversity Information Facility. Available online: https://www.gbif.org/ (accessed on 10 February 2020).
13. Kingston, C.; Jeeva, S.; Jeeva, G.M.; Kiruba, S.; Mishra, B.P.; Kannan, D. Indigenous knowledge of using medicinal plants in treating skin diseases in Kanyakumari district, Southern India. *Indian J. Tradit. Knowl.* **2009**, *8*, 196–200.
14. Pradhan, B.K.; Badola, H.K. Ethnomedicinal plant use by Lepcha tribe of Dzongu valley, bordering Khangchendzonga Biosphere Reserve, in north Sikkim India. *J. Ethnobiol. Ethnomed.* **2008**, *4*, 1–18. [CrossRef] [PubMed]
15. Sharma, P.K.; Chauhan, N.S.; Lal, B. Observations on the traditional phytotherapy among the inhabitants of Parvati valley in western Himalaya, India. *J. Ethnopharmacol.* **2004**, *92*, 167–176. [CrossRef] [PubMed]

16. Dwivedi, S.N.; Dwivedi, S.; Patel, P.C. Medicinal plants used by the tribal and rural people of Satna district, Madhya Pradesh for the treatment of gastrointestinal diseases and disorders. *Nat. Prod. Rad.* **2006**, *5*, 60–63.
17. Usher, G. *Spilanthes Acmella, a Dictionary of Plants Used by Man*; CBS Publishers and Distributers: New Delhi, India, 1984; p. 38.
18. Ghosh, A. Ethnomedicinal plants used in West Rarrh region of West Bengal. *Nat. Prod. Rad.* **2008**, *7*, 461–465.
19. Natarajan, B.; Paulsen, B.S.; Korneliussen, V. An ethnopharmacological study from Kulu District, Himachal Pradesh, India: Traditional knowledge compared with modern biological science. *Pharm. Biol.* **2000**, *38*, 129–138. [CrossRef]
20. Nisha, M.C.; Rajeshkumar, S. Survey of crude drugs from Coimbatore city. *Indian J. Nat. Prod. Resour.* **2010**, *1*, 376–383.
21. Ragupathy, S.; Steven, N.G.; Maruthakkutti, M.; Velusamy, B.; Ul-Huda, M.M. Consensus of the 'Malasars' traditional aboriginal knowledge of medicinal plants in the Velliangiri holy hills, India. *J. Ethnobiol. Ethnomed.* **2008**, *4*, 8–16. [CrossRef]
22. Tomar, A. Folk medicinal uses of plant roots from Meerut district, Uttar Pradesh. *Indian J. Tradit. Knowl.* **2009**, *8*, 298–301.
23. Rajith, N.P.; Ramachandran, V.S. Ethnomedicines of Kurichyas, Kannur district, Western Ghats, Kerala. *Indian J. Nat. Prod. Resour.* **2010**, *1*, 249–253.
24. Barbhuiya, A.R.; Sharma, G.D.; Arunachalam, A.; Deb, S. Diversity and conservation of medicinal plants in Barak valley, Northeast India. *Indian J. Tradit. Knowl.* **2009**, *8*, 169–175.
25. Kadel, C.; Jain, A.K. Folklore claims on snakebite among some tribal communities of Central India. *Indian J. Tradit. Knowl.* **2008**, *7*, 296–299.
26. Boktapa, N.R.; Sharma, A.K. Wild medicinal plants used by local communities of Manali, Himachal Pradesh, India. *Ethnobot. Leafl.* **2010**, *3*, 259–267.
27. Kingston, C.; Nisha, B.S.; Kiruba, S.; Jeeva, S. Ethnomedicinal plants used by indigenous community in a traditional healthcare system. *Ethnobot. Leafl.* **2007**, *11*, 32–37.
28. Jain, A.; Roshnibala, S.; Kanjilal, P.B.; Singh, R.S.; Singh, H.B. Aquatic /semi-aquatic plants used in herbal remedies in the wetlands of Manipur, Northeastern India. *Indian J. Tradit. Knowl.* **2007**, *6*, 346–351.
29. Yabesh, J.M.; Prabhu, S.; Vijayakumar, S. An ethnobotanical study of medicinal plants used by traditional healers in silent valley of Kerala, India. *J. Ethnopharmacol.* **2014**, *154*, 774–789. [CrossRef]
30. Sher, Z.; Khan, Z.; Hussain, F. Ethnobotanical studies of some plants of Chagharzai valley, district Buner, Pakistan. *Pak. J. Bot.* **2011**, *43*, 1445–1452.
31. Poonam, K.; Singh, G.S. Ethnobotanical study of medicinal plants used by the Taungya community in Terai Arc Landscape, India. *J. Ethnopharmacol.* **2009**, *123*, 167–176. [CrossRef]
32. Shrestha, P.M.; Dhillion, S.S. Medicinal plant diversity and use in the highlands of Dolakha district Nepal. *J. Ethnopharmacol.* **2003**, *86*, 81–96. [CrossRef]
33. Khatun, M.A.; Harun-Or-Rashid, M.; Rahmatullah, M. Scientific validation of eight medicinal plants used in traditional medicinal systems of Malaysia: A review. *Am. Eurasian J. Sustain. Agric.* **2011**, *5*, 67–75.
34. Dastur, J.F. *Medicinal Plants of India and Pakistan*; D. B. Taraporevala Sons and Co. Ltd: Bombay, India, 1951; p. 12.
35. Satyavati, G.V.; Raina, M.K.; Sharmal, M. *Medicinal Plants of India*; Indian Council of Medical Research: New Delhi, India, 1976; Volume I, pp. 14–16.
36. Jain, S.K. *Medicinal Plants*; National Book Trust: New Delhi, India, 1968.
37. Malhi, B.S.; Trivedi, V.P. Vegetable antifertility drugs of India. *Q. J. Crude Drug Res.* **1972**, *12*, 19–22.
38. Singh, M.P.; Malla, S.B.; Rajbhandari, S.B.; Manandhar, A. Medicinal plants of Nepal retrospect's and prospects. *Econ. Bot.* **1979**, *33*, 185–198. [CrossRef]
39. Kirtikar, K.R.; Basu, B.D. *Indian Medicinal Plants*; M/S. Bishen Singh Mahendra Pal Singh: Dehradun, India, 1975; Volume IV.
40. Lama, S.; Santra, S.C. Development of Tibetan plant medicine. *Sci. Cult.* **1979**, *45*, 262–265. [PubMed]
41. Burang, T. Cancer therapy of Tibetan healers. *Comp. Med. East West* **1979**, *7*, 294–296. [CrossRef] [PubMed]
42. Wallnofer, H.; Rottauscher, A. *Chinese Folk Medicine and Acupuncture*; Bell Publishing Co, Inc: New York, NY, USA, 1965.
43. Agarwal, S.L.; Dandiya, P.C.; Singh, K.P.; Arora, R.B. A note on the preliminary studies of certain pharmacological actions of *Acorus calamus*. *J. Am. Pharm. Assoc.* **1956**, *45*, 655–656. [CrossRef]
44. Duke, J.A.; Ayensu, E.S. *Medicinal Plants of China*; Reference Publications, Inc: Algonac, MI, USA, 1985.

45. Perry, L.M.; Metzger, J. *Medicinal Plants of East and Southeast Asia*; MIT Press: Cambridge, UK, 1980.
46. Boissya, C.L.; Majumder, R. Some folklore claims from the Brahmaputra Valley (Assam). *Ethnomedicine* **1980**, *6*, 139–145.
47. Dragendorff, G. *Die Heilpflanzen der Verschie Denen Volker und Zeiten*; F. Enke: Stuttgart, Germany, 1898.
48. Li, H.L. Hallucinogenic plants in Chinese herbals. *Harv. Univ. Bot. Mus. Leafl.* **1977**, *25*, 161–177.
49. Shih-Chen, L. *Chinese Medicinal Herbs*; Georgetown Press: San Francisco, CA, USA, 1973.
50. Hirschhorn, H.H. Botanical remedies of the former Dutch East Indies (Indonesia) I: Eumycetes, Pteridophyta, Gymnospermae, Angiospermae (Monocotyledones only). *J. Ethnopharmacol.* **1983**, *7*, 123–156. [CrossRef]
51. Wren, R.C. *Potter's New Cyclopaedia of Botanical Drugs and Preparations*; Sir Isaac Pitman and Sons, Ltd: London, UK, 1956.
52. Grieve, M. *A Modern Herbal*; Dover Publications, Inc: New York, NY, USA, 1971; Volume II.
53. Wheelwright, E.G. *Medicinal Plants and Their Stor*; Dover Publications, Inc: New York, NY, USA, 1974.
54. Moerman, D.E. *Geraniums for the Iroquois*; Reference Publications, Inc: Algonac, MI, USA, 1981.
55. Jochle, W. Menses-inducing drugs: Their role in antique, medieval and renaissance gynecology and birth control. *Contraception* **1974**, *10*, 425–439. [CrossRef]
56. Watt, J.M.; Breyer-Brandwijk, M.G. *The Medicinal and Poisonous Plants of Southern and Eastern Africa*; E. & S. Livingstone Ltd.: London, UK, 1962.
57. Kantor, W. Quack abortifacients and declining birth rate. *Therap. Monatsh.* **1916**, *30*, 561–568.
58. Herrmann, G. Therapy with medicinal plants in present medicine. *Med. Monatsschr. Pharm.* **1956**, *10*, 79.
59. Burkill, I.H. *Dictionary of the Economic Products of the Malay Peninsula*; Ministry of Agriculture and Cooperatives: Kuala Lumpur, Malaysia, 1966; Volume 1.
60. Motley, T.J. The Ethnobotany of Sweet Flag, *Acorus calamus* (Araceae). *Econ. Bot.* **1994**, *48*, 397–412. [CrossRef]
61. Krochmal, A.; Krochmal, C. *A Guide to the Medicinal Plants of the United States*; Quadrangle/The New York Times Book Co: New York, NY, USA, 1975.
62. El'Yashevych, O.H.; Cholii, R. Some means of treatment in the folk medicine of L'Vov. *Farmatsevtychnyi Zhurnal* **1972**, *27*, 78.
63. Barton, B.H.; Castle, T. *The British Flora Medica*; Chatto and Windus: Piccadilly, London, UK, 1877.
64. Mokkhasamit, M.; Ngarmwathana, W.; Sawasdimongkol, K.; Permphiphat, U. Pharmacological evaluation of Thai medicinal plants. (Continued). *J. Med. Assoc. Thail.* **1971**, *54*, 490–504.
65. Harris, B.C. *The Complete Herbal*; Barre Publishers: Barre, MA, USA, 1972.
66. Lindley, J. *Flora Medica*; Paternoster-Row: London, UK, 1838.
67. Caius, J.F. *The Medicinal and Poisonous Plants of India*; Scientific Publishers: Jodhpur, India, 1986.
68. Clymer, R.S. *Nature's Healing Agents*; Dorrance and Company: Philadelphia, PA, USA, 1963.
69. Manfred, L. *Siete Mil Recetas Botanicas a Base de Mil Trescientas Plantas*; Edit Kier: Buenos Aires, Argentina, 1947.
70. Dobelis, I.N. *Magic and Medicine of Plants*; The Reader's Digest Association, Inc.: Pleasantville, New York, NY, USA, 1986.
71. Kumar, H.; Song, S.Y.; More, S.V.; Kang, S.M.; Kim, B.Y. Traditional Korean East Asian Medicines and Herbal Formulations for Cognitive Impairment. *Molecules* **2013**, *18*, 14670–14693. [CrossRef]
72. Napagoda, M.T.; Sundarapperuma, T.; Fonseka, D.; Amarasiri, S.; Gunaratna, P. Traditional Uses of Medicinal Plants in Polonnaruwa District in North Central Province of Sri Lanka. *Scientifica* **2019**, *2019*, 1–12. [CrossRef]
73. Chaudhury, S.S.; Gautam, S.K.; Handa, K.L. Composition of calamus oil from calamus roots growing in Jammu and Kashmir. *Indian J. Pharm. Sci.* **1957**, *19*, 183–186.
74. Mukherjee, P.K. *Quality Control of Herbal Drugs: An Approach to Evaluation of Botanicals*; Business Horizons: New Delhi, India, 2002; pp. 692–694.
75. Soledade, M.; Pedras, C.; Zheng, Q. The Chemistry of Arabidopsis thaliana. *Comp. Nat. Prod.* **2010**, *3*, 1297–1315.
76. Sharma, J.D.; Dandiya, P.C.; Baxter, R.M.; Kandel, S.I. Pharmacodynamical effects of asarone and β-asarone. *Nature* **1961**, *192*, 1299–1300. [CrossRef]
77. Sharma, P.K.; Dandiya, P.C. Synthesis and some pharmacological actions of asarone. *Indian J. Appl. Chem.* **1969**, *32*, 236–238.
78. Nigam, M.C.; Ateeque, A.; Misra, L.N. GC-MS examination of essential oil of *Acorus calamus*. *Indian Perfum.* **1990**, *34*, 282–285.
79. Matejić, J.; Šarac, Z.; Ranđelović, V. Pharmacological activity of sesquiterpene lactones. *Biotech. Biotechnol. Equip.* **2010**, *24*, S95–S100. [CrossRef]

80. Benaiges, A.; Guillén, P. Botanical Extracts. *Anal. Cosmet. Prod.* **2007**, 345–363. [CrossRef]
81. Sparg, S.; Light, M.E.; Van Staden, J. Biological activities and distribution of plant saponins. *J. Ethnopharmacol.* **2007**, *94*, 219–243. [CrossRef]
82. Rai, R.; Siddiqui, I.R.; Singh, J. Triterpenoid Saponins from *Acorus calamus*. *ChemInform* **1998**, *29*, 473–476.
83. Rai, R.; Gupta, A.; Siddiqui, I.R.; Singh, J. Xanthone Glycoside from rhizome of *Acorus calamus*. *Indian J. Chem.* **1999**, *38*, 1143–1144.
84. Kumar, S.S.; Akram, A.S.; Ahmed, T.F.; Jaabir, M.M. Phytochemical analysis and antimicrobial activity of the ethanolic extract of *Acorus calamus* rhizome. *Orient. J. Chem.* **2010**, *26*, 223–227.
85. Wu, H.S.; Li, Y.Y.; Weng, L.J.; Zhou, C.X.; He, Q.J.; Lou, Y.J. A Fraction of *Acorus calamus* L. extract devoid of β-asarone Enhances adipocyte differentiation in 3T3-L1 cells. *Phytother. Res.* **2007**, *21*, 562–564. [CrossRef]
86. Vashi, I.G.; Patel, H.C. Chemical constituents and antimicrobial activity of *Acorus calamus* Linn. *Comp. Physiol. Ecol.* **1987**, *12*, 49–51.
87. Weber, M.; Brändle, R. Dynamics of nitrogen-rich compounds in roots, rhizomes, and leaves of the Sweet Flag (*Acorus calamus* L.) at its natural site. *Flora* **1994**, *189*, 63–68. [CrossRef]
88. Asif, M.; Siddiqi, M.T.A.; Ahmad, M.U. Fatty acid and sugar composition of *Acorus calamus* Linn. *Fette Seifen Anstrichm.* **1984**, *86*, 24–25. [CrossRef]
89. Lee, M.H.; Chen, Y.Y.; Tsai, J.W.; Wang, S.C.; Watanabe, T.; Tsai, Y.C. Inhibitory effect of β-asarone, a component of *Acorus calamus* essential oil, on inhibition of adipogenesis in 3T3-L1 cells. *Food Chem.* **2011**, *126*, 1–7. [CrossRef]
90. Padalia, R.C.; Chauhan, A.; Verma, R.S.; Bisht, M.; Thul, S.; Sundaresan, V. Variability in rhizome volatile constituents of *Acorus calamus* L. from Western Himalaya. *J. Essent. Oil Bear. Plants* **2014**, *17*, 32–41. [CrossRef]
91. Kumar, S.N.; Aravind, S.R.; Sreelekha, T.T.; Jacob, J.; Kumar, B.D. Asarones from *Acorus calamus* in combination with azoles and amphotericin b: A novel synergistic combination to compete against human pathogenic candida species In-vitro. *Appl. Biochem. Biotech.* **2015**, *175*, 3683–3695. [CrossRef]
92. Srivastava, V.K.; Singh, B.M.; Negi, K.S.; Pant, K.C.; Suneja, P. Gas chromatographic examination of some aromatic plants of Uttar Pradesh hills. *Indian Perfum.* **1997**, *41*, 129–139.
93. Özcan, M.; Akgül, A.; Chalchat, J.C. Volatile constituents of the essential oil of *Acorus calamus* L. grown in Konya province (Turkey). *J. Essent. Oil Res.* **2002**, *14*, 366–368. [CrossRef]
94. Kim, W.J.; Hwang, K.H.; Park, D.G.; Kim, T.J.; Kim, D.W.; Choi, D.K.; Lee, K.H. Major constituents and antimicrobial activity of Korean herb *Acorus calamus*. *Nat. Prod. Res.* **2011**, *25*, 1278–1281. [CrossRef]
95. Patra, A.; Mitra, A.K. Constituents of *Acorus calamus*: Structure of acoramone. Carbon-13 NMR spectra of cis-and trans-asarone. *J. Nat. Prod.* **1981**, *44*, 668–669. [CrossRef]
96. Saxena, D.B. Phenyl indane from *Acorus calamus*. *Phytochemistry* **1986**, *25*, 553–555. [CrossRef]
97. Radušienė, J.; Judžentienė, A.; Pečiulytė, D.; Janulis, V. Essential oil composition and antimicrobial assay of *Acorus calamus* leaves from different wild populations. *Plant Genet. Resour.* **2007**, *5*, 37–44. [CrossRef]
98. Haghighi, S.R.; Asadi, M.H.; Akrami, H.; Baghizadeh, A. Anti-carcinogenic and anti-angiogenic properties of the extracts of *Acorus calamus* on gastric cancer cells. *Avicenna J. Phytomed.* **2017**, *7*, 145.
99. Nawamaki, K.; Kuroyanagi, M. Sesquiterpenoids from *Acorus calamus* as germination inhibitors. *Phytochemistry* **1996**, *43*, 1175–1182. [CrossRef]
100. Zaugg, J.; Eickmeier, E.; Ebrahimi, S.N.; Baburin, I.; Hering, S.; Hamburger, M. Positive GABAA receptor modulators from *Acorus calamus* and structural analysis of (+)-dioxosarcoguaiacol by 1D and 2D NMR and molecular modeling. *J. Nat. Prod.* **2011**, *74*, 1437–1443. [CrossRef] [PubMed]
101. Yamamura, S.; Iguchi, M.; Nishiyama, A.; Niwa, M.; Koyama, H.; Hirata, Y. Sesquiterpenes from *Acorus calamus* L. *Tetrahedron* **1971**, *27*, 5419–5431. [CrossRef]
102. Li, J.; Zhao, J.; Wang, W.; Li, L.; Zhang, L.; Zhao, X.F.; Li, S.X. New Acorane-Type Sesquiterpene from *Acorus calamus* L. *Molecules* **2017**, *22*, 529. [CrossRef]
103. Zhou, C.X.; Qiao, D.; Yan, Y.Y.; Wu, H.S.; Mo, J.X.; Gan, L.S. A new anti-diabetic sesquiterpenoid from *Acorus calamus*. *Chin. Chem. Lett.* **2012**, *23*, 1165–1168. [CrossRef]
104. Yao, X.; Ling, Y.; Guo, S.; Wu, W.; He, S.; Zhang, Q.; Zou, M.; Nandakumar, K.S.; Chen, X.; Liu, S. Tatanan A from the *Acorus calamus* L. root inhibited dengue virus proliferation and infections. *Phytomedicine* **2018**, *42*, 258–267. [CrossRef]
105. Prisilla, D.H.; Balamurugan, R.; Shah, H.R. Antidiabetic activity of methanol extract of *Acorus calamus* in STZ induced diabetic rats. *Asian Pac. J. Trop. Biomed.* **2012**, *2*, S941–S946. [CrossRef]

106. Prashanth, D.; Ahmed, F.Z. Evaluation of hypoglycemic activity of methanolic extract of *Acorus calamus* (linn). roots in alloxan induced diabetes rat model. *Int. J. Basic Clin. Pharmacol.* **2017**, *6*, 2665–2670.
107. Wu, H.S.; Zhu, D.F.; Zhou, C.X.; Feng, C.R.; Lou, Y.J.; Yang, B.; He, Q.J. Insulin sensitizing activity of ethyl acetate fraction of *Acorus calamus* L. In-vitro and in-vivo. *J. Ethnopharmacol.* **2009**, *123*, 288–292. [CrossRef]
108. Liu, Y.X.; Si, M.M.; Lu, W.; Zhang, L.X.; Zhou, C.X.; Deng, S.L.; Wu, H.S. Effects and molecular mechanisms of the antidiabetic fraction of *Acorus calamus* L. on GLP-1 expression and secretion in-vivo and In-vitro. *J. Ethnopharmacol.* **2015**, *166*, 168–175. [CrossRef] [PubMed]
109. Si, M.M.; Lou, J.S.; Zhou, C.X.; Shen, J.N.; Wu, H.H.; Yang, B.; Wu, H.S. Insulin releasing and alpha-glucosidase inhibitory activity of ethyl acetate fraction of *Acorus calamus* In-vitro and in-vivo. *J. Ethnopharmacol.* **2010**, *128*, 154–159. [CrossRef] [PubMed]
110. Parab, R.S.; Mengi, S.A. Hypolipidemic activity of *Acorus calamus* L. in rats. *Fitoterapia* **2002**, *73*, 451–455. [CrossRef]
111. D'Souza, T.; Mengi, S.A.; Hassarajani, S.; Chattopadhayay, S. Efficacy study of the bioactive fraction (F-3) of *Acorus calamus* in hyperlipidemia. *Indian J. Pharmacol.* **2007**, *39*, 196–200.
112. Kumar, G.; Nagaraju, V.; Kulkarni, M.; Kumar, B.S.; Raju, S. Evaluation of Antihyperlipidemic Activity of Methanolic Extract of Acorus Calamus in fat diet Induced Rats. *Asian J. Med. Pharm. Sci.* **2016**, *4*, 71–76.
113. Arun, K.S.; Augustine, A. Hypolipidemic Effect of Methanol Fraction of *Acorus calamus* Linn. in Diet-Induced Obese Rats. In *Prospects in Bioscience: Addressing the Issues*; Springer, Springer Science & Business Media: New Delhi, India, 2012; pp. 399–404.
114. Athesh, K.; Jothi, G. Pharmacological screening of anti-obesity potential of *Acorus calamus* linn. In high fat cafeteria diet fed obese rats. *Asian J. Pharm. Clin. Res.* **2017**, *10*, 384–390.
115. Patel, P.; Vaghasiya, J.; Thakor, A.; Jariwala, J. Antihypertensive effect of rhizome part of *Acorus calamus* on renal artery occlusion induced hypertension in rats. *Asian Pac. J. Trop. Dis.* **2012**, *2*, S6–S10. [CrossRef]
116. Shah, A.J.; Gilani, A.H. Blood pressure-lowering and vascular modulator effects of *Acorus calamus* extract are mediated through multiple pathways. *J. Cardiovasc. Pharmacol.* **2009**, *54*, 38–46. [CrossRef]
117. Sundaramahalingam, M.; Ramasundaram, S.; Rathinasamy, S.D.; Natarajan, R.P.; Somasundaram, T. Role of *Acorus calamus* and alpha-asarone on hippocampal dependent memory in noise stress exposed rats. *Pak. J. Biol. Sci.* **2013**, *16*, 770–778. [CrossRef]
118. Jain, D.K.; Gupta, S.; Jain, R.; Jain, N. Anti-inflammatory Activity of 80% Ethanolic Extract of *Acorus calamus* Linn. Leaves in Albino Rats. *Res. J. Pharm. Tech.* **2010**, *3*, 882–884.
119. Manikandan, S.; Devi, R.S. Antioxidant property of α-asarone against noise-stress-induced changes in different regions of rat brain. *Pharmacol. Res.* **2005**, *52*, 467–474. [CrossRef] [PubMed]
120. Devi, S.A.; Ganjewala, D. Antioxidant activities of methanolic extracts of sweet-flag (*Acorus calamus*) leaves and rhizomes. *J. Herbs Spices Med. Plants* **2011**, *1*, 1–11. [CrossRef]
121. Acuña, U.M.; Atha, D.E.; Ma, J.; Nee, M.H.; Kennelly, E.J. Antioxidant capacities of ten edible North American plants. *Phytother. Res.* **2002**, *16*, 63–65. [CrossRef] [PubMed]
122. Palani, S.; Raja, S.; Kumar, R.P.; Parameswaran, P.; Kumar, B.S. Therapeutic efficacy of *Acorus calamus* on acetaminophen induced nephrotoxicity and oxidative stress in male albino rats. *Acta Pharm. Sci.* **2010**, *52*, 89–100.
123. Venkatramaniah, C.; Praba, A.M.A. Effect of Beta Asarone–The Active Principle of Acorus Calamus in Neuroprotection and Nerve Cell Regeneration on the Pyramidal Region of Hippocampus in Mesial Temporal Lobe Epileptic Rat Models. *J. Neurosci.* **2019**, *5*, 19–24.
124. Jayaraman, R.; Anitha, T.; Joshi, V.D. Analgesic and anticonvulsant effects of *Acorus calamus* roots in mice. *Int. J. PharmTech Res.* **2010**, *2*, 552–555.
125. Kaushik, R.; Jain, J.; Yadav, R.; Singh, L.; Gupta, D.; Gupta, A. Isolation of β-Asarone from *Acorus calamus* Linn. and Evaluation of its Anticonvulsant Activity using MES and PTZ Models in Mice. *Pharmacol. Toxicol. Biomed. Rep.* **2017**, *3*, 21–26. [CrossRef]
126. Chandrashekar, R.; Adake, P.; Rao, S.N. Anticonvulsant activity of ethanolic extract of *Acorus calamus* rhizome in swiss albino mice. *J. Sci. Innov. Res.* **2013**, *2*, 846–851.
127. Yende, S.R.; Harle, U.N.; Bore, V.V.; Bajaj, A.O.; Shroff, K.K.; Vetal, Y.D. Reversal of neurotoxicity induced cognitive impairment associated with phenytoin and phenobarbital by *Acorus calamus* in mice. *J. Herb. Med. Toxicol.* **2009**, *3*, 111–115.
128. Pawar, V.S.; Anup, A.; Shrikrishna, B.; Shivakumar, H. Antidepressant–like effects of *Acorus calamus* in forced swimming and tail suspension test in mice. *Asian Pac. J. Trop. Biomed.* **2011**, *1*, S17–S19. [CrossRef]

129. Pushpa, V.H.; Padmaja, S.K.; Suresha, R.N.; Vaibhavi, P.S.; Kalabharathi, H.L.; Satish, A.M.; Naidu, S. Antidepressant Activity of Methanolic Extract of Acorus Calamus Leaves in Albino Mice. *Int. J. Pharm. Tech.* **2013**, *5*, 5458–5465.
130. Shashikala, G.H.; Prashanth, D.; Jyothi, C.H.; Maniyar, I.; Manjunath, H. Evaluation of antidepressant activity of aqueous extract of roots of acorus calamus in albino mice. *World J. Pharm. Res.* **2015**, *4*, 1357–1365.
131. De, A.; Singh, M.S. *Acorus calamus* linn. Rhizomes extract for antidepressant activity in mice model. *Adv. Res. Pharm. Biol.* **2013**, *3*, 520–525.
132. Tripathi, A.K.; Singh, R.H. Experimental evaluation of antidepressant effect of Vacha (*Acorus calamus*) in animal models of depression. *Ayu* **2010**, *31*, 153–158. [CrossRef] [PubMed]
133. Pandy, V.; Jose, N.; Subhash, H. CNS activity of methanol and acetone extracts of *Acorus calamus* leaves in mice. *J. Pharmacol. Toxicol.* **2009**, *4*, 79–86. [CrossRef]
134. Tiwari, N.; Mishra, A.; Bhatt, G.; Chaudhary, A. Isolation of Principle Active Compound of Acorus Calamus. In-vivo assessment of pharmacological activity in the treatment of neurobiological disorder (stress). *J. Med. Clin. Res.* **2014**, *2*, 2201–2212.
135. Muthuraman, A.; Singh, N. Neuroprotective effect of saponin rich extract of *Acorus calamus* L. in rat model of chronic constriction injury (CCI) of sciatic nerve-induced neuropathic pain. *J. Ethnopharmacol.* **2012**, *142*, 723–731. [CrossRef]
136. Muthuraman, A.; Singh, N. Attenuating effect of *Acorus calamus* extract in chronic constriction injury induced neuropathic pain in rats: An evidence of anti-oxidative, anti-inflammatory, neuroprotective and calcium inhibitory effects. *BMC Complement. Altern. Med.* **2011**, *11*, 1–14. [CrossRef]
137. Vengadesh Prabu, K.; George, T.; Vinoth Kumar, R.; Nancy, J.; Kalaivani, M.; Vijayapandi, P. Neuromodulatory effect of Acrous calamus leaves extract on dopaminergic system in mice. *Int. J. PharmTech Res.* **2009**, *1*, 1255–1259.
138. Hazra, R.; Guha, D. Effect of chronic administration of *Acorus calamus* on electrical activity and regional monoamine levels in rat brain. *Biog. Amines* **2003**, *17*, 161–170. [CrossRef]
139. Shukla, P.K.; Khanna, V.K.; Ali, M.M.; Maurya, R.; Khan, M.Y.; Srimal, R.C. Neuroprotective effect of *Acorus calamus* against middle cerebral artery occlusion–induced ischaemia in rat. *Hum. Exp. Toxicol.* **2006**, *25*, 187–194. [CrossRef] [PubMed]
140. Fathima, A.; Patil, H.V.; Kumar, S. Suppression of elevated reactive oxygen species by acorus calamus (vacha) a sweet flag in drosophila melanogaster under stress full conditions. *Int. J. Pharm. Sci. Res.* **2014**, *5*, 1431–1439.
141. Kumar, M.S.; Hiremath, V.S.M.A. Cardioprotective effect of *Acorus calamus* against doxorubicin-induced myocardial toxicity in albino Wistar rats. *Indian J. Health Sci. Biomed. Res.* **2016**, *9*, 225–234.
142. Shah, A.J.; Gilani, A.H. Bronchodilatory effect of *Acorus calamus* (Linn.) is mediated through multiple pathways. *J. Ethnopharmacol.* **2010**, *131*, 471–477. [CrossRef] [PubMed]
143. Thakare, M.M.; Surana, S.J. β-Asarone modulate adipokines and attenuates high fat diet-induced metabolic abnormalities in Wistar rats. *Pharmacol. Res.* **2016**, *103*, 227–235. [CrossRef] [PubMed]
144. Karthiga, T.; Venkatalakshmi, P.; Vadivel, V.; Brindha, P. In-vitro anti-obesity, antioxidant and anti-inflammatory studies on the selected medicinal plants. *Int. J. Toxicol. Pharmacol. Res.* **2016**, *8*, 332–340.
145. Singh, D.K.; Kumar, N.; Sachan, A.; Lakhani, P.; Tutu, S.; Shankar, P.; Dixit, R.K. An experimental study to see the antihypertensive effects of gymnema sylvestre and acorus calamus in wistar rats and its comparison with amlodipine. *Asian J. Med. Sci.* **2017**, *8*, 11–15. [CrossRef]
146. Tanaka, S.; Yoichi, S.; Ao, L.; Matumoto, M.; Morimoto, K.; Akimoto, N.; Zaini bin Asmawi, M. Potential immunosuppressive and anti-inflammatory activities of Malaysian medicinal plants characterized by reduced cell surface expression of cell adhesion molecules. *Phytother. Res.* **2001**, *15*, 681–686. [CrossRef]
147. Kim, H.; Han, T.H.; Lee, S.G. Anti-inflammatory activity of a water extract of *Acorus calamus* L. leaves on keratinocyte HaCaT cells. *J. Ethnopharmacol.* **2009**, *122*, 149–156. [CrossRef]
148. Ahmed, S.; Gul, S.; Zia-Ul-Haq, M.; Stanković, M.S. Pharmacological basis of the use of *Acorus calamus* L. in inflammatory diseases and underlying signal transduction pathways. *Bol. Latinoam. Caribe Plantas Med. Aromát.* **2014**, *13*, 38–46.
149. Loying, R.; Gogoi, R.; Sarma, N.; Borah, A.; Munda, S.; Pandey, S.K.; Lal, M. Chemical Compositions, In-vitro Antioxidant, Anti-microbial, Anti-inflammatory and Cytotoxic Activities of Essential Oil of *Acorus calamus* L. Rhizome from North-East India. *J. Essent. Oil Bear. Plants* **2019**, *22*, 1299–1312. [CrossRef]

150. Bahukhandi, A.; Rawat, S.; Bhatt, I.D.; Rawal, R.S. Influence of solvent types and source of collection on total phenolic content and antioxidant activities of *Acorus calamus* L. *Natl. Acad. Sci. Lett.* **2013**, *36*, 93–99. [CrossRef]
151. Manju, S.; Chandran, R.P.; Shaji, P.K.; Nair, G.A. In-vitro free radical scavenging potential of Acorus Calamus L. rhizome from Kuttanad Wetlands, Kerala, India. *Int. J. Pharm. Pharm. Sci.* **2013**, *5*, 376–380.
152. Barua, C.C.; Sen, S.; Das, A.S.; Talukdar, A.; Hazarika, N.J.; Barua, A.G.; Barua, I. A comparative study of the In-vitro antioxidant property of different extracts of *Acorus calamus* Linn. *J. Nat. Prod. Plant Resour.* **2014**, *4*, 8–18.
153. Elayaraja, A.; Vijayalakshmi, M.; Devalarao, G. In-vitro free radical scavenging activity of various root and rhizome extracts of *Acorus calamus* Linn. *Int. J. Pharm. Biol. Sci.* **2010**, *1*, 301–304.
154. Govindarajan, R.; Agnihotri, A.K.; Khatoon, S.; Rawat, A.K.S.; Mehrotra, S. Pharmacognostical evaluation of an antioxidant plant-*Acorus calamus* Linn. *Nat. Prod. Sci.* **2003**, *9*, 264–269.
155. Sujitha, R.; Bhimba, B.V.; Sindhu, M.S.; Arumugham, P. Phytochemical Evaluation and Antioxidant Activity of *Nelumbo nucifera*, *Acorus calamus* and *Piper longum*. *Int. J. Pharm. Chem. Sci.* **2013**, *2*, 1573–1578.
156. Shukla, R.; Singh, P.; Prakash, B.; Dubey, N.K. Efficacy of *Acorus calamus* L. essential oil as a safe plant-based antioxidant, A flatoxin B 1 suppressor and broad-spectrum antimicrobial against food-infesting fungi. *Int. J. Food Sci. Tech.* **2013**, *48*, 128–135. [CrossRef]
157. Ahmeda, F.; Urooja, A.; KS, R. In-vitro antioxidant and anticholinesterase activity of *Acorus calamus* and Nardostachys jatamansi rhizomes. *J. Pharm. Res.* **2009**, *2*, 830–833.
158. Bhat, S.D.; Ashok, B.K.; Acharya, R.N.; Ravishankar, B. Anticonvulsant activity of raw and classically processed Vacha (*Acorus calamus* Linn.) rhizomes. *Ayu* **2012**, *33*, 119–122. [CrossRef]
159. Patel, S.; Rajshree, N.; Shah, P. Evaluation of antidepressant activity of herbomineral formulation. *Int. J. Pharm. Pharm. Sci.* **2016**, *8*, 145–147.
160. Rauniar, G.P.; Deo, S.; Bhattacharya, S.K. Evaluation of anxiolytic activity of tensarin in mice. *Kathman. Univ. Med. J.* **2007**, *5*, 188–194.
161. Naderi, G.A.; Khalili, M.; Karimi, M.; Soltani, M. The effect of oral and intraperitoneal administration of *Acorus calamus* L. extract on learning and memory in male rats. *J. Med. Plant* **2010**, *2*, 46–56.
162. Vohora, S.B.; Shah, S.A.; Dandiya, P.C. Central nervous system studies on an ethanol extract of *Acorus calamus* rhizomes. *J. Ethnopharmacol.* **1990**, *28*, 53–62. [CrossRef]
163. Singh, B.K.; Pillai, K.K.; Kohli, K.; Haque, S.E. Isoproterenol-Induced Cardiomyopathy in Rats: Influence of *Acorus calamus* Linn. *Cardiovasc. Toxicol.* **2011**, *11*, 263–271. [CrossRef] [PubMed]
164. Shah, A.J.; Gilani, A.H. Aqueous-methanolic extract of sweet flag (*Acorus calamus*) possesses cardiac depressant and endothelial-derived hyperpolarizing factor-mediated coronary vasodilator effects. *J. Nat. Med.* **2012**, *66*, 119–126. [CrossRef]
165. Hasheminejad, G.; Caldwell, J. Genotoxicity of the alkenylbenzenes α− and β-asarone, myristicin and elemicin as determined by the UDS assay in cultured rat hepatocytes. *Food Chem. Toxicol.* **1994**, *32*, 223–231. [CrossRef]
166. Cartus, A.T.; Schrenk, D. Metabolism of the carcinogen alpha-asarone in liver microsomes. *Food Chem. Toxicol.* **2016**, *87*, 103–112. [CrossRef]
167. Cartus, A.T.; Stegmuller, S.; Simson, N.; Wahl, A.; Neef, S.; Kelm, H.; Schrenk, D. Hepatic metabolism of carcinogenic betaasarone. *Chem. Res. Toxicol.* **2015**, *28*, 1760–1773. [CrossRef]
168. Cartus, A.T.; Schrenk, D. Metabolism of carcinogenic alpha-asarone by human cytochrome P450 enzymes. *Naunyn-Schmiedeberg's Arch. Pharmacol.* **2020**, *393*, 213–223. [CrossRef]
169. Pandit, S.; Mukherjee, P.K.; Ponnusankar, S.; Venkatesh, M.; Srikanth, N. Metabolism mediated interaction of α-asarone and *Acorus calamus* with CYP3A4 and CYP2D6. *Fitoterapia* **2011**, *82*, 369–374. [CrossRef] [PubMed]
170. Muthuraman, A.; Singh, N. Acute and sub-acute oral toxicity profile of *Acorus calamus* (Sweet flag) in rodents. *Asian Pac. J. Trop Biomed.* **2012**, *2*, S1017–S1023. [CrossRef]
171. Areekul, S.; Sinchaisri, P.; Tigvatananon, S. Effects of Thai plant extracts on the oriental fruit fly III. *Nat. Sci.* **1988**, *22*, 160–164.
172. Shah, P.D.; Ghag, M.; Deshmukh, P.B.; Kulkarni, Y.; Joshi, S.V.; Vyas, B.A.; Shah, D.R. Toxicity study of ethanolic extract of *Acorus calamus* rhizome. *Int. J. Green Pharm.* **2012**, *6*, 29–35. [CrossRef]
173. Bhat, S.D.; Ashok, B.K.; Acharya, R.; Ravishankar, B. A comparative acute toxicity evaluation of raw and classically processed rhizomes of Vacha (*Acorus calamus* Linn.). *Indian J. Nat. Prod. Resour.* **2012**, *3*, 506–511.
174. Keller, K.; Stahl, E. Composition of the essential oil from beta-Asarone free calamus. *Planta Med.* **1983**, *47*, 71–74. [CrossRef]

175. JECFA (Joint FAO/WHO Expert Committee on Food Additives). Monograph on -asarone. In *WHO Food Additive Series No. 16*; WHO Food Additives Series; JECFA, WHO Press: Geneva, Switzerland, 1981.
176. Opdyke, D.L.J. Monographs on fragrance raw materials. *Food Cosmet. Toxicol.* **1973**, *11*, 855–876. [CrossRef]
177. Jenner, P.M.; Hagan, E.C.; Taylor, J.M.; Cook, E.L.; Fitzhugh, O.G. Food flavourings and compounds of related structure I. Acute oral toxicity. *Food Cosmet. Toxicol.* **1964**, *2*, 327–343. [CrossRef]
178. Singh, A.K.; Ravishankar, B.; Sharma, P.P.; Pandaya, T. Clinical study of anti-hyperlipidaemic activity of vacha (*Acorus calamus* linn) w.s.r to sthaulya. *Int. Ayurvedic Med. J.* **2017**, *5*, 1–8.
179. Tajadini, H.; Saifadini, R.; Choopani, R.; Mehrabani, M.; Kamalinejad, M.; Haghdoost, A.A. Herbal medicine Davaie Loban in mild to moderate Alzheimer's disease: A 12-week randomized double-blind placebo-controlled clinical trial. *Complement. Ther. Med.* **2015**, *23*, 767–772. [CrossRef]
180. Bhattacharyya, D.; Sur, T.K.; Lyle, N.; Jana, U.; Debnath, P.K. A clinical study on the management of generalized anxiety disorder with Vaca (*Acorus calamus*). *Indian J. Tradit. Knowl.* **2011**, *10*, 668–671.
181. Soni1, P.; Sharma, C. A clinical study of Vachadi Churna in the management of obesity. *Int. J. Ayurveda Allied Sci.* **2012**, *1*, 179–186.
182. Kulatunga, R.D.H.; Dave, A.R.; Baghel, M.S. Clinical efficacy of Guduchyadi Medhya Rasayana on senile memory impairment. *Ayu* **2012**, *33*, 202–208. [CrossRef] [PubMed]
183. Pande, D.N.; Mishra, S.K. Vacha (Acorus Calamus) as an ayurvedic premedicant. *Ayu* **2009**, *30*, 279–283.
184. Mishra, J.; Joshi, N.P.; Pandya, D.M. A comparative study of Shankhapushpyadi Ghana Vati and Sarpagandhadi Ghana Vati in the management of "Essential Hypertension". *Ayu* **2012**, *33*, 54–61. [CrossRef]
185. Ramu, M.G.; Senapati, H.M.; Janakiramaiah, N.; Shankara, M.R.; Chaturvedi, D.D.; Murthy, N.N. A pilot study of role of brahmyadiyoga in chronic unmada (schizophrenia). *Anc. Sci. Life* **1983**, *2*, 205–207.
186. Appaji, R.R.; Sharma, R.D.; Katiyar, G.P.; Sai, P.A. Clinical study of the Immunoglobululin Enhancing Effect of "Bala compound" on Infants. *Anc. Sci. Life* **2009**, *28*, 18–22.
187. Pawar, M.; Magdum, P. Clinical study of assessment of therapeutic potential of Vachadi ghrita, a medicated ghee formulation on healthy individual's cognition. *Int. J. Pharm. Sci. Res.* **2018**, *9*, 3408–3413.
188. Mishra, D.; Tubaki, B.R. Effect of Brahmi vati and Sarpagandha Ghana vati in management of essential hypertension–A randomized, double blind, clinical study. *J. Ayurveda Integr. Med.* **2019**, *10*, 269–276. [CrossRef]
189. Sharma, Y.; Upadhyay, A.; Sharma, Y.K.; Chaudhary, V. A randomized clinical study to evaluate the effect of Tagaradi yoga in the management of insomnia. *Indian J. Tradit. Knowl.* **2017**, *16*, S75–S80.
190. Paradkar, S.R.; Pardhi, S.N. Clinical evaluation of lekhaniya effect of vacha (acorus calamus) and musta (cyperus rotundus) in medoroga wsr to obesity: A comparative study. *Res. Rev. J. Pharmacogn.* **2019**, *3*, 1–8.
191. Mamgain, P.; Singh, R.H. Control clinical trial of the lekhaniya drug vaca (*Acorus calamus*) in case of ischemic heart diseases. *J. Res. Ayurveda Siddha* **1994**, *15*, 35–51.
192. Ning, B.; Zhang, Q.; Wang, N.; Deng, M.; Fang, Y. β-Asarone Regulates ER Stress and Autophagy Via Inhibition of the PERK/CHOP/Bcl-2/Beclin-1 Pathway in 6-OHDA-Induced Parkinsonian Rats. *Neurochem. Res.* **2019**, *44*, 1159–1166. [CrossRef]
193. Ning, B.; Deng, M.; Zhang, Q.; Wang, N.; Fang, Y. β-Asarone inhibits IRE1/XBP1 endoplasmic reticulum stress pathway in 6-OHDA-induced parkinsonian rats. *Neurochem. Res.* **2016**, *41*, 2097–2101. [CrossRef] [PubMed]
194. Huang, L.; Deng, M.; Zhang, S.; Fang, Y.; Li, L. Coadministration of β-asarone and levodopa increases dopamine in rat brain by accelerating transformation of levodopa: A different mechanism from M adopar. *Clin. Exp. Pharmacol. Physiol.* **2014**, *41*, 685–690. [PubMed]
195. Huang, L.; Deng, M.; He, Y.; Lu, S.; Ma, R.; Fang, Y. β-asarone and levodopa co-administration increase striatal dopamine level in 6-hydroxydopamine induced rats by modulating P-glycoprotein and tight junction proteins at the blood-brain barrier and promoting levodopa into the brain. *Clin. Exp. Pharmacol. Physiol.* **2016**, *43*, 634–643. [CrossRef]
196. Chang, W.; Teng, J. β-asarone prevents Aβ25-35-induced inflammatory responses and autophagy in SH-SY5Y cells: Down expression Beclin-1, LC3B and up expression Bcl-2. *Int. J. Clin. Exp. Med.* **2015**, *8*, 20658.
197. Liu, S.J.; Yang, C.; Zhang, Y.; Su, R.Y.; Chen, J.L.; Jiao, M.M.; Quan, S.J. Neuroprotective effect of β-asarone against Alzheimer's disease: Regulation of synaptic plasticity by increased expression of SYP and GluR1. *Drug Des. Dev. Ther.* **2016**, *10*, 1461. [CrossRef]
198. Li, C.; Xing, G.; Dong, M.; Zhou, L.; Li, J.; Wang, G.; Niu, Y. Beta-asarone protection against beta-amyloid-induced neurotoxicity in PC12 cells via JNK signaling and modulation of Bcl-2 family proteins. *Eur. J. Pharmacol.* **2010**, *635*, 96–102. [CrossRef]

199. Xue, Z.; Guo, Y.; Zhang, S.; Huang, L.; He, Y.; Fang, R.; Fang, Y. Beta-asarone attenuates amyloid beta-induced autophagy via Akt/mTOR pathway in PC12 cells. *Eur. J. Pharmacol.* **2014**, *741*, 195–204. [CrossRef]
200. Yang, Q.Q.; Xue, W.Z.; Zou, R.X.; Xu, Y.; Du, Y.; Wang, S.; Chen, X.T. β-Asarone rescues Pb-induced impairments of spatial memory and synaptogenesis in rats. *PLoS ONE* **2016**, *11*, e0167401. [CrossRef] [PubMed]
201. Guo, J.H.; Chen, Y.; Wei, G.; Nei, H.; Zhou, Y.; Cheng, S. Effects of active components of Rhizoma Acori Tatarinowii and their compatibility at different ratios on learning and memory abilities in dementia mice. *Tradit. Chin. Drug Res. Clin. Pharmacol.* **2012**, *23*, 144–147.
202. Li, J.; Li, Z.X.; Zhao, J.P.; Wang, W.; Zhao, X.F.; Xu, B.; Li, S.X. A Novel Tropoloisoquinoline Alkaloid, Neotatarine, from *Acorus calamus* L. *Chem. Biodivers.* **2017**, *14*, e1700201. [CrossRef] [PubMed]
203. He, X.; Cai, Q.; Li, J.; Guo, W. Involvement of brain-gut axis in treatment of cerebral infarction by β-asaron and paeonol. *Neurosci. Lett.* **2018**, *666*, 78–84. [CrossRef]
204. Gao, E.; Zhou, Z.Q.; Zou, J.; Yu, Y.; Feng, X.L.; Chen, G.D.; Gao, H. Bioactive Asarone-derived phenylpropanoids from the rhizome of Acorus tatarinowii Schott. *J. Nat. Prod.* **2017**, *80*, 2923–2929. [CrossRef]
205. Zhang, S.; Gui, X.H.; Huang, L.P.; Deng, M.Z.; Fang, R.M.; Ke, X.H.; Fang, Y.Q. Neuroprotective effects of β-asarone against 6-hydroxy dopamine-induced parkinsonism via JNK/Bcl-2/Beclin-1 pathway. *Mol. Neurobiol.* **2016**, *53*, 83–94. [CrossRef]
206. Liang, S.; Ying, S.S.; Wu, H.H.; Liu, Y.T.; Dong, P.Z.; Zhu, Y.; Xu, Y.T. A novel sesquiterpene and three new phenolic compounds from the rhizomes of Acorus tatarinowii Schott. *Bioorg. Med. Chem. Lett.* **2015**, *25*, 4214–4218. [CrossRef]
207. Xu, F.; Wu, H.; Zhang, K.; Lv, P.; Zheng, L.; Zhao, J. Pro-neurogenic effect of β-asarone on RSC96 Schwann cells in vitro. *In Vitro Cell. Dev. Biol. Anim.* **2016**, *52*, 278–286. [CrossRef]
208. Deng, M.; Huang, L.; Ning, B.; Wang, N.; Zhang, Q.; Zhu, C.; Fang, Y. β-asarone improves learning and memory and reduces Acetyl Cholinesterase and Beta-amyloid 42 levels in APP/PS1 transgenic mice by regulating Beclin-1-dependent autophagy. *Brain Res.* **2016**, *1652*, 188–194. [CrossRef]
209. Yang, Y.; Xuan, L.; Chen, H.; Dai, S.; Ji, L.; Bao, Y.; Li, C. Neuroprotective Effects and Mechanism of β-Asarone against Aβ1–42-Induced Injury in Astrocytes. *Evid.-Based Complement. Altern. Med.* **2017**, *2017*, 8516518. [CrossRef]
210. Dong, H.; Gao, Z.; Rong, H.; Jin, M.; Zhang, X. β-asarone reverses chronic unpredictable mild stress-induced depression-like behavior and promotes hippocampal neurogenesis in rats. *Molecules* **2014**, *19*, 5634–5649. [CrossRef] [PubMed]
211. Chellian, R.; Pandy, V.; Mohamed, Z. Biphasic effects of α-asarone on immobility in the tail suspension test: Evidence for the involvement of the noradrenergic and serotonergic systems in its antidepressant-like activity. *Front. Pharmacol.* **2016**, *7*, 72. [CrossRef] [PubMed]
212. Liu, H.; Song, Z.; Liao, D.G.; Zhang, T.Y.; Liu, F.; Zhuang, K.; Lei, J.P. Anticonvulsant and sedative effects of eudesmin isolated from Acorus tatarinowii on mice and rats. *Phytother. Res.* **2015**, *29*, 996–1003. [CrossRef] [PubMed]
213. Tian, J.; Tian, Z.; Qin, S.L.; Zhao, P.Y.; Jiang, X. Anxiolytic-like effects of α-asarone in a mouse model of chronic pain. *Metab. Brain Dis.* **2017**, *32*, 2119–2129. [CrossRef] [PubMed]
214. Miao, J.K.; Chen, Q.X.; Li, C.; Li, X.W.; Wu, X.M.; Zhang, X.P. Modulation Effects of α-Asarone on the GABA homeostasis in the Lithium-Pilocarpine Model of Temporal Lobe Epilepsy. *Pharmacology* **2013**, *9*, 24–32.
215. Wang, Z.J.; Levinson, S.R.; Sun, L.; Heinbockel, T. Identification of both GABAA receptors and voltage-activated Na+ channels as molecular targets of anticonvulsant α-asarone. *Front. Pharmacol.* **2014**, *5*, 40. [CrossRef]
216. Chen, L.; Liao, W.P. Changes of amino acid content in hippocampus of epileptic rats treated with volatile oil of Acorus tatarinowii. *Zhongguo ZhongYao ZaZhi* **2004**, *29*, 670–673.
217. Jo, M.J.; Kumar, H.; Joshi, H.P.; Choi, H.; Ko, W.K.; Kim, J.M.; Kim, K.T. Oral administration of α-Asarone promotes functional recovery in rats with spinal cord injury. *Front. Pharmacol.* **2018**, *9*, 445. [CrossRef]
218. Lam, K.Y.; Yao, P.; Wang, H.; Duan, R.; Dong, T.T.; Tsim, K.W. Asarone from Acori Tatarinowii Rhizome prevents oxidative stress-induced cell injury in cultured astrocytes: A signaling triggered by Akt activation. *PLoS ONE* **2017**, *12*, e0179077. [CrossRef]
219. Wu, Q.D.; Yuan, D.J.; Wang, Q.W.; Wu, X.R. Effects of volatile oil of Rhizoma Acori Tatarinowii on morphology and cell viability in cultured cardiac myocytes. *Zhong Yao Cai* **2009**, *32*, 242–245.
220. Yong, H.Y.F.Y.J.; Shuying, L.Y.W. In-vitro Observation of β-asarone for Counteracting Arteriosclerosis. *J. Guangzhou Univ. Tradit. Chin. Med.* **2008**, *3*, 14.

221. Yang, Y.X.; Chen, Y.T.; Zhou, X.J.; Hong, C.L.; Li, C.Y.; Guo, J.Y. Beta-asarone, a major component of Acorus tatarinowii Schott, attenuates focal cerebral ischemia induced by middle cerebral artery occlusion in rats. *BMC Complement. Altern. Med.* **2013**, *13*, 236. [CrossRef] [PubMed]
222. Das, B.K.; Choukimath, S.M.; Gadad, P.C. Asarone and metformin delays experimentally induced hepatocellular carcinoma in diabetic milieu. *Life Sci.* **2019**, *230*, 10–18. [CrossRef] [PubMed]
223. Lee, S.H.; Kim, K.Y.; Ryu, S.Y.; Yoon, Y.O.O.S.I.K.; Hahm, D.H.; Kang, S.A.; Lee, H.G. Asarone inhibits adipogenesis and stimulates lipolysis in 3T3-L1 adipocytes. *Cell. Mol. Biol.* **2010**, *56*, 1215–1222.

Journal of
Clinical Medicine

MDPI

Review

Pharmacological Therapeutics Targeting RNA-Dependent RNA Polymerase, Proteinase and Spike Protein: From Mechanistic Studies to Clinical Trials for COVID-19

Jiansheng Huang [1,3,*], Wenliang Song [1], Hui Huang [2] and Quancai Sun [3,*]

[1] Department of Medicine, Vanderbilt University Medical Center, 318 Preston Research Building, 2200 Pierce Avenue, Nashville, TN 37232, USA
[2] Center of Structural Biology, Vanderbilt University, 2200 Pierce Avenue, Nashville, TN 37232, USA
[3] School of Food and Biological Engineering, Jiangsu University, Zhenjiang 212013, Jiangsu, China
* Correspondence: Jiansheng.huang@vumc.org (J.H.); sqctp8@ujs.edu.cn (Q.S.)

Received: 28 March 2020; Accepted: 13 April 2020; Published: 15 April 2020

Abstract: An outbreak of novel coronavirus-related pneumonia COVID-19, that was identified in December 2019, has expanded rapidly, with cases now confirmed in more than 211 countries or areas. This constant transmission of a novel coronavirus and its ability to spread from human to human have prompted scientists to develop new approaches for treatment of COVID-19. A recent study has shown that remdesivir and chloroquine effectively inhibit the replication and infection of severe acute respiratory syndrome coronavirus-2 (SARS-CoV-2, 2019-nCov) in vitro. In the United States, one case of COVID-19 was successfully treated with compassionate use of remdesivir in January of 2020. In addition, a clinically proven protease inhibitor, camostat mesylate, has been demonstrated to inhibit Calu-3 infection with SARS-CoV-2 and prevent SARS-2-spike protein (S protein)-mediated entry into primary human lung cells. Here, we systemically discuss the pharmacological therapeutics targeting RNA-dependent RNA polymerase (RdRp), proteinase and S protein for treatment of SARS-CoV-2 infection. This review should shed light on the fundamental rationale behind inhibition of SARS-CoV-2 enzymes RdRp as new therapeutic approaches for management of patients with COVID-19. In addition, we will discuss the viability and challenges in targeting RdRp and proteinase, and application of natural product quinoline and its analog chloroquine for treatment of coronavirus infection. Finally, determining the structural-functional relationships of the S protein of SARS-CoV-2 will provide new insights into inhibition of interactions between S protein and angiotensin-converting enzyme 2 (ACE2) and enable us to develop novel therapeutic approaches for novel coronavirus SARS-CoV-2.

Keywords: RNA-dependent RNA polymerase; remdesivir; chloroquine; SARS-CoV-2; COVID-19; spike glycoproteins

1. Introduction

Since its discovery in December 2019, the novel coronavirus-related pneumonia COVID-19 has continued to disseminate, with the current case count close to 1,214,466 cases, and more than 67,767 deaths according to the World Health Organization (WHO) as of 7 April 2020 [1,2]. Epidemiological studies suggest that the incubation period was estimated to be 1–14 days, whereas the serial interval was estimated to be 4–8 days. It takes about 3–7 days for the epidemic to double in the number of infections [3]. In addition, recent study demonstrated that there was about 5% of severe acute respiratory syndrome coronavirus-2 (SARS-CoV-2) among other patients with mild influenza-like symptom without risk factors [4]. These patients had only mild or moderate symptoms, so they are still active in the community during infection, which promotes the possibility of constant transmission. To have a better understanding of respiratory infectious disease transmission for pathogenesis and epidemiological spread of disease, a model for respiratory emissions was established and it was found that droplets containing the virus can be as small as 1 micron and a multiphase turbulent gas cloud from a human sneeze exhibited the property to travel great distance (7–8 m) [5]. This suggests that the gas cloud with its pathogen payload can span a certain space in a few seconds [5]. Giving a high rate of community spread, there is a need to change the public health policy from containment to mitigation of transmission, and determine the extent to which mild disease is contagious in the community, particularly among less vulnerable young adults for acquisition of SARS-CoV-2 infection [4]. This study also stresses the importance of close cooperation between clinicians, pharmaceutical companies and public health authorities [6]. Increase of clinical knowledge sharing will facilitate the rapid diagnosis and development of pharmacological approaches for treatment of SARS-CoV-2 infection [7,8]. The constant and rapid spread of novel coronavirus SARS-CoV-2 and its ability to disseminate from human to human has prompted scientists to develop new approaches for treatment of the novel coronavirus-related pneumonia COVID-19.

2. Coronavirus

Respiratory viral infection is a global health concern because the virus is contagious and may cause life-threatening respiratory infection and severe pneumonia in humans [9]. Currently, there are three single strand RNA (ssRNA) beta-coronavirus that have been identified, including severe acute respiratory syndrome (SARS) virus, Middle East respiratory syndrome (MERS) virus and SARS-CoV-2 [9]. Full-length genome sequence has identified that the genome sequences of SARS-CoV-2 obtained from five patients at the early stage of the outbreak were almost identical to each other and exhibited about 79.5% sequence identify to SARS-CoV [10,11]. Furthermore, it is found that SARS-CoV-2 is 96% identical at the whole-genome level to a bat coronavirus, which indicates that bats might be the intermediate host of this virus [12].There are several symptoms of coronavirus infection, such as sore throat, running nose, cough, sneezing, fever, viral conjunctivitis, loss of smell and taste and severe pneumonia [7,9,13–16]. It is also very challenging to make an accurate and timely diagnosis and it is not easy to distinguish when diagnosing between coronavirus and the influenza respiratory syndromes without RT-PCR diagnosis assay [17–19]. The number of deaths from COVID-19 is already more than the number of lives lost to SARS. There is a high rate of infection resulting from viral pneumonia, consequent inflammation and acute respiratory distress syndrome (ARDS) caused by SARS-CoV-2 [8,12]. Severe pneumonia, secondary infections and cardiovascular events were the major reason for death [13,20]. The pathological features of one case of death from severe infection with SARS-CoV-2 was investigated, and it was found that the pathological features of COVID-19 substantially resembled characteristics observed in SARS and Middle Eastern respiratory syndrome (MERS) coronavirus infection [21–23]. Recent study has shown that remdesivir and chloroquine efficiently suppressed the replication of SARS-CoV-2 in vitro [24]. One case of COVID-19 was treated with remdesivir in the United States [25]. After successful treatment, there was no detectable nucleic acid of SARS-CoV-2 from serum and oropharyngeal swab specimens and there was no gene mutation after comparing it with the previously reported genome sequence of SARS-CoV-2 [10,25]. This will be useful in understanding the pathogenesis of COVID-19 and discovering new therapies and clinical strategies against the infection.

3. Potential Mechanisms of Coronavirus Invasion

3.1. Molecular Mechanisms of Coronavirus Invasion

The coronavirus (CoV) family has a large homogeneous "spike protein". This spike protein (S protein) is responsible for interacting with the host cells, such as the pulmonary and parabronchial epithelial cell, and helps the coronavirus get through the epithelial cell membrane [26]. In addition, the alveolar epithelial cells have abundant expression of angiotensin-converting enzyme 2 (ACE2), which is targeted by the virus. The recognition of ACE2 by the S protein of the virus enables the invasion of the coronavirus into the human circulation system [27]. Recent study demonstrates that ACE2 is the SARS-CoV-2 receptor, which is required for cell entry [28]. Single-strand RNA (ssRNA) viruses such as the coronavirus family replicate the virus genomes by taking advantage of host cells. For example, after coronavirus approaches the ribosome of the epithelial cells or other host cells, it uses the ribosome of the host cell to replicate polyproteins. The replication and subsequent processes of precursor polyproteins can occur in the epithelial cells [29]. After the coronavirus' polyproteins are expressed, two enzymes—specifically, coronavirus main proteinase (3CLpro) and the papain-like protease (PLpro)—are thought to be involved in cleaving the polyproteins into smaller products used for replicating new viruses [30]. In order to generate the daughter RNA genome, the coronavirus expresses an RNA-dependent RNA polymerase (RdRp), which is a crucial replicase that catalyzes the synthesis of a complementary RNA strand using the virus RNA template as shown in Figure 1 [31].

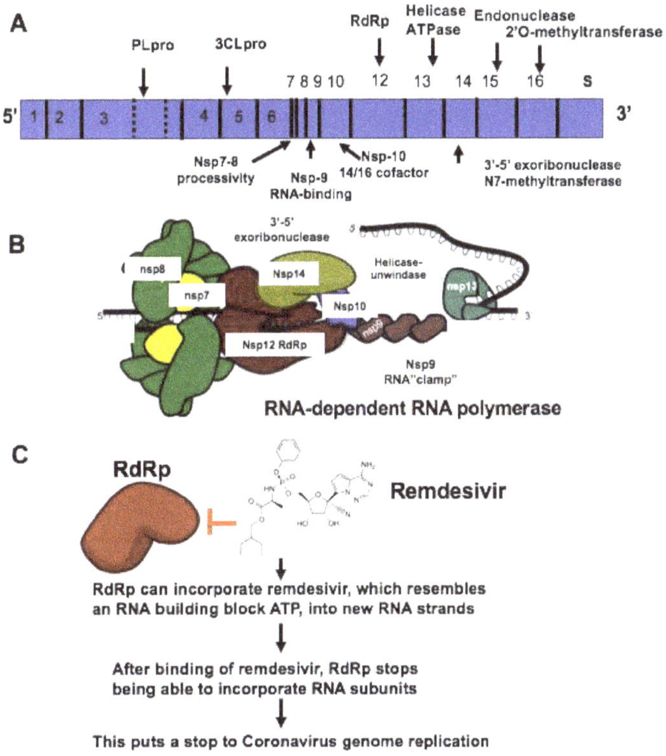

Figure 1. Mechanisms of remdesivir to inhibit RNA-dependent RNA polymerase (RdRp). (**A**) The genome composition model of single strand RNA (ssRNA) of coronavirus. (**B**) The RNA-dependent RNA polymerase RdRp mediated RNA replication during coronavirus infection. (**C**) Remdesivir functions as the ATP analog to inhibit RdRp.

3.2. Factors Involved in Transcription and Release of Coronavirus Particles

Although genome replication and transcription are well known to be regulated by the viral RdRp, several host factors have been implicated in this process. RNA chaperones are usually nonspecific nucleic acid binding proteins, which have long disordered structures that promote RNA molecules to adjust conformational changes. For example, coronavirus nucleoproteins (N protein) have RNA chaperone activity and function as an RNA chaperone, which could help template switching [32–34]. In addition, recent studies demonstrate that glycogen synthase kinase 3 (GSK3) phosphorylates the N protein of SARS-CoV and further inhibition of GSK3 can effectively inhibit viral replication in Vero E6 cells infected with SARS-CoV [35]. Furthermore, heterogeneous nuclear ribonucleoprotein A1 (hnRNP A1) is involved in the pre-mRNA splicing in the nucleus and translation regulation in the host cells. Importantly, it has been shown that the nucleocapsid protein of SARS-CoV had binding ability to human hnRNP A1 with high affinity by using kinetic analyses with a surface plasmon resonance (SPR) approach. These studies suggest that hnRNPA1 is able to bind to SARS-CoV N protein to form a replication/transcription complex and control viral RNA synthesis [36].

In addition, several virus proteins and host factors are essential for the assembly and release of coronavirus. Homotypic interaction of M protein serves as the scaffold for the virus assembly and morphogenesis in the infected cells, specifically, both the interaction between the membrane (M) and S protein and the interaction between M and N protein promote the recruitment of structural components to the assembly location of host cells [37,38]. For example, both envelope (E) protein and N proteins are required to be co-expressed with M protein for the formation and release of virus-like particles (VLPs) after transfection of Vero E6 cells. Two crucial structural proteins, the M protein and E protein, play important roles in the coronavirus assembly. In addition, the E protein is involved in particle assembly by binding with M and further inducing membrane curvature [39]. Subsequently, coronavirus particles can be budded into the ER-Golgi intermediate compartment (ERGIC) of host cells, then trafficked in a smooth-wall vesicle and transported through the secretory pathway for assembly and release by exocytosis [40,41].

4. Current Treatment of Coronavirus

There are two subunits of S protein, including the S1 subunit with a receptor-binding domain that engages with the host cell receptor ACE2, and the S2 subunit involved in regulating fusion between the viral and host cell membranes [42]. The S protein plays important roles in the induction of neutralizing-antibody and leads to T cell responses, so it is involved in protective immunity during infection with SARS-CoV [42]. Vaccines can be developed to specifically recognize the spike protein for SARS and ACE2 receptor [42]. However, mutations of the virus gene and the antibody-dependent enhancement (ADE) effect might affect the efficacy of previously developed biological vaccines, or even spur a counterproductive immune response, although spike protein sequences in SARS-CoV-2 and SARS exhibit some overlap [43–45]. Although it is of importance to develop vaccines and biological therapeutics to prevent the expansion of the SARS-CoV-2, a careful evaluation of possible immune complications is required before applying the vaccine to the public. Therefore, it may take several months or a few years to generate effective vaccines to prevent outbreak. Recent study demonstrates that SARS-CoV-2 has very similar genome sequence identity with severe acute respiratory syndrome-related coronavirus (SARS-CoV) and there is more than 90% sequence similarity in several essential enzymes, such as RNA-dependent RNA polymerase, papain-like proteinase (PLpro), 3CL-protease (3CL-pro) and spike glycoproteins [31]. Dissecting the structure of RdRp may provide new insights into the mechanisms of RNA replication as shown in Figure 2 [23]. Several drug candidates including ribavirin, lopinavir-ritonavir, and favipiravir, have been used previously to treat SARS or MERS, and these compounds may have potential in treating patients with SARS-CoV-2 from this current outbreak [31].

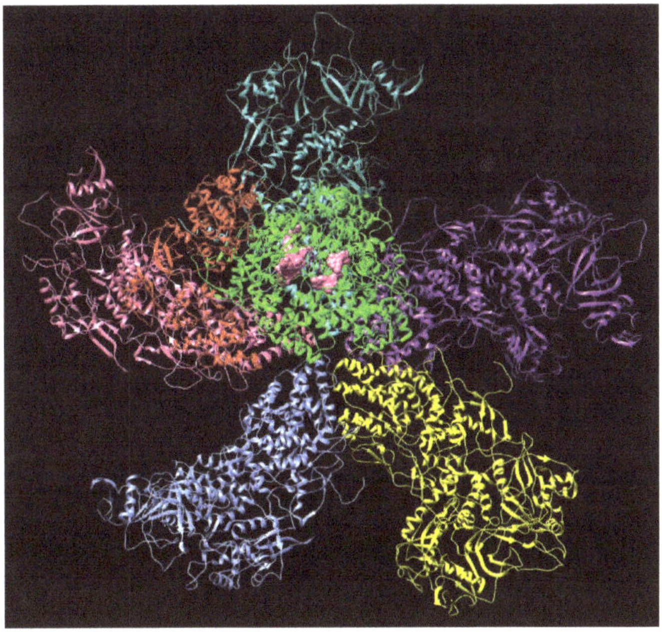

Figure 2. The structure of the RNA-dependent RNA polymerase (RdRp) complexes in the dinucleotide primed state a dsRNA virus (PDB: 6K32 RdRp complex). Chain A is shown as green, chain B is shown as red, chain C is highlighted in cyan, chain D is highlighted in pink, chain E is highlighted in blue, chain F is highlighted in yellow, chain G is highlighted in purple, chain P is highlighted in magenta and chain T is highlighted in orange. The structures demonstrate the interaction between the nucleotide substrates shown in pink and the conserved residues during the RdRp initiation, and the coordinated conformational changes preceding the elongation stage during replication.

5. Current Diagnosis and Treatment of COVID-19

5.1. Current Molecular Diagnostic Assays

Researchers have posted the genome sequence information of SARS-CoV-2 isolated from pneumonia patients on the USCS Genome Browser [10,46]. This helps scientists to establish a real-time reverse transcription PCR (real time RT-PCR) diagnostic assay [47]. It is of importance to detect nucleic acids of SARS-CoV-2 in clinical diagnostics and biotechnology. Clustered regularly interspaced short palindromic repeats (CRISPR) technology, a simple and powerful tool, was initially developed to edit the genome of mammalian cells. Development of rapid, low-cost, and sensitive RNA detection may enhance point-of-care virus detection, genotyping, and disease progression monitoring. The RNA-targeting clustered regularly interspaced short palindromic repeats (CRISPR) effector Cas13a/C2c2 displays an unintentional effect of promiscuous ribonuclease activity along with specific RNA gene target recognition. Recently, a CRISPR-based diagnostic assay, that makes use of nucleic acid pre-amplification and CRISPR–Cas enzymology targeting either spike gene or Orf1ab gene, was established to specifically recognize desired RNA sequences [48]. Effective CRISPR guide RNAs (gRNA) and isothermal amplification primers can be designed to specifically target spike gene and Orf1ab gene. In the specific high-sensitivity enzymatic reporter unlocking (SHERLOCK) assays, coronavirus RNA can be amplified by using recombinase-mediated polymerase amplification with isothermal primers to boost the sensitivity at 37–42 °C. Subsequent Cas13a-mediated recognition of nucleic acid of coronavirus then cleaves the fluorescent RNA probe to separate a fluorophore from its quencher after Cas13a/C2c2 finds its target coronavirus RNA [49]. The cleaved fluorescent products can be readily detected and measured. This rapid CRISPR diagnostic assay can provide specific results in 1 h and will provide timely virus RNA detection with super-high sensitivity and the ability of single-base pair mismatch [48]. Therefore, development of rapid and robust diagnostic assay to measure the nucleic acid of SARS-CoV-2 is crucial for the accurate diagnosis of moderate and severe patients and screening of asymptomatic patients, especially under the current serious health care situation.

5.2. Treatment of COVID-19 with Remdesivir

Currently, there is no effective drug for treating COVID-19 although there was one case reported as having been treated successfully with compassionate use of remdsivir in the US. Recent studies have found that small molecules of remdesivir and chloroquine effectively suppress the replication of SARS-CoV-2 in vitro [24]. According to comparison of genome sequences of SARS-Cov-2 with SARS sequence, the catalytic domains of enzymes such as RdRp are highly conserved in these coronaviruses as shown in Figures 3 and 4. More importantly, it is predictable that the protein sequence of the drug binding pocket of the enzymes is highly conserved [56]. Therefore, these enzymes and spike protein could be very promising drug targets for developing a therapeutic approach for COVID-19 as shown in Table 1 [57,58]. RdRp, also known as nsp12, which catalyzes the synthesis of coronavirus RNA, is an essential enzyme of the coronaviral replication/transcription machinery complex. Recent study revealed the structure of SARS-CoV-2 full-length nsp12 in complex with cofactors nsp7 and nsp8 using cryo-EM [59]. Excepting the conserved features of the polymerase component of the viral polymerase family and key domains for the coronavirus replication shown in RdRp, SARS-CoV-2 nsp12 has a newly featured β-hairpin domain at the N-terminal (PDB: 6M71) as shown in Figure 4. Further comparative analysis has shown how remdesivir binds to the binding pocket of RdRp of SARS-CoV-2 [59]. This structure provides new insight into the key enzyme of the coronaviral replication/transcription complex and lays a solid foundation for the design of new antiviral therapeutics targeting RdRp of SARS-CoV-2.

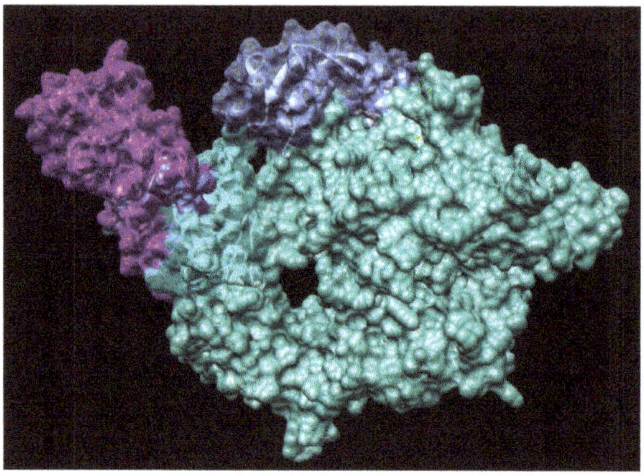

Figure 3. Structure of SARS-Coronavirus RNA polymerase NSP12 complex with NSP7 and NSP8 co-factors (PDB: 6NUR). Chain A is highlighted in light sea green, chain B is shown as blue, chain C is highlighted in cyan, chain D is highlighted in purple.

Remdesivir (GS-5734, Gilead) was initially developed to examine its effect on inhibition of Ebola virus (EBOV) replication [60]. RdRp can incorporate remdesivir, which resembles an RNA building block ATP, into new RNA strands. After binding of remdesivir, RdRp stops being able to incorporate RNA subunits. This puts a stop to the coronavirus genome replication. Enzyme kinetics demonstrated that EBOV RdRp incorporated ATP and remdesivir-TP with comparable efficiencies. The selectivity of

ATP for EBOV RdRp is four times against remdesivir-TP. In comparison, purified human mitochondrial RNA polymerase (h-mtRNAP) effectively distinguished against remdesivir-TP with a selectivity value of about 500-fold [60].

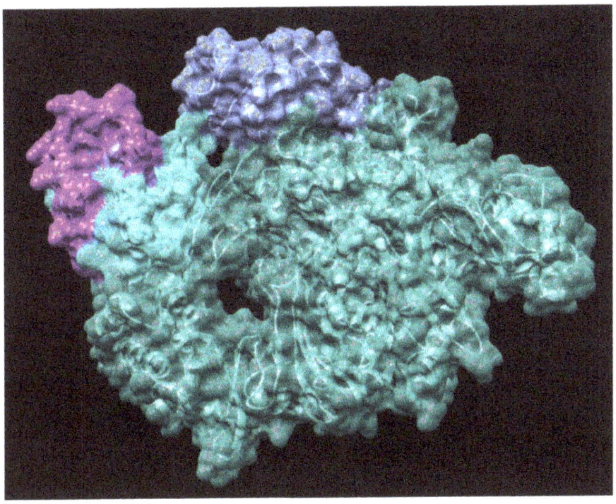

Figure 4. Structure of SARS-CoV-2 RNA polymerase NSP12 complex with NSP7 and NSP8 co-factors (PDB: 6M71). Chain A is highlighted in light sea green, chain B is shown as blue, chain C is highlighted in cyan, chain D is highlighted in purple.

Table 1. Potential pharmacological therapeutics for COVID-19.

Therapeutic Targets	Functions	Potential Drug Candidates	References
RNA-dependent RNA polymerase, RdRp	An RNA-dependent RNA polymerase for replicating coronavirus genome	Remdesivir, Ribavirin and Favipiravir can inhibit viral RdRp	[24]
Papain-like protease, PLpro	A protease for the conversion of viral polyprotein into functional enzyme	Lopinavir, protease inhibitors that may inhibit the viral proteases: 3CLpro or Plpro. Darunavir inhibits the proteolysis activity of 3-chymotrypsin-like protease.	[50]
Main protease 3CLproteinase, 3CLpro	A protease for the conversion of viral polyprotein into functional protein	Lopinavir, protease inhibitors that may inhibit the viral proteases: 3CLpro or Plpro.	[51,52]
S protein and TMPRSS2	A viral surface protein for binding to host cell receptor ACE2. TMPRSS2, a host cell-produced protease that primes S protein to facilitate its binding to ACE2	Arbidol can prevent S protein/ACE2 interaction and inhibit membrane fusion of the viral envelope by preventing the binding of viral envelope protein to host cells and preventing viral entry to the target cell. Camostat mesylate inhibits TMPRSS2 and viral cell entry	[28,53]
ACE2	A viral receptor protein on the host cells which binds to viral S protein	Chloroquine and hydroxychloroquine can inhibits vial entry and endocytosis by increasing endosomal pH, interfere with ACE2 glycosylation as well as host immunomodulatory effects	[54,55]

Remdesivir has been recently developed as a potential antiviral drug candidate against a wide array of RNA virus such as SARS-CoV and MERS-CoV5 infections in both in vitro cell experiment and preclinical studies with mice and nonhuman primate (NHP) models [61]. Recent study examined the efficacy of the broad-acting antiviral remdesivir in the rhesus macaque model of MERS-CoV infection. Interestingly, it was found that administration of remdesivir initiated 24 h prior to inoculation completely restrained MERS-CoV–caused respiratory disease, remarkably suppressed MERS-CoV virus replication in the respiratory system and abolished the progression of lung lesions [62]. These results demonstrated that remdesivir was a potential antiviral therapeutic against MERS and its efficacy could be further examined in clinical trials. Subsequently, recent study has tested the efficacy of remdesivir on inhibition of SARS-CoV-2 replication in vitro [24]. Vero E6 cells were infected with SARS-CoV-2. Different doses of the indicated antivirals were added to treat cells for 48 h. The viral yield from the cell supernatant was then detected by qRT-PCR. It is worth noting that two compounds, remdesivir significantly abolished virus infection at high affinity [24]. This also suggests the possibility that remdesivir has efficacy for related coronaviruses such as the novel coronavirus SARS-CoV-2 [62]. More importantly, administration to patients with COVID-19 of remdesivir has been shown to be effective in treating one patient for the purpose of compassionate use in the US, and there was no adverse event observed in association with infusion of remdesivir.

5.3. *Pharmacological Therapeutics Targeting Proteinase of SARS-Cov-2*

Due to the COVID-19 pandemic and global health concern, it is urgent to develop effective broad-spectrum virus replication inhibitors to manage patients with COVID-19. Drug targets among coronaviruses include the main protease 3CL(pro) and papain-like protease(PLpro). These proteinase play essential roles in processing polyproteins and viral replication. The structures of the unliganded SARS-CoV-2 M(pro) and its complex with an alpha-ketoamide inhibitor have been recently revealed [52]. Comparison of genome sequences of SARS-CoV-2 with SARS sequence indicates that the catalytic domains of proteinase are highly conserved in these coronaviruses. Therefore, it is plausible to repurpose the compound library for treatment of SARS-CoV for developing potential therapeutics for SARS-CoV-2. Computational analysis was also used to screen the effective and potent cysteine protease inhibitors for malaria and SARS infection [63–65]. Recently, a series of N-(tert-Butyl)-2-(N-arylamido)-2-(pyridin-3-yl) acetamides (ML188) were identified as potent noncovalent small molecule inhibitors targeting SARS-CoV 3CL protease [66,67]. In addition, the analogues of keto-glutamine were developed as potent inhibitors for treatment of SARS infection [68,69]. Furthermore, recent study has shown that compounds containing electrophilic arylketone moiety were designed and synthesized as new SARS-Cov 3CL protease inhibitors [70]. The anilide derived from 2-chloro-4-nitroaniline, l-phenylalanine and 4-(dimethylamino)benzoic acid was found to be a competitive inhibitor of the SARS-CoV 3CL protease with K(i) = 0.03 uM by using a fluorogenic tetradecapeptide substrate [70,71]. It is demonstrated that trioxa-adamantane-triols (TATs) (BN, IBNCA, VANBA, euBN), trivially termed bananins, were identified to be effective inhibitors of SARS-CoV NSP10/nsp13 RNA/DNA helicase/NTPase protein ATPase enzymatic function. Bananin (BN) effectively suppresses both SARS-CoV RNA/DNA helicase nucleic acid unwinding function and SARS-CoV RNA-viral replication in cell culture [72]. In addition, high-throughput screening (HTS) approaches were used to screen potent inhibitors of the SARS-CoV main proteinase [73,74]. Recent computational studies found that lopinavir, oseltamivir and ritonavir are able to bind with SARS-CoV-2 protease [75]. Potential therapeutic options targeting the main protease 3CLpro were identified for SARS-CoV-2, including covalent drugs (approved or clinically tested). There were at least six hits among the total of 11 potential hits identified by using the SCAR protocol [76]. Therefore, it will be intriguing to determine whether these compounds might be effective for inhibiting the activity of proteinase of SARS-CoV-2 in vitro and reducing the replication of the virus in treating novel coronavirus SARS-CoV-2 infection.

5.4. *Broad-Spectrum Antiviral Compounds NHC and EIDD-2801*

No therapies specific or effective for human coronavirus SARS-CoV-2 have been approved by Food and Drug Administration (FDA). β-D-N4-hydroxycytidine (NHC, EIDD-1931) was initially synthesized as an orally bioavailable ribonucleoside analog with broad-spectrum antiviral activity against various RNA viruses such as Ebola [77]. Recent study discovered that NHC effectively inhibited MERS-CoV and newly emerging SARS-CoV-2 replication using antiviral assays in the human lung epithelial cell line Calu-3 2B4 ("Calu3" cells) [78]. NHC has shown potent antiviral activity with an average half-maximum effective concentration (IC50) of 0.15 μM for cells with a recombinant MERS-CoV expressing nanoluciferase (MERS-nLUC), and there is no observed cytotoxicity. In addition, NHC was potently antiviral with an IC50 of 0.3 μM and CC50 of >10 μM when using a clinically isolated strain of SARS-CoV2 infected African green monkey kidney (Vero) cells [78]. Furthermore, NHC is highly effective for preventing the virus replication of SARS-CoV-2, MERS-CoV as well as SARS-CoV infection in primary human airway epithelial cell cultures [78]. More importantly, NHC inhibited the replication of remdesivir (RDV)-resistant virus and multiple distinct zoonotic CoV [77]. EIDD-2801, an orally bioavailable prodrug of NHC (β-D-N4-hydroxycytidine-5′-isopropyl ester) designed for improved in vivo pharmacokinetics, remarkably reduced SARS-CoV replication and pathogenesis, significantly decreased MERS-CoV infectious titers, and reduced viral RNA and pathogenesis under both prophylactic and early therapeutic conditions in mice [78]. These studies indicate that EIDD-2801 could not only provide effective treatment of SARS-CoV-2 infection, but also enable the prevention of the spread of SARS-CoV-2 and control future outbreaks of other emerging coronaviruses. It is worth noting that animal experiments and human clinical trials are needed to examine its efficacy for treatment of COVID-19.

5.5. Application of Anti-Viral Natural Products for Treatment of COVID-19

Under the current outbreak of COVID-19, it is necessary to repurpose natural products to manage patients with COVID-19. Recent studies have shown that hydroxychloroquine can improve the outcomes of COVID-19 patients in small clinical trials although it should be used with caution on humans due to its toxicity. There are a large number of natural products with known safety profiles, such as isoflavones and artemisinin. Recent study has shown that several isoflavones and related flavonoid compounds have potent antiviral properties. In this regards, natural products that have been repurposed for broad-spectrum anti-viral therapy can offer safe and inexpensive platforms for discovery of efficient and novel agents for treatment of SARS-CoV-2. It will be of significance if these FDA-approved drugs could be repurposed for treatment of COVID-19.

Recent studies found that naturally occurring flavonoids exhibit a broad-spectrum of antiviral effects against RNA virus such as polio-virus type 1, parainfluenza virus type 3 (Pf-3), and respiratory syncytial virus (RSV) by inhibiting their replication [79]. Computational drug design methods were used to identify Chymotrypsin-like protease inhibitors from FDA approved natural and drug-like compounds [80]. It has been shown that two natural compounds including flavone and coumarine derivatives were identified as promising hits of proteinase inhibitors of SARS-CoV-2 [80]. In addition, recent study has shown that hydroxychloroquine, an anti-malarial drug, significantly abolished SARS-CoV-2 infection [77]. Consistent with this, hydroxychloroquine in combination with azithromycin treatment improved the outcomes of COVID-19 patients in a small clinical study although it should be cautious due to its adverse effects. [81]. Quinine bark was one of the most extensively used therapeutic approached for malaria during the mid-1800s, which provides evidence that chemical compounds from natural products can be used successfully to treat an infectious disease [82,83]. In addition, 36 alkaloids, alcohol extracts and chloroquine are effective in blocking the polymerization process in parasites. One of the main derivatives of quinine, mefloquine, was discovered to suppress the uptake of chloroquine in infected cells by blocking ingestion of hemoglobin to prevent parasite infection [82,83]. Previous study demonstrated that chloroquine inhibited the replication of severe acute respiratory syndrome coronavirus in vitro [84]. Because there is no effective treatment of COVID-19, the extensive outbreak of constant human to human transmission prompts us to apply broad-spectrum anti-viral natural products to prevent or improve the condition of patients with SARS-CoV-2 [43,85].

Recent study revealed that the protein sequence of the drug binding pocket of the enzymes is highly homogeneous between SARS-CoV and SARS-CoV-2 [86]. Much progress has been made in the application of natural products and the development of novel therapy for SARS infection [87–90], for example, a new type of effective inhibitor was identified for inhibition of SARS-CoV proteinase by using substrate specificity profiling [72,91,92]. In addition to chloroquine, an anti-malaria natural product artemisinin has anti-viral activity although the mechanism of artemisinin to in inhibiting virus infection is unknown [93–95]. Natural products Tordylium persicum Boiss & Hausskn extract have also been identified for treatment of HIV [96]. Consistent with this, Cuscuta campestris crude extracts have been demonstrated to be effective for inhibition of HIV replication [97]. Cell-based screening assay has been developed to screen virus-specific and broad-spectrum inhibitors for treatment of coronavirus infection [98–100]. Therefore, it is necessary to examine the efficacy of artemisinin and other natural products on COVID-19 replication and infection. Another study has shown that the administration of hydroxychloroquine reduced the morbidity of COVID-19 pneumonia [101–103]. Chloroquine in clinical trials with a large number of patients will be further examined for treatment of COVID-19 [104]. Some traditional Chinese medicines such as Polygonum cuspidatum that may consist of components with efficacy against COVID-19 have been examined in clinical trials [105]. The pro-inflammatory metabolites of arachidonic acid (AA) and eicosapentaenoic acid (EPA) such as leukotrienes and thromboxanes promote inflammation, whereas lipoxins, resolvins, protectins and maresins derived from AA, EPA and DHA facilitate wound healing, promote phagocytosis of macrophages and other immunocytes and decrease microbial load [106]. It is implicated that these unsaturated fatty acids and pro-inflammatory metabolites may serve as endogenous anti-viral compounds. It is intriguing to determine the efficacy of the metabolites on prevention of SARS-CoV-2 infection [107]. In addition, using structure-based drug selection for identification of SARS-CoV-2 protease inhibitors, old drugs such as macrolides were predicted to be effective against COVID-19 [108]. Therefore, treatments with macrolides alone or in combination with other drugs may be promising and provide the possibility of a new strategy to fight this emerging SARS-CoV-2 infection.

6. Spike Glycoproteins of SARS-CoV-2 and ACE2

Revealing the structural-functional relationships of the S protein of SARS-CoV-2 will provide new insights into inhibition of interactions between S protein and angiotensin-converting enzyme 2 (ACE2) to develop novel therapeutic approaches for coronavirus. More studies are focused on investigating the mechanism of coronavirus invasion into host cells. Similar to SARS–CoV and MERS-CoV, the novel coronavirus SARS-CoV-2 is armed with a large "spike protein", which is used to interact with host cells and then gain entry through the cell membrane [109,110]. Recent study has discovered the structure of MERS-CoV spike glycoprotein in complex with sialoside attachment receptors (PDB: 4KR0) [111]. MERS-CoV Spike glycoprotein is composed of an N-terminal S1 subunit, which is assembled as four domains (A–D) and controls attachment to dipeptidyl-peptidase 4 (DPP4, the host receptor), and a C-terminal S2 subunit that combines the viral and cellular membranes to initiate infection, as shown in Figure 5 [111].

Angiotensin-converting enzyme 2 (ACE2) is required for coronavirus invasion into host cells. The viral spike glycoprotein utilizes ACE2 as a host protein receptor and mediates merging of the viral and host membranes. This allows viral entry into host epithelial cells and host species tropism [112]. Given that the structure of S protein (PDB ID:6VSB) of SARS-CoV-2 is revealed [30,86], more computational analysis and virtual screening could be performed to identify the potential inhibitors of S protein and ACE2 interaction as shown in Figure 6. In addition, recent study has shown that S-phase kinase-associated protein 2 (SKP2) is necessary for lysine-48-linked poly-ubiquitination of beclin 1, leading to its proteasomal degradation. Suppression of SKP2 promotes autophagy and decreases MERS coronavirus replication [113]. Recent study demonstrate that SARS-CoV-2 uses the SARS-CoV receptor ACE2 for invasion and the transmembrane protease serine 2 (TMPRSS2) for S protein priming [28]. A clinically proven protease inhibitor, camostat mesylate, has been demonstrated to inhibit Calu-3 infection with SARS-CoV-2 and prevent SARS-2-Spike protein (S protein)-mediated entry into primary human lung cells [28]. In addition, recent study demonstrated that a neutralizing antibody CR3022 targets a highly conserved epitope, distal from the receptor-binding site, that enables cross-reactive binding between SARS-CoV-2 and SARS-CoV. The structure of CR3022 in complex with the receptor-binding domain (RBD) of the SARS-CoV-2 spike (S) protein has been revealed. The modeling study further proved that the binding epitope can only be targeted by CR3022 when the conformational changes with two RBD on the trimeric S protein are in the "up" orientation. This provides a molecular mechanism in the binding of the antibody with S protein of SARS-CoV-2 [114]. In line with this result, recent study demonstrates a highly potent pan-coronavirus fusion inhibitor targeting its spike protein that harbors a high capacity to mediate membrane fusion, and inhibited SARS-CoV-2 infection [115]. The molecular mechanisms of coronavirus invasion into host cells will provide new insights into the development of therapeutic approaches for COVID-19 by targeting spike proteins and ACE2 [116–118].

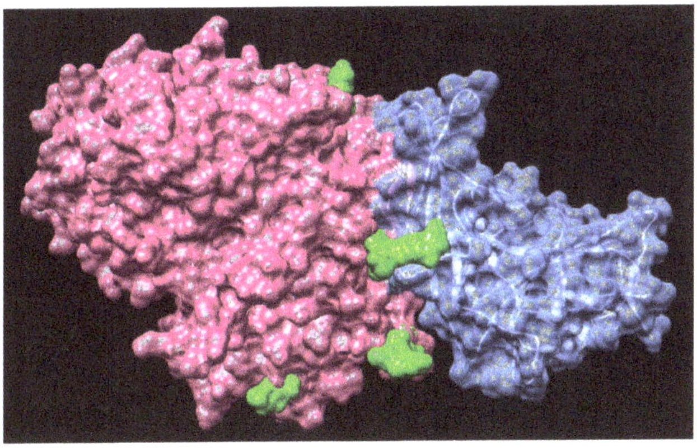

Figure 5. Structures of MERS-CoV spike glycoprotein in complex with sialoside attachment receptors (PDB: 4KR0). MERS-CoV Spike glycoprotein is composed of an N-terminal S1 subunit, which is assembled as four domains (A–D) and controls attachment to dipeptidyl-peptidase 4 (DPP4, the host receptor), and a C-terminal S2 subunit that combines the viral and cellular membranes to initiate infection. Spike glycoprotein is highlighted in pink, DPP4 is highlighted in blue and the ligand Neu5Ac is highlighted in green.

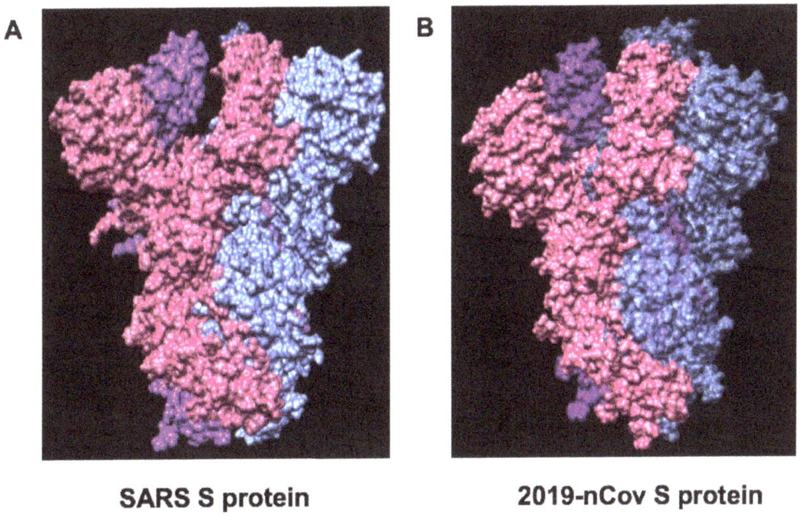

Figure 6. Comparison of Spike glycoprotein structures between SARS (PDB ID:6CRZ) and SARS-Cov-2 (PDB ID:6VSB). (**A**) SARS Spike glycoprotein is composed of NTD, RBD, SD1 and SD2, S2 subunit. The SARS-CoV S trimer is highlighted as a molecular surface with each protomer colored blue, pink or purple. (**B**) SARS-CoV-2 trimer is highlighted as a molecular surface with each protomer colored blue, pink or purple.

7. Clinical trials of Remdesivir for Treatment of COVID-19 in China

The outbreak of COVID-19, and previous devastating SARS and MERS-CoV, highlight the importance for developing effective approaches for treatment of human coronavirus infections (SARS coronavirus anti-infectives). This will decrease risk of disease dissemination, ameliorate disease progression, and bring down the need for intensive supportive care. Furthermore, treatments for moderate cases to decrease the time span of illness and infectivity may also be of significance for preventing COVID19 from becoming more wide-spread. Recent study demonstrated that there was no observed benefit with lopinavir–ritonavir treatment in hospitalized adult patients with severe COVID-19 [119]. Future trials in patients with severe illness may help to confirm or exclude the possibility of treatment benefit. We mainly compare two ongoing clinical trials with remdesivir for treatment of SARS-CoV-2 infection. The first one targets mild/moderate patients, the second severe cases with SARS-CoV-2 infection.

7.1. Treatment of Mild/Moderate Case of COVID-19 with Remdesivir RCT (ClinicalTrials.gov Identifier: NCT04252664)

Because there is no specific antiviral treatment for COVID-19 infection, the widely investigated small molecule compound remdesvir could be a potential antiviral agent, based on pre-clinical studies in SARS-CoV and MERS-CoV infections. Remdesivir is a 1′-cyano-substituted adenosine nucleotide analogue prodrug that can be metabolized into its active form to exhibit broad-spectrum antiviral activity against coronavirus as shown in Figure 7. A phase 3 randomized, double-blind, placebo-controlled study was designed to examine the efficacy of remdsivir in adult patients with mild/moderate COVID-19 respiratory disease. The inclusion criteria include: (1) laboratory RT-PCR confirmed patients infected with SARS-CoV-2; (2) lung involvement confirmed with CT imaging. The exclusion criteria include: patients with SaO2/SPO2≤94% in room air condition; severe liver disease and severe renal impairment; and patients with any experimental treatment for COVID-19 (off-label, compassionate use, or trial related). 308 participants have been recruited and the clinical trial outcome will be released at the end of April 2020.

Remdesivir (GS-5734, Gilead)	**Formula: C27H35N6O8P MW:602.6g/mole Nucleotide analogs, Gilead**	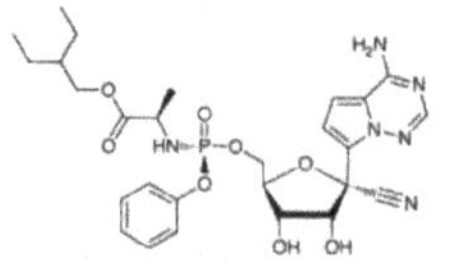
Ribavirin an adenosine analog, nucleoside inhibitor	**Formula: C8H12N4O5 MW: 244.21g/mole International Chemical and Nuclear Corporation**	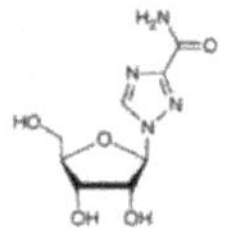
Galidesivir (BCX-4430) an adenosine analog	**Formula: C11H15N5O3 MW: 256.27 BioCryst Pharmaceuticals**	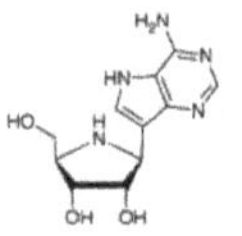
Favipiravir (T705)	**Formula: C5H4FN3O2 MW: 157.1 6-fluoro-3-hydroxy-2-pyrazinecarboxamide, Toyama Chemical of Japan**	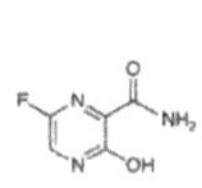

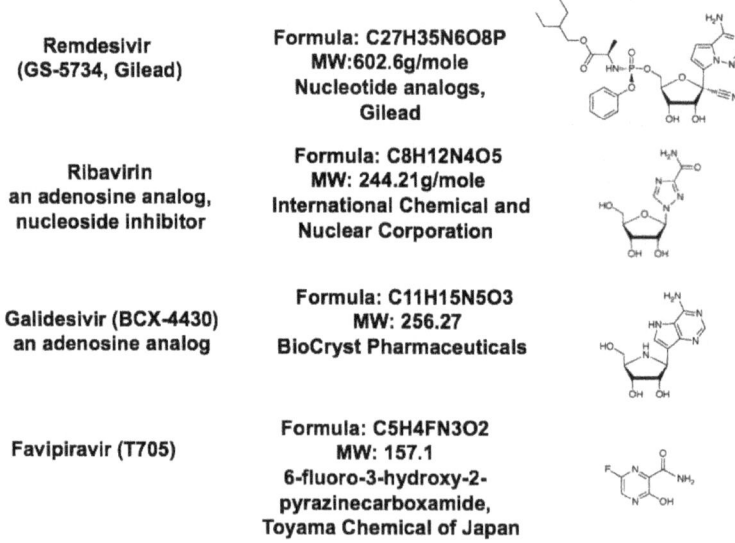

Figure 7. Structures of nucleotide substrate analogues.

7.2. Treatment of Severe Case of COVID-19 with Remdesivir RCT (ClinicalTrials.gov Identifier: NCT04257656)

There are no therapeutics proven effective for the treatment of severe illness caused by SARS-CoV-2, so a phase 3 randomized, double-blind, placebo-controlled study was designed to examine the efficacy of remdsivir in adult patients with severe COVID-19 respiratory disease. The clinical trial is sponsored by Capital Medical University and China-Japan Friendship Hospital. The inclusion criteria include: (1) confirmation of COVID-19 by using laboratory RT-PCR; (2) less than 12 days since symptom; (3) lung involvement confirmed with CT chest imaging; (4) patients with a SaO2/SPO2 ≤ 94% in room air condition. The exclusion criteria include: severe liver disease and severe renal impairment; and patients with any experimental treatment for COVID-19 (off-label, compassionate use, or trial related). 452 participants will be recruited and the clinical trial outcome will be released in May 2020. In adults presenting with hypoxic respiratory failure or acute respiratory distress syndrome (ARDS) from COVID-19, invasive mechanical ventilation, a conservative fluid strategy over a liberal fluid strategy, and intermittent boluses of neuromuscular blocking agents (NMBA) to facilitate protective lung ventilation are necessary for supporting treatment [120]. For severe ARDS cases, the routine use of inhaled nitric oxide is recommended [120]. A randomized, controlled clinical trial to evaluate the safety and efficacy of the investigation of antiviral remdesivir in hospitalized patients with COVID-19 has also initiated at the University of Nebraska Medical Center (UNMC) in Omaha. These clinical trials will be of significance for therapy involving severe cases of COVID-19 after completion of examining the efficacy of remdesivir to treat COVID-19.

Recent studies have shown that SARS-CoV-2 receptor ACE2 and transmembrane protease serine 2 (TMPRSS2) are primarily expressed in bronchial transient secretory cells, which provides the rationale that supporting treatment on lung should be emphasized [121]. The expression of ACE2 can be upregulated by smoking in humans [122], therefore, smoking status should be included for information of identified cases of COVID-19. In addition, it is crucial to manage patients with inherited arrhythmia syndromes such as long QT syndrome and short QT syndrome in the setting of the COVID-19 pandemic [123]. Patients with inherited arrhythmia may be susceptible to pro-arrhythmic factors of COVID-19 such as use of antiviral drugs, fever, stress, and electrolyte imbalance [123,124]. The current studies on potential therapeutic agents, such as lopinavir/ritonavir, favipiravir, chloroquine, hydroxychloroquine, interferon, ribavirin, tocilizumab and sarilumab are important for management of COVID-19 [51,125]. More clinical trials are being conducted for further confirmation of the efficacy and safety of these agents in treating COVID-19 [126].

8. Coronavirus and Host Interaction

Several host factors regulate the replication of coronavirus and induce dramatic changes in the host cellular structure and function, simultaneously. Induction of critical signaling proteins is crucial for the pathogenesis of CoV and is also involved in the activation of the innate immune response during CoV infection. Neutrophils are the first immune cells recruited to sites of viral infection. Recent studies demonstrate that excessive recruitment of neutrophils and formation of neutrophil extracellular traps results in acute lung injury of influenza pneumonitis [127]. In addition, neutrophil-derived myeloperoxidase (MPO) serves as a potent tissue damage factor and also contributes to influenza pneumonia in mice infected with influenza virus [128–131]. In addition, coronavirus infection is able to induce stress response, autophagy, apoptosis, and activate innate immunity [40]. Host cell apoptosis caused by CoV infection has been extensively studied, for example, SARS-CoV and MERS-CoV infect and induce apoptosis in a variety of tissues including lung, spleen, thyroid tissues, and a variety of cell types, such as respiratory epithelial cells, neuronal cells, primary T lymphocytes, and dendritic cells [132,133]. In addition, overexpression of SARS-CoV S was shown to induce a potent ER stress response, and the re-arrangement of DMV production and membrane alteration for the assembly of the virus may contribute to endoplasmic reticulum (ER) stress during CoV infection [40]. Unfolded protein response (UPR) -mediated signaling pathway was induced to maintain ER homeostasis [134,135]. The IRE1 branch of UPR promotes cell survival during CoV infection and CoV infection activates

JNK to modulate apoptosis induction [136,137]. Induction of cell apoptosis provided the possible explanations for the fact that lymphopenia was observed in some patients with CoV infection, such as SARS-CoV and SARS-CoV-2. Immune cell apoptosis may lead to the suppression of host immune response and promote the occurring of ARDS.

Coronavirus infection promotes the activation of inflammasome in host cells and activates innate immunity [138,139]. In macrophages, ORF8b provides a potent signal 2 required for activation of inflammasome and activates the NLRP3 (NOD-, LRR- and pyrin domain-containing protein 3) to form the inflammasome complex. Specifically, ORF8b is able to interact directly with the Leucine Rich Repeat (LRR) domain of NLRP3 and bind with apoptosis-associated speck-like protein containing a CARD (ASC) in cytosolic dot-like structures [140]. ORF8b induces cell apoptosis and pyroptotic cell death in macrophages, while in those cells lacking NLRP3, accumulating ORF8b cytosolic substances lead to mitochondrial dysfunction, activation of inflammasome and caspase-independent cell death [140,141]. Recent genome-wide and transcriptome-wide complementary network analysis of SARS-CoV-2/human interaction provided a new network of host proteins affected by the SARS-CoV-2 infection [141]. It has been shown that ACE2 is downregulated in the presence of viral infection, therefore application of recombinant ACE2 has been shown to be effective in treating severe pulmonary infections and acute respiratory distress syndrome [142]. Recent studies demonstrate that soluble forms of ACE2 are beneficial to SARS patients, due to its competitive binders of SARS-CoV Spike proteins, preventing binding to the host cell ACE2 [143].

9. Concluding Remarks

Recent study indicate that there is a substantial number of undocumented infections and this facilitates the rapid dissemination of SARS-CoV2 [144]. These findings explain the rapid geographic spread of SARS-CoV2 and indicate containment of this virus will be particularly challenging. It is also informative to help understand the potential for infection by non-symptomatic subjects. Therefore, one of the most important strategies of management of COVID-19 infection is to effectively reduce the possibility of constant human-to-human viral transmission [145]. Keeping social distancing, contact tracing and quarantine are necessary for preventing substantial human to human transmission of COVID-19 [146–148]. Recent study demonstrated that the affinity of the SARS-CoV-2 S protein with ACE2 was 10- to 20-fold higher than the SARS-CoV S protein as shown in Figure 5 [30], which explains the observations of rapid transmission from human-to-human in COVID-19 infection. Genetic analyses of hundreds of SARS-CoV-2 genomes revealed that there were two major types, L type and S type [149]. It seems that the L type (~70%) was more dominant than the S type (~30%). The L type was more common in the early stages of the outbreak in China. Artificial intervention may have put selective pressure on the L type, which might be more susceptible to mutate and spread more widely [149]. It is very challenging to makes an effective vaccine because of the rapid mutation of ssRNA and the antibody-dependent enhancement (ADE) effect [149]. Therefore, it is urgent to develop effective medicine for treatment of moderate and severe patients with low SpO2. Remdsivir may be potentially developed for treatment of COVID-19 after completing the phase 3 randomized, double-blind, placebo-controlled study to examine its efficacy in patients with COVID-19. In addition, better understanding of the mechanisms of coronavirus invasion into host cells could accelerate discovery of new inhibitors of interaction of spike glycoproteins and ACE2 and promote the development of therapeutic approaches for COVID-19. Finally, by drawing lessons from mechanisms of replication of SARS-CoV-2 RNA-dependent RNA polymerase, development of potent and effective RdRp inhibitors will provide new insights required for putting RdRp targeted therapeutics into full gear.

Author Contributions: J.H., Q.S., wrote this review. H.H dealt with the figures and edited the review. W.S. edited the review and made critical comments throughout. All authors have read and agreed to the published version of the manuscript.

Funding: This research was based upon work funded by Jiangsu University talent cultivation program:18JDG023 (Q.S.) and the Jiangsu "Mass Innovation and Entrepreneurship" (Shuang Chuang Ph.Ds) Talent Program (Q.S.).

Conflicts of Interest: The authors declare no conflict of interest.

Abbreviations

ARDS	Acute respiratory distress syndrome
ADE	Antibody-dependent enhancement
SARS-Cov-2	Severe acute respiratory syndrome coronavirus 2
COVID-19	Novel Coronavirus disease-2019
3CLpro	Coronavirus main proteinase
ACE2	Angiotensin-converting Enzyme 2
CRISPR	Clustered Regularly Interspaced Short Palindromic Repeats
Cov	Coronavirus
dsRNA	Double strand RNA
DPP4	Dipeptidyl-peptidase 4
ERGIC	ER-Golgi intermediate compartment
EBOV	Ebola virus
gRNA	Guide RNA
GSK3	Glycogen synthase kinase 3
hM-RNAP	Human mitochondrial RNA polymerase
Orf1	Open reading frame 1
PLpro	Papain-like protease
MERS	Middle East Respiratory Syndrome
MPO	Myeloperoxidase
NTD	N-terminal domain
NMBA	Neuromuscular blocking agents
NHC	β-D-N4-hydroxycytidine
N protein	Coronavirus nucleoproteins
NLRP3	NOD-, LRR- and pyrin domain-containing protein 3
RBD	Receptor-binding domain
RT-PCR	Reverse transcription PCR
SARS	Severe Acute Respiratory Syndrome
S protein	Spike glycoprotein
ssRNA	Single strand RNA
SPR	Surface plasmon resonance
SKP2	S-phase kinase-associated protein 2
SpO2	Peripheral capillary oxygen saturation
RdRp	RNA-dependent RNA Polymerase
RBD	Receptor-binding domain
TMPSS2	Transmembrane protease serine 2
TATs	Trioxa-adamantane-triols
UPR	Unfolded protein response
VLPs	Virus-like particles

References

1. Service, R.F. Coronavirus epidemic snarls science worldwide. *Science* **2020**, *367*, 836–837. [CrossRef] [PubMed]
2. WHO. *Coronavirus Disease (COVID-19) Pandemic*; World Health Organization: Geneva, Switzerland, 2020.
3. Park, M.; Cook, A.; Lim, J.T.; Sun, Y.; Dickens, B. A Systematic Review of COVID-19 Epidemiology Based on Current Evidence. *J. Clin. Med.* **2020**, *9*, 967. [CrossRef] [PubMed]
4. Spellberg, B.; Haddix, M.; Lee, R.; Butler-Wu, S.; Holtom, P.; Yee, H.; Gounder, P. Community Prevalence of SARS-CoV-2 Among Patients With Influenzalike Illnesses Presenting to a Los Angeles Medical Center in March 2020. *JAMA* **2020**. [CrossRef] [PubMed]
5. Bourouiba, L. Turbulent Gas Clouds and Respiratory Pathogen Emissions: Potential Implications for Reducing Transmission of COVID-19. *JAMA* **2020**. [CrossRef] [PubMed]

6. Del Rio, C.; Malani, P.N. 2019 Novel Coronavirus—Important Information for Clinicians. *JAMA* **2020**, *323*, 1039. [CrossRef]
7. Chan, J.F.-W.; Yuan, S.; Kok, K.-H.; To, K.K.-W.; Chu, H.; Yang, J.; Xing, F.; Liu, J.; Yip, C.C.-Y.; Poon, R.W.-S.; et al. A familial cluster of pneumonia associated with the 2019 novel coronavirus indicating person-to-person transmission: A study of a family cluster. *Lancet* **2020**, *395*, 514–523. [CrossRef]
8. Heymann, D.L. Data sharing and outbreaks: Best practice exemplified. *Lancet* **2020**, *395*, 469–470. [CrossRef]
9. Huang, C.; Wang, Y.; Li, X.; Ren, L.; Zhao, J.; Hu, Y.; Zhang, L.; Fan, G.; Xu, J.; Gu, X.; et al. Clinical features of patients infected with 2019 novel coronavirus in Wuhan, China. *Lancet* **2020**, *395*, 497–506. [CrossRef]
10. Lu, R.; Zhao, X.; Li, J.; Niu, P.; Yang, B.; Wu, H.; Wang, W.; Song, H.; Huang, B.; Zhu, N.; et al. Genomic characterisation and epidemiology of 2019 novel coronavirus: Implications for virus origins and receptor binding. *Lancet* **2020**, *395*, 565–574. [CrossRef]
11. Cao, Y.-C.; Deng, Q.-X.; Dai, S.-X. Remdesivir for severe acute respiratory syndrome coronavirus 2 causing COVID-19: An evaluation of the evidence. *Travel Med. Infect. Dis.* **2020**. [CrossRef]
12. Zhou, P.; Yang, X.-L.; Wang, X.-G.; Hu, B.; Zhang, L.; Zhang, W.; Si, H.-R.; Zhu, Y.; Li, B.; Huang, C.-L.; et al. A pneumonia outbreak associated with a new coronavirus of probable bat origin. *Nature* **2020**, *579*, 270–273. [CrossRef] [PubMed]
13. Li, Q.; Guan, X.; Wu, P.; Wang, X.; Zhou, L.; Tong, Y.; Ren, R.; Leung, K.S.; Lau, E.H.; Wong, J.Y.; et al. Early Transmission Dynamics in Wuhan, China, of Novel Coronavirus–Infected Pneumonia. *N. Engl. J. Med.* **2020**, *382*, 1199–1207. [CrossRef] [PubMed]
14. Xia, J.; Tong, J.; Liu, M.; Shen, Y.; Guo, D. Evaluation of coronavirus in tears and conjunctival secretions of patients with SARS-CoV-2 infection. *J. Med. Virol.* **2020**. [CrossRef] [PubMed]
15. Yang, W.; Cao, Q.; Qin, L.; Wang, X.; Cheng, Z.; Pan, A.; Dai, J.; Sun, Q.; Zhao, F.; Qu, J.; et al. Clinical characteristics and imaging manifestations of the 2019 novel coronavirus disease (COVID-19):A multi-center study in Wenzhou city, Zhejiang, China. *J. Infect.* **2020**, *80*, 388–393. [CrossRef] [PubMed]
16. Guan, W.-J.; Ni, Z.-Y.; Hu, Y.; Liang, W.-H.; Ou, C.-Q.; He, J.-X.; Liu, L.; Shan, H.; Lei, C.-L.; Hui, D.S.; et al. Clinical Characteristics of Coronavirus Disease 2019 in China. *N. Engl. J. Med.* **2020**. [CrossRef] [PubMed]
17. Wu, F.; Zhao, S.; Yu, B.; Chen, Y.-M.; Wang, W.; Song, Z.-G.; Hu, Y.; Tao, Z.-W.; Tian, J.-H.; Pei, Y.-Y.; et al. A new coronavirus associated with human respiratory disease in China. *Nature* **2020**, *579*, 265–269. [CrossRef]
18. Lei, J.; Li, J.; Li, X.; Qi, X. CT Imaging of the 2019 Novel Coronavirus (2019-nCoV) Pneumonia. *Radiology* **2020**, *295*, 18. [CrossRef]
19. Wu, P.; Duan, F.; Luo, C.; Liu, Q.; Qu, X.; Liang, L.; Wu, K. Characteristics of Ocular Findings of Patients With Coronavirus Disease 2019 (COVID-19) in Hubei Province, China. *JAMA Ophthalmol.* **2020**. [CrossRef]
20. Chen, N.; Zhou, M.; Dong, X.; Qu, J.; Gong, F.; Han, Y.; Qiu, Y.; Wang, J.; Liu, Y.; Wei, Y.; et al. Epidemiological and clinical characteristics of 99 cases of 2019 novel coronavirus pneumonia in Wuhan, China: A descriptive study. *Lancet* **2020**, *395*, 507–513. [CrossRef]
21. Xu, Z.; Shi, L.; Wang, Y.; Zhang, J.; Huang, L.; Zhang, C.; Liu, S.; Zhao, P.; Liu, H.; Zhu, L.; et al. Pathological findings of COVID-19 associated with acute respiratory distress syndrome. *Lancet Respir. Med.* **2020**, *8*, 420–422. [CrossRef]
22. Liu, J.; Zheng, X.; Tong, Q.; Li, W.; Wang, B.; Sutter, K.; Trilling, M.; Lu, M.; Dittmer, U.; Yang, D. Overlapping and discrete aspects of the pathology and pathogenesis of the emerging human pathogenic coronaviruses SARS-CoV, MERS-CoV, and 2019-nCoV. *J. Med.Virol.* **2020**. [CrossRef] [PubMed]
23. Xu, X.-W.; Wu, X.-X.; Jiang, X.-G.; Xu, K.-J.; Ying, L.-J.; Ma, C.-L.; Li, S.-B.; Wang, H.-Y.; Zhang, S.; Gao, H.-N.; et al. Clinical findings in a group of patients infected with the 2019 novel coronavirus (SARS-Cov-2) outside of Wuhan, China: Retrospective case series. *BMJ* **2020**, *368*, 606. [CrossRef] [PubMed]
24. Wang, M.; Cao, R.; Zhang, L.; Yang, X.; Liu, J.; Xu, M.; Shi, Z.; Hu, Z.; Zhong, W.; Xiao, G. Remdesivir and chloroquine effectively inhibit the recently emerged novel coronavirus (2019-nCoV) in vitro. *Cell Res.* **2020**, *30*, 269–271. [CrossRef]
25. Holshue, M.L.; DeBolt, C.; Lindquist, S.; Lofy, K.H.; Wiesman, J.; Bruce, H.; Spitters, C.; Ericson, K.; Wilkerson, S.; Tural, A.; et al. First Case of 2019 Novel Coronavirus in the United States. *N. Engl. J. Med.* **2020**, *382*, 929–936. [CrossRef]
26. Xia, S.; Zhu, Y.; Liu, M.; Lan, Q.; Xu, W.; Wu, Y.; Ying, T.; Liu, S.; Shi, Z.; Jiang, S.; et al. Fusion mechanism of 2019-nCoV and fusion inhibitors targeting HR1 domain in spike protein. *Cell. Mol. Immunol.* **2020**, 1–3. [CrossRef] [PubMed]

27. Belouzard, S.; Chu, V.C.; Whittaker, G.R. Activation of the SARS coronavirus spike protein via sequential proteolytic cleavage at two distinct sites. *Proc. Natl. Acad. Sci. USA* **2009**, *106*, 5871–5876. [CrossRef] [PubMed]
28. Hoffmann, M.; Kleine-Weber, H.; Schroeder, S.; Krüger, N.; Herrler, T.; Erichsen, S.; Schiergens, T.S.; Herrler, G.; Wu, N.-H.; Nitsche, A.; et al. SARS-CoV-2 Cell Entry Depends on ACE2 and TMPRSS2 and Is Blocked by a Clinically Proven Protease Inhibitor. *Cell* **2020**. [CrossRef]
29. Hoffmann, M.; Kleine-Weber, H.; Krüger, N.; Müller, M.; Drosten, C.; Pöhlmann, S.; A Muller, M. The novel coronavirus 2019 (2019-nCoV) uses the SARS-coronavirus receptor ACE2 and the cellular protease TMPRSS2 for entry into target cells. *BioRxiv* **2020**. [CrossRef]
30. Wrapp, D.; Wang, N.; Corbett, K.S.; Goldsmith, J.A.; Hsieh, C.-L.; Abiona, O.; Graham, B.S.; McLellan, J.S. Cryo-EM structure of the 2019-nCoV spike in the prefusion conformation. *Science* **2020**, *367*, 1260–1263. [CrossRef]
31. Mullard, A. Ebola outbreak prompts experimental drug rollout. *Nat. Rev. Drug Discov.* **2018**, *17*, 460. [CrossRef]
32. Zuñiga, S.; Cruz, J.L.G.; Sola, I.; Mateos-Gómez, P.; Palacio, L.; Enjuanes, L. Coronavirus Nucleocapsid Protein Facilitates Template Switching and Is Required for Efficient Transcription. *J. Virol.* **2009**, *84*, 2169–2175. [CrossRef] [PubMed]
33. Spencer, K.-A.; Dee, M.; Britton, P.; Hiscox, J.A. Role of phosphorylation clusters in the biology of the coronavirus infectious bronchitis virus nucleocapsid protein. *Virology* **2008**, *370*, 373–381. [CrossRef] [PubMed]
34. Zuñiga, S.; Sola, I.; Moreno, J.L.; Sabella, P.; Plana-Durán, J.; Enjuanes, L. Coronavirus nucleocapsid protein is an RNA chaperone. *Virology* **2007**, *357*, 215–227. [CrossRef] [PubMed]
35. Wu, C.-H.; Yeh, S.-H.; Tsay, Y.-G.; Shieh, Y.-H.; Kao, C.-L.; Chen, Y.-S.; Wang, S.-H.; Kuo, T.-J.; Chen, P.-J.; Chen, P.-J. Glycogen Synthase Kinase-3 Regulates the Phosphorylation of Severe Acute Respiratory Syndrome Coronavirus Nucleocapsid Protein and Viral Replication. *J. Boil. Chem.* **2008**, *284*, 5229–5239. [CrossRef]
36. Luo, H.; Chen, Q.; Chen, J.; Chen, K.; Shen, X.; Jiang, H. The nucleocapsid protein of SARS coronavirus has a high binding affinity to the human cellular heterogeneous nuclear ribonucleoprotein A1. *FEBS Lett.* **2005**, *579*, 2623–2628. [CrossRef]
37. Nakauchi, M.; Kariwa, H.; Kon, Y.; Yoshii, K.; Maeda, A.; Takashima, I. Analysis of severe acute respiratory syndrome coronavirus structural proteins in virus-like particle assembly. *Microbiol. Immunol.* **2008**, *52*, 625–630. [CrossRef]
38. Siu, Y.L.; Teoh, K.T.; Lo, J.; Chan, C.M.; Kien, F.; Escriou, N.; Tsao, S.W.; Nicholls, J.M.; Altmeyer, R.; Peiris, J.S.M.; et al. The M, E, and N Structural Proteins of the Severe Acute Respiratory Syndrome Coronavirus Are Required for Efficient Assembly, Trafficking, and Release of Virus-Like Particles. *J. Virol.* **2008**, *82*, 11318–11330. [CrossRef]
39. Lim, K.P.; Liu, D.X. The missing link in coronavirus assembly. Retention of the avian coronavirus infectious bronchitis virus envelope protein in the pre-Golgi compartments and physical interaction between the envelope and membrane proteins. *J. Biol. Chem.* **2001**, *276*, 17515–17523. [CrossRef]
40. Fung, T.S.; Liu, D.X. Human Coronavirus: Host-Pathogen Interaction. *Annu. Rev. Microbiol.* **2019**, *73*, 529–557. [CrossRef]
41. Brandizzi, F.; Barlowe, C. Organization of the ER-Golgi interface for membrane traffic control. *Nat. Rev. Mol. Cell Boil.* **2013**, *14*, 382–392. [CrossRef]
42. Du, L.; He, Y.; Zhou, Y.; Liu, S.; Zheng, B.-J.; Jiang, S. The spike protein of SARS-CoV—A target for vaccine and therapeutic development. *Nat. Rev. Genet.* **2009**, *7*, 226–236. [CrossRef] [PubMed]
43. Pyrc, K.; Berkhout, B.; Van Der Hoek, L. Antiviral strategies against human coronaviruses. *Infect. Disord.-Drug Targets* **2007**, *7*, 59–66. [CrossRef] [PubMed]
44. Tetro, J.A. Is COVID-19 receiving ADE from other coronaviruses? *Microbes Infect.* **2020**, *22*, 72–73. [CrossRef] [PubMed]
45. Peeples, L. News Feature: Avoiding pitfalls in the pursuit of a COVID-19 vaccine. *Proc. Natl. Acad. Sci. USA* **2020**, 202005456. [CrossRef]
46. Wu, A.; Peng, Y.; Huang, B.; Ding, X.; Wang, X.; Niu, P.; Meng, J.; Zhu, Z.; Zhang, Z.; Wang, J.; et al. Genome Composition and Divergence of the Novel Coronavirus (2019-nCoV) Originating in China. *Cell Host Microbe* **2020**, *27*, 325–328. [CrossRef]

47. Chudhary, S.A.; Imtiaz, S.; Iqbal, N. Laboratory Detection of Novel Corona Virus 2019 using Polymerase Chain Reaction. *Int. J. Front. Sci.* **2020**, *4*. [CrossRef]
48. Kellner, M.J.; Koob, J.G.; Gootenberg, J.S.; Abudayyeh, O.O.; Zhang, F. SHERLOCK: Nucleic acid detection with CRISPR nucleases. *Nat. Protoc.* **2019**, *14*, 2986–3012. [CrossRef]
49. Seletsky, A.; O'Connell, M.; Knight, S.C.; Burstein, D.; Cate, J.H.D.; Tjian, R.; Doudna, J.A. Two distinct RNase activities of CRISPR-C2c2 enable guide-RNA processing and RNA detection. *Nature* **2016**, *538*, 270–273. [CrossRef]
50. Sheahan, T.P.; Sims, A.C.; Leist, S.R.; Schäfer, A.; Won, J.; Brown, A.J.; Montgomery, S.A.; Hogg, A.; Babusis, D.; Clarke, M.O.; et al. Comparative therapeutic efficacy of remdesivir and combination lopinavir, ritonavir, and interferon beta against MERS-CoV. *Nat. Commun.* **2020**, *11*, 222–224. [CrossRef]
51. Li, G.; De Clercq, E. Therapeutic options for the 2019 novel coronavirus (2019-nCoV). *Nat. Rev. Drug Discov.* **2020**, *19*, 149–150. [CrossRef]
52. Zhang, L.; Lin, D.; Sun, X.; Curth, U.; Drosten, C.; Sauerhering, L.; Becker, S.; Rox, K.; Hilgenfeld, R. Crystal structure of SARS-CoV-2 main protease provides a basis for design of improved α-ketoamide inhibitors. *Science* **2020**, eabb3405. [CrossRef] [PubMed]
53. Kadam, R.U.; Wilson, I.A. Structural basis of influenza virus fusion inhibition by the antiviral drug Arbidol. *Proc. Natl. Acad. Sci. USA* **2016**, *114*, 206–214. [CrossRef] [PubMed]
54. Rosa, S.G.V.; Santos, W.C. Clinical trials on drug repositioning for COVID-19 treatment. *Rev. Panam. Salud Pública* **2020**, *44*. [CrossRef]
55. Liu, J.; Cao, R.; Xu, M.; Wang, X.; Zhang, H.; Hu, H.; Li, Y.; Hu, Z.; Zhong, W.; Wang, M. Hydroxychloroquine, a less toxic derivative of chloroquine, is effective in inhibiting SARS-CoV-2 infection in vitro. *Cell Discov.* **2020**, *6*, 1–4. [CrossRef]
56. Venkataraman, S.; Prasad, B.V.L.S.; Selvaraj, V. RNA Dependent RNA Polymerases: Insights from Structure, Function and Evolution. *Viruses* **2018**, *10*, 76. [CrossRef] [PubMed]
57. Letko, M.; Marzi, A.; Munster, V. Functional assessment of cell entry and receptor usage for SARS-CoV-2 and other lineage B betacoronaviruses. *Nat. Microbiol.* **2020**, *5*, 562–569. [CrossRef] [PubMed]
58. Lundin, A.; Dijkman, R.; Bergström, T.; Kann, N.; Adamiak, B.; Hannoun, C.; Kindler, E.; Jonsdottir, H.; Muth, D.; Kint, J.; et al. Targeting Membrane-Bound Viral RNA Synthesis Reveals Potent Inhibition of Diverse Coronaviruses Including the Middle East Respiratory Syndrome Virus. *PLoS Pathog.* **2014**, *10*, e1004166. [CrossRef] [PubMed]
59. Gao, Y.; Yan, L.; Huang, Y.; Liu, F.; Zhao, Y.; Cao, L.; Wang, T.; Sun, Q.; Ming, Z.; Zhang, L.; et al. Structure of RNA-dependent RNA polymerase from 2019-nCoV, a major antiviral drug target. *BioRxiv* **2020**. [CrossRef]
60. Tchesnokov, E.P.; Feng, J.Y.; Porter, D.P.; Gotte, M. Mechanism of Inhibition of Ebola Virus RNA-Dependent RNA Polymerase by Remdesivir. *Viruses* **2019**, *11*, 326. [CrossRef]
61. Agostini, M.L.; Andres, E.L.; Sims, A.C.; Graham, R.L.; Sheahan, T.P.; Lu, X.; Smith, E.C.; Case, J.B.; Feng, J.Y.; Jordan, R.; et al. Coronavirus Susceptibility to the Antiviral Remdesivir (GS-5734) Is Mediated by the Viral Polymerase and the Proofreading Exoribonuclease. *MBio* **2018**, *9*, e00221-18. [CrossRef]
62. de Wit, E.; Feldmann, F.; Cronin, J.; Jordan, R.; Okumura, A.; Thomas, T.; Scott, D.; Cihlar, T.; Feldmann, H. Prophylactic and therapeutic remdesivir (GS-5734) treatment in the rhesus macaque model of MERS-CoV infection. *Proc. Natl. Acad. Sci. USA* **2020**, *117*, 6771–6776. [CrossRef] [PubMed]
63. Kaeppler, U.; Stiefl, N.; Schiller, M.; Vicik, R.; Breuning, A.; Schmitz, W.; Rupprecht, D.; Schmuck, C.; Baumann, K.; Ziebuhr, J.; et al. A New Lead for Nonpeptidic Active-Site-Directed Inhibitors of the Severe Acute Respiratory Syndrome Coronavirus Main Protease Discovered by a Combination of Screening and Docking Methods||. *J. Med. Chem.* **2005**, *48*, 6832–6842. [CrossRef] [PubMed]
64. Shah, F.; Mukherjee, P.; Desai, P.; Avery, M. Computational approaches for the discovery of cysteine protease inhibitors against malaria and SARS. *Curr. Comput. Drug Des.* **2010**, *6*, 1–23. [CrossRef] [PubMed]
65. Martina, E.; Stiefl, N.; Degel, B.; Schulz, F.; Breuning, A.; Schiller, M.; Vicik, R.; Baumann, K.; Ziebuhr, J.; Schirmeister, T. Screening of electrophilic compounds yields an aziridinyl peptide as new active-site directed SARS-CoV main protease inhibitor. *Bioorganic Med. Chem. Lett.* **2005**, *15*, 5365–5369. [CrossRef]

66. Jacobs, J.; Grum-Tokars, V.; Zhou, Y.; Turlington, M.; Saldanha, S.A.; Chase, P.; Eggler, A.; Dawson, E.S.; Baez-Santos, Y.M.; Tomar, S.; et al. Discovery, Synthesis, And Structure-Based Optimization of a Series ofN-(tert-Butyl)-2-(N-arylamido)-2-(pyridin-3-yl) Acetamides (ML188) as Potent Noncovalent Small Molecule Inhibitors of the Severe Acute Respiratory Syndrome Coronavirus (SARS-CoV) 3CL Protease. *J. Med. Chem.* **2013**, *56*, 534–546.
67. Shie, J.J.; Fang, J.M.; Kuo, T.H.; Kuo, C.J.; Liang, P.H.; Huang, H.J.; Wu, Y.T.; Jan, J.T.; Cheng, Y.S.; Wong, C.H. Inhibition of the severe acute respiratory syndrome 3CL protease by peptidomimetic alpha,beta-unsaturated esters. *Bioorg. Med. Chem.* **2005**, *13*, 5240–5252. [CrossRef]
68. Zhang, H.-Z.; Zhang, H.; Kemnitzer, W.; Tseng, B.; Cinatl, J.; Michaelis, M.; Doerr, H.W.; Cai, S.X. Design and Synthesis of Dipeptidyl Glutaminyl Fluoromethyl Ketones as Potent Severe Acute Respiratory Syndrome Coronovirus (SARS-CoV) Inhibitors. *J. Med. Chem.* **2006**, *49*, 1198–1201. [CrossRef]
69. Severson, W.E.; Shindo, N.; Sosa, M.; Fletcher, T.; White, E.L.; Ananthan, S.; Jonsson, C.B. Development and Validation of a High-Throughput Screen for Inhibitors of SARS CoV and Its Application in Screening of a 100,000-Compound Library. *J. Biomol. Screen.* **2007**, *12*, 33–40. [CrossRef]
70. Konno, S.; Thanigaimalai, P.; Yamamoto, T.; Nakada, K.; Kakiuchi, R.; Takayama, K.; Yamazaki, Y.; Yakushiji, F.; Akaji, K.; Kiso, Y.; et al. Design and synthesis of new tripeptide-type SARS-CoV 3CL protease inhibitors containing an electrophilic arylketone moiety. *Bioorganic Med. Chem.* **2013**, *21*, 412–424. [CrossRef]
71. Shie, J.-J.; Fang, J.-M.; Kuo, C.-J.; Kuo, T.-H.; Liang, P.-H.; Huang, H.-J.; Yang, W.-B.; Lin, C.-H.; Chen, J.-L.; Wu, Y.-T.; et al. Discovery of Potent Anilide Inhibitors against the Severe Acute Respiratory Syndrome 3CL Protease. *J. Med. Chem.* **2005**, *48*, 4469–4473. [CrossRef]
72. Kesel, A.J. Synthesis of novel test compounds for antiviral chemotherapy of severe acute respiratory syndrome (SARS). *Curr. Med. Chem.* **2005**, *12*, 2095–2162. [CrossRef] [PubMed]
73. Blanchard, J.E.; Elowe, N.H.; Huitema, C.; Fortin, P.D.; Cechetto, J.D.; Eltis, L.D.; Brown, E.D. High-throughput screening identifies inhibitors of the SARS coronavirus main proteinase. *Chem. Boil.* **2004**, *11*, 1445–1453. [CrossRef] [PubMed]
74. Zhou, J.; Fang, L.; Yang, Z.; Xu, S.; Lv, M.; Sun, Z.; Chen, J.; Wang, D.; Gao, J.; Xiao, S. Identification of novel proteolytically inactive mutations in coronavirus 3C-like protease using a combined approach. *FASEB J.* **2019**, *33*, 14575–14587. [CrossRef] [PubMed]
75. Muralidharan, N.; Sakthivel, R.; Velmurugan, D.; Gromiha, M.M. Computational studies of drug repurposing and synergism of lopinavir, oseltamivir and ritonavir binding with SARS-CoV-2 Protease against COVID-19. *J. Biomol. Struct. Dyn.* **2020**, 1–7. [CrossRef]
76. Liu, S.; Zheng, Q.; Wang, Z. Potential covalent drugs targeting the main protease of the SARS-CoV-2 coronavirus. *Bioinformatic* **2020**. [CrossRef]
77. Yoon, J.-J.; Toots, M.; Lee, S.; Lee, M.-E.; Ludeke, B.; Luczo, J.; Ganti, K.; Cox, R.M.; Sticher, Z.M.; Edpuganti, V.; et al. Orally Efficacious Broad-Spectrum Ribonucleoside Analog Inhibitor of Influenza and Respiratory Syncytial Viruses. *Antimicrob. Agents Chemother.* **2018**, *62*. [CrossRef]
78. Sheahan, T.P.; Sims, A.C.; Zhou, S.; Graham, R.L.; Pruijssers, A.J.; Agostini, M.L.; Leist, S.R.; Schäfer, A.; Dinnon, K.H.; Stevens, L.J.; et al. An orally bioavailable broad-spectrum antiviral inhibits SARS-CoV-2 in human airway epithelial cell cultures and multiple coronaviruses in mice. *Sci. Transl. Med.* **2020**, eabb5883. [CrossRef]
79. Kaul, T.N.; Middleton, E.; Ogra, P.L. Antiviral effect of flavonoids on human viruses. *J. Med. Virol.* **1985**, *15*, 71–79. [CrossRef]
80. Khan, S.A.; Zia, K.; Ashraf, S.; Uddin, R.; Ul-Haq, Z. Identification of Chymotrypsin-like Protease Inhibitors of SARS-CoV-2 Via Integrated Computational Approach. *J. Biomol. Struct. Dyn.* **2020**, 1–13. [CrossRef]
81. Gautret, P.; Lagier, J.-C.; Parola, P.; Hoang, V.T.; Meddeb, L.; Mailhe, M.; Doudier, B.; Courjon, J.; Giordanengo, V.; Vieira, V.E.; et al. Hydroxychloroquine and azithromycin as a treatment of COVID-19: Results of an open-label non-randomized clinical trial. *Int. J. Antimicrob. Agents* **2020**, 105949. [CrossRef]
82. Weinreb, S.M. Synthetic lessons from quinine. *Nature* **2001**, *411*, 429–431. [CrossRef] [PubMed]
83. Lin, L.-T.; Hsu, W.-C.; Lin, C.-C. Antiviral Natural Products and Herbal Medicines. *J. Tradit. Complement. Med.* **2014**, *4*, 24–35. [CrossRef]
84. Keyaerts, E.; Vijgen, L.; Maes, P.; Neyts, J.; Van Ranst, M. In vitro inhibition of severe acute respiratory syndrome coronavirus by chloroquine. *Biochem. Biophys. Res. Commun.* **2004**, *323*, 264–268. [CrossRef] [PubMed]

85. Tsai, K.-C.; Chen, S.-Y.; Liang, P.-H.; Lu, I.-L.; Mahindroo, N.; Hsieh, H.-P.; Chao, Y.-S.; Liu, L.; Liu, N.; Lien, W.; et al. Discovery of a Novel Family of SARS-CoV Protease Inhibitors by Virtual Screening and 3D-QSAR Studies. *J. Med. Chem.* **2006**, *49*, 3485–3495. [CrossRef] [PubMed]
86. Coutard, B.; Valle, C.; De Lamballerie, X.; Canard, B.; Seidah, N.; Decroly, E. The spike glycoprotein of the new coronavirus 2019-nCoV contains a furin-like cleavage site absent in CoV of the same clade. *Antivir. Res.* **2020**, *176*, 104742. [CrossRef]
87. Tong, T.R. Drug targets in severe acute respiratory syndrome (SARS) virus and other coronavirus infections. *Infect. Disord. Drug Targets* **2009**, *9*, 223–245. [CrossRef]
88. Mukherjee, P.; Desai, P.; Ross, L.; White, E.L.; Avery, M.A. Structure-based virtual screening against SARS-3CL(pro) to identify novel non-peptidic hits. *Bioorg. Med. Chem.* **2008**, *16*, 4138–4149. [CrossRef]
89. Lee, T.-W.; Cherney, M.M.; Liu, J.; James, K.E.; Powers, J.C.; Eltis, L.D.; James, M.N. Crystal Structures Reveal an Induced-fit Binding of a Substrate-like Aza-peptide Epoxide to SARS Coronavirus Main Peptidase. *J. Mol. Boil.* **2007**, *366*, 916–932. [CrossRef]
90. Wang, D.; Huang, J.; Gui, T.; Yang, Y.; Feng, T.; Tzvetkov, N.T.; Xu, T.; Gai, Z.; Zhou, Y.; Zhang, J.; et al. SR-BI as a target of natural products and its significance in cancer. *Semin. Cancer Boil.* **2020**. [CrossRef]
91. Goetz, D.H.; Choe, Y.; Hansell, E.; Chen, Y.T.; McDowell, M.; Jonsson, C.B.; Roush, W.R.; McKerrow, J.; Craik, C.S. Substrate Specificity Profiling and Identification of a New Class of Inhibitor for the Major Protease of the SARS Coronavirus. *Biochemistry* **2007**, *46*, 8744–8752. [CrossRef]
92. Dooley, A.J.; Shindo, N.; Taggart, B.; Park, J.G.; Pang, Y.P. From genome to drug lead: Identification of a small-molecule inhibitor of the SARS virus. *Bioorg. Med. Chem. Lett.* **2006**, *16*, 830–833. [CrossRef] [PubMed]
93. He, R.; Mott, B.T.; Rosenthal, A.S.; Genna, D.T.; Posner, G.H.; Arav-Boger, R. An artemisinin-derived dimer has highly potent anti-cytomegalovirus (CMV) and anti-cancer activities. *PLoS ONE* **2011**, *6*, e24334. [CrossRef] [PubMed]
94. D'Alessandro, S.; Scaccabarozzi, D.; Signorini, L.; Perego, F.; Ilboudo, D.; Ferrante, P.; Delbue, S. The Use of Antimalarial Drugs against Viral Infection. *Microorganisms* **2020**, *8*, 85. [CrossRef]
95. Reiter, C.; Fröhlich, T.; Gruber, L.; Hutterer, C.; Marschall, M.; Voigtländer, C.; Friedrich, O.; Kappes, B.; Efferth, T.; Tsogoeva, S.B. Highly potent artemisinin-derived dimers and trimers: Synthesis and evaluation of their antimalarial, antileukemia and antiviral activities. *Bioorg. Med. Chem.* **2015**, *23*, 5452–5458. [CrossRef]
96. Sharifi-Rad, J.; Fallah, F.; Setzer, W.N.; Heravi, R.E.; Sharifi-Rad, M. Tordylium persicum Boiss. & Hausskn extract: A possible alternative for treatment of pediatric infectious diseases. *Cell Mol. Biol.* **2016**, *62*, 20–26.
97. Park, I.-W.; Han, C.; Song, X.-P.; A Green, L.; Wang, T.; Liu, Y.; Cen, C.; Song, X.; Yang, B.; Chen, G.; et al. Inhibition of HIV-1 entry by extracts derived from traditional Chinese medicinal herbal plants. *BMC Complement. Altern. Med.* **2009**, *9*, 29. [CrossRef]
98. Kilianski, A.; Baker, S.C. Cell-based antiviral screening against coronaviruses: Developing virus-specific and broad-spectrum inhibitors. *Antivir. Res.* **2013**, *101*, 105–112. [CrossRef]
99. Sharifi-Rad, M.; Nazaruk, J.; Polito, L.; Morais-Braga, M.F.B.; Rocha, J.E.; Coutinho, H.; Salehi, B.; Tabanelli, G.; Montanari, C.; Contreras, M.D.M.; et al. Matricaria genus as a source of antimicrobial agents: From farm to pharmacy and food applications. *Microbiol. Res.* **2018**, *215*, 76–88. [CrossRef]
100. Chen, L.; Li, J.; Luo, C.; Liu, H.; Xu, W.; Chen, G.; Liew, O.W.; Zhu, W.; Puah, C.M.; Shen, X.; et al. Binding interaction of quercetin-3-beta-galactoside and its synthetic derivatives with SARS-CoV 3CL(pro): Structure-activity relationship studies reveal salient pharmacophore features. *Bioorg. Med. Chem.* **2006**, *14*, 8295–8306. [CrossRef]
101. Gao, J.; Tian, Z.; Yang, X. Breakthrough: Chloroquine phosphate has shown apparent efficacy in treatment of COVID-19 associated pneumonia in clinical studies. *Biosci. Trends* **2020**, *14*, 72–73. [CrossRef]
102. Lai, C.-C.; Shih, T.-P.; Ko, W.-C.; Tang, H.-J.; Hsueh, P.-R. Severe acute respiratory syndrome coronavirus 2 (SARS-CoV-2) and coronavirus disease-2019 (COVID-19): The epidemic and the challenges. *Int. J. Antimicrob. Agents* **2020**, *55*, 105924. [CrossRef] [PubMed]
103. Colson, P.; Rolain, J.-M.; Lagier, J.-C.; Brouqui, P.; Raoult, D. Chloroquine and hydroxychloroquine as available weapons to fight COVID-19. *Int. J. Antimicrob. Agents* **2020**, 105932. [CrossRef] [PubMed]
104. Sharifi-Rad, J.; Iriti, M.; Setzer, W.N.; Sharifi-Rad, M.; Roointan, A.; Salehi, B. Antiviral activity of Veronica persica Poir. on herpes virus infection. *Cell. Mol. Boil.* **2018**, *64*, 11–17. [CrossRef]
105. Coronavirus: Chinese Scientists to Test 30 Therapeutic Candidates 2020. Available online: https://www.pharmaceutical-technology.com/news/china-tests-30-drug-candidates/ (accessed on 21 February 2020).

106. Huang, J.; Wang, D.; Huang, L.-H.; Huang, H. Huang Roles of Reconstituted High-Density Lipoprotein Nanoparticles in Cardiovascular Disease: A New Paradigm for Drug Discovery. *Int. J. Mol. Sci.* **2020**, *21*, 739. [CrossRef] [PubMed]
107. Das, U.N. Can Bioactive Lipids Inactivate Coronavirus (COVID-19)? *Arch. Med. Res.* **2020**. [CrossRef] [PubMed]
108. Ohe, M.; Shida, H.; Jodo, S.; Kusunoki, Y.; Seki, M.; Furuya, K.; Goudarzi, H. Macrolide treatment for COVID-19: Will this be the way forward? *Biosci. Trends* **2020**, 2020.03058. [CrossRef]
109. Chen, S.; Luo, H.; Chen, L.; Chen, J.; Shen, J.; Zhu, W.; Chen, K.; Shen, X.; Jiang, H. An overall picture of SARS coronavirus (SARS-CoV) genome-encoded major proteins: Structures, functions and drug development. *Curr. Pharm. Des.* **2006**, *12*, 4539–4553. [CrossRef]
110. Walls, A.C.; Park, Y.-J.; Tortorici, M.A.; Wall, A.; McGuire, A.T.; Veesler, D. Structure, Function, and Antigenicity of the SARS-CoV-2 Spike Glycoprotein. *Cell* **2020**. [CrossRef]
111. Park, Y.-J.; Walls, A.C.; Wang, Z.; Sauer, M.M.; Li, W.; Tortorici, M.A.; Bosch, B.-J.; DiMaio, F.; Veesler, D. Structures of MERS-CoV spike glycoprotein in complex with sialoside attachment receptors. *Nat. Struct. Mol. Boil.* **2019**, *26*, 1151–1157. [CrossRef]
112. Kirchdoerfer, R.N.; Wang, N.; Pallesen, J.; Wrapp, D.; Turner, H.L.; Cottrell, C.A.; Corbett, K.S.; Graham, B.S.; McLellan, J.S.; Ward, A. BStabilized coronavirus spikes are resistant to conformational changes induced by receptor recognition or proteolysis. *Sci. Rep.* **2018**, *8*, 15701. [CrossRef]
113. Gassen, N.C.; Niemeyer, D.; Muth, D.; Corman, V.M.; Martinelli, S.; Gassen, A.; Hafner, K.; Papies, J.; Mösbauer, K.; Zellner, A.; et al. SKP2 attenuates autophagy through Beclin1-ubiquitination and its inhibition reduces MERS-Coronavirus infection. *Nat. Commun.* **2019**, *10*, 5570. [CrossRef] [PubMed]
114. Yuan, M.; Wu, N.C.; Zhu, X.; Lee, C.-C.D.; So, R.T.Y.; Lv, H.; Mok, C.K.P.; Wilson, I.A. A highly conserved cryptic epitope in the receptor-binding domains of SARS-CoV-2 and SARS-CoV. *Science* **2020**, eabb7269. [CrossRef] [PubMed]
115. Xia, S.; Liu, M.; Wang, C.; Xu, W.; Lan, Q.; Feng, S.; Qi, F.; Bao, L.; Du, L.; Liu, S.; et al. Inhibition of SARS-CoV-2 (previously 2019-nCoV) infection by a highly potent pan-coronavirus fusion inhibitor targeting its spike protein that harbors a high capacity to mediate membrane fusion. *Cell Res.* **2020**, *30*, 343–355. [CrossRef] [PubMed]
116. Ortega, J.T.; Serrano, M.L.; Pujol, F.H.; Rangel, H.R. Role of changes in SARS-CoV-2 spike protein in the interaction with the human ACE2 receptor: An in silico analysis. *EXCLI J.* **2020**, *19*, 410–417.
117. Tai, W.; He, L.; Zhang, X.; Pu, J.; Voronin, D.; Jiang, S.; Zhou, Y.; Du, L. Characterization of the receptor-binding domain (RBD) of 2019 novel coronavirus: Implication for development of RBD protein as a viral attachment inhibitor and vaccine. *Cell. Mol. Immunol.* **2020**, 1–8. [CrossRef] [PubMed]
118. Luan, J.; Lu, Y.; Jin, X.; Zhang, L. Spike protein recognition of mammalian ACE2 predicts the host range and an optimized ACE2 for SARS-CoV-2 infection. *Biochem. Biophys. Res. Commun.* **2020**. [CrossRef]
119. Cao, B.; Wang, Y.; Wen, D.; Liu, W.; Wang, J.; Fan, G.; Ruan, L.; Song, B.; Cai, Y.; Wei, M.; et al. A Trial of Lopinavir–Ritonavir in Adults Hospitalized with Severe Covid-19. *N. Engl. J. Med.* **2020**. [CrossRef]
120. Alhazzani, W.; Møller, M.H.; Arabi, Y.M.; Loeb, M.; Gong, M.N.; Fan, E.; Oczkowski, S.; Levy, M.M.; Derde, L.; Dzierba, A.; et al. Surviving Sepsis Campaign: Guidelines on the management of critically ill adults with Coronavirus Disease 2019 (COVID-19). *Intensive Care Med.* **2020**, 1–34. [CrossRef]
121. Lukassen, S.; Chua, R.L.; Trefzer, T.; Kahn, N.C.; A Schneider, M.; Muley, T.; Winter, H.; Meister, M.; Veith, C.; Boots, A.W.; et al. SARS-CoV-2 receptor ACE2 and TMPRSS2 are primarily expressed in bronchial transient secretory cells. *EMBO J.* **2020**. [CrossRef]
122. Brake, S.; Barnsley, K.; Lu, W.; McAlinden, K.; Eapen, M.S.; Sohal, S. Smoking Upregulates Angiotensin-Converting Enzyme-2 Receptor: A Potential Adhesion Site for Novel Coronavirus SARS-CoV-2 (Covid-19). *J. Clin. Med.* **2020**, *9*, 841. [CrossRef]
123. Wu, C.-I.; Postema, P.G.; Arbelo, E.; Behr, E.R.; Bezzina, C.R.; Napolitano, C.; Robyns, T.; Probst, V.; Schulze-Bahr, E.; Remme, C.A.; et al. SARS-CoV-2, COVID-19 and inherited arrhythmia syndromes. *Heart Rhythm* **2020**. [CrossRef] [PubMed]
124. Huang, H.; Kuenze, G.; Smith, J.; Taylor, K.C.; Duran, A.M.; Hadziselimovic, A.; Meiler, J.; Vanoye, C.G.; George, A.L.; Sanders, C.R. Mechanisms of KCNQ1 channel dysfunction in long QT syndrome involving voltage sensor domain mutations. *Sci. Adv.* **2018**, *4*, eaar2631. [CrossRef] [PubMed]

125. Sarma, P.; Prajapat, M.; Avti, P.; Kaur, H.; Kumar, S.; Medhi, B. Therapeutic options for the treatment of 2019-novel coronavirus: An evidence-based approach. *Indian J. Pharmacol.* **2020**, *52*, 1–5. [CrossRef] [PubMed]
126. Lu, C.-C.; Chen, M.-Y.; Chang, Y.-L. Potential therapeutic agents against COVID-19: What we know so far. *J. Chin. Med. Assoc.* **2020**. [CrossRef]
127. Narasaraju, T.; Yang, E.; Samy, R.P.; Ng, H.H.; Poh, W.P.; Liew, A.-A.; Phoon, M.C.; Van Rooijen, N.; Chow, V.T. Excessive Neutrophils and Neutrophil Extracellular Traps Contribute to Acute Lung Injury of Influenza Pneumonitis. *Am. J. Pathol.* **2011**, *179*, 199–210. [CrossRef]
128. Sugamata, R.; Dobashi, H.; Nagao, T.; Yamamoto, K.-I.; Nakajima, N.; Sato, Y.; Aratani, Y.; Oshima, M.; Sata, T.; Kobayashi, K.; et al. Contribution of neutrophil-derived myeloperoxidase in the early phase of fulminant acute respiratory distress syndrome induced by influenza virus infection. *Microbiol. Immunol.* **2012**, *56*, 171–182. [CrossRef]
129. Camp, J.V.; Jonsson, C.B. A Role for Neutrophils in Viral Respiratory Disease. *Front. Immunol.* **2017**, *8*, 11. [CrossRef]
130. Huang, J.; Smith, F.; Panizzi, J.R.; Goodwin, D.C.; Panizzi, P. Inactivation of myeloperoxidase by benzoic acid hydrazide. *Arch. Biochem. Biophys.* **2015**, *570*, 14–22. [CrossRef]
131. Huang, J.; Milton, A.; Arnold, R.; Huang, H.; Smith, F.; Panizzi, J.R.; Panizzi, P. Methods for measuring myeloperoxidase activity toward assessing inhibitor efficacy in living systems. *J. Leukoc. Boil.* **2016**, *99*, 541–548. [CrossRef]
132. Favreau, D.J.; Meessen-Pinard, M.; Desforges, M.; Talbot, P.J. Human Coronavirus-Induced Neuronal Programmed Cell Death Is Cyclophilin D Dependent and Potentially Caspase Dispensable. *J. Virol.* **2011**, *86*, 81–93. [CrossRef]
133. Chu, H.; Zhou, J.; Wong, B.H.-Y.; Li, C.; Chan, J.F.-W.; Cheng, Z.-S.; Yang, D.; Wang, D.; Lee, A.C.-Y.; Li, C.; et al. Middle East Respiratory Syndrome Coronavirus Efficiently Infects Human Primary T Lymphocytes and Activates the Extrinsic and Intrinsic Apoptosis Pathways. *J. Infect. Dis.* **2015**, *213*, 904–914. [CrossRef] [PubMed]
134. Marinko, J.T.; Huang, H.; Penn, W.D.; Capra, J.A.; Schlebach, J.P.; Sanders, C.R. Folding and Misfolding of Human Membrane Proteins in Health and Disease: From Single Molecules to Cellular Proteostasis. *Chem. Rev.* **2019**, *119*, 5537–5606. [CrossRef]
135. Hung, A.M.; Tsuchida, Y.; Nowak, K.L.; Sarkar, S.; Chonchol, M.; Whitfield, V. IL-1 Inhibition and Function of the HDL-Containing Fraction of Plasma in Patients with Stages 3 to 5 CKD. *Clin. J. Am. Soc. Nephrol.* **2019**, *14*, 702–711. [CrossRef]
136. Fung, T.S.; Liao, Y.; Liu, D.X. The Endoplasmic Reticulum Stress Sensor IRE1α Protects Cells from Apoptosis Induced by the Coronavirus Infectious Bronchitis Virus. *J. Virol.* **2014**, *88*, 12752–12764. [CrossRef]
137. Fung, T.S.; Liu, D.X. Activation of the c-Jun NH2-terminal kinase pathway by coronavirus infectious bronchitis virus promotes apoptosis independently of c-Jun. *Cell Death Dis.* **2017**, *8*, 3215. [CrossRef] [PubMed]
138. Fung, T.S.; Liu, D.X. Coronavirus infection, ER stress, apoptosis and innate immunity. *Front. Microbiol.* **2014**, *5*, 296. [CrossRef] [PubMed]
139. Fung, T.S.; Liao, Y.; Liu, D.X. Regulation of Stress Responses and Translational Control by Coronavirus. *Viruses* **2016**, *8*, 18. [CrossRef]
140. Shi, C.-S.; Nabar, N.; Huang, N.-N.; Kehrl, J.H. SARS-Coronavirus Open Reading Frame-8b triggers intracellular stress pathways and activates NLRP3 inflammasomes. *Cell Death Discov.* **2019**, *5*, 101. [CrossRef]
141. Zhou, Y.; Hou, Y.; Shen, J.; Huang, Y.; Martin, W.; Cheng, F. Network-based drug repurposing for novel coronavirus 2019-nCoV/SARS-CoV-2. *Cell Discov.* **2020**, *6*, 14–18. [CrossRef]
142. Zhang, H.; Baker, A.J. Recombinant human ACE2: Acing out angiotensin II in ARDS therapy. *Crit. Care* **2017**, *21*, 305. [CrossRef]
143. Batlle, D.; Wysocki, J.; Satchell, K. Soluble angiotensin-converting enzyme 2: A potential approach for coronavirus infection therapy? *Clin. Sci.* **2020**, *134*, 543–545. [CrossRef] [PubMed]
144. Li, R.; Pei, S.; Chen, B.; Song, Y.; Zhang, T.; Yang, W.; Shaman, J. Substantial undocumented infection facilitates the rapid dissemination of novel coronavirus (SARS-CoV2). *Science* **2020**, eabb3221. [CrossRef] [PubMed]
145. Poland, G.A. SARS-CoV-2: A time for clear and immediate action. *Lancet Infect. Dis.* **2020**. [CrossRef]

146. Thompson, R. Novel Coronavirus Outbreak in Wuhan, China, 2020: Intense Surveillance Is Vital for Preventing Sustained Transmission in New Locations. *J. Clin. Med.* **2020**, *9*, 498. [CrossRef] [PubMed]
147. Nishiura, H.; Linton, N.M.; Akhmetzhanov, A.R. Initial Cluster of Novel Coronavirus (2019-nCoV) Infections in Wuhan, China Is Consistent with Substantial Human-to-Human Transmission. *J. Clin. Med.* **2020**, *9*, 488. [CrossRef] [PubMed]
148. Nishiura, H.; Kobayashi, T.; Yang, Y.; Hayashi, K.; Miyama, T.; Kinoshita, R.; Linton, N.M.; Jung, S.-M.; Yuan, B.; Suzuki, A.; et al. The Rate of Underascertainment of Novel Coronavirus (2019-nCoV) Infection: Estimation Using Japanese Passengers Data on Evacuation Flights. *J. Clin. Med.* **2020**, *9*, 419. [CrossRef]
149. Tang, X.; Wu, C.; Li, X.; Song, Y.; Yao, X.; Wu, X.; Duan, Y.; Zhang, H.; Wang, Y.; Qian, Z.; et al. On the origin and continuing evolution of SARS-CoV-2. *Natl. Sci. Rev.* **2020**. [CrossRef]

Journal of
Clinical Medicine

MDPI

Review

Therapeutic Applications of Curcumin Nanomedicine Formulations in Cardiovascular Diseases

Bahare Salehi [1], María L. Del Prado-Audelo [2,3], Hernán Cortés [4], Gerardo Leyva-Gómez [2], Zorica Stojanović-Radić [5], Yengkhom Disco Singh [6], Jayanta Kumar Patra [7], Gitishree Das [7], Natália Martins [8,9,*], Miquel Martorell [10,11,*], Marzieh Sharifi-Rad [12], William C. Cho [13,*] and Javad Sharifi-Rad [14,*]

1 Student Research Committee, School of Medicine, Bam University of Medical Sciences, Bam 44340847, Iran; bahar.salehi007@gmail.com
2 Departamento de Farmacia, Facultad de Química, Universidad Nacional Autónoma de México, Ciudad Universitaria, Circuito Exterior S/N, Del. Coyoacán, Mexico City 04510, Mexico; luisa.delpradoa@gmail.com (M.L.D.P.-A.); gerardoleyva@hotmail.com (G.L.-G.)
3 Laboratorio de Posgrado en Tecnología Farmacéutica, FES-Cuautitlán, Universidad Nacional Autónoma de México, Cuautitlán Izcalli 54740, Mexico
4 Laboratorio de Medicina Genómica, Departamento de Genética, Instituto Nacional de Rehabilitación Luis Guillermo Ibarra Ibarra, Mexico City 14389, Mexico; hcortes_c@hotmail.com
5 Department of Biology and Ecology, Faculty of Science and Mathematics, University of Niš, 18000 Niš, Serbia; zstojanovicradic@yahoo.com
6 Department of Post-Harvest Technology, College of Horticulture and Forestry, Central Agricultural University, Pasighat 791102, Arunachal Pradesh, India; disco.iitg@gmail.com
7 Research Institute of Biotechnology & Medical Converged Science, Dongguk University-Seoul, Goyangsi 10326, Korea; jkpatra.cet@gmail.com (J.K.P.); gitishreedas@gmail.com (G.D.)
8 Faculty of Medicine, University of Porto, 4200-319 Porto, Portugal
9 Institute for Research and Innovation in Health (i3S), University of Porto, 4200-135 Porto, Portugal
10 Department of Nutrition and Dietetics, Faculty of Pharmacy, University of Concepcion, Concepcion 4070386, Chile
11 Unidad de Desarrollo Tecnológico, Universidad de Concepción UDT, Concepcion 4070386, Chile
12 Research Department of Agronomy and Plant Breeding, Agricultural Research Institute, University of Zabol, Zabol 3585698613, Iran; marzieh.sharifirad@gmail.com
13 Department of Clinical Oncology, Queen Elizabeth Hospital, 30 Gascoigne Road, Hong Kong, China
14 Phytochemistry Research Center, Shahid Beheshti University of Medical Sciences, Tehran 1991953381, Iran
* Correspondence: ncmartins@med.up.pt (N.M.); mmartorell@udec.cl (M.M.); chocs@ha.org.hk (W.C.C.); javad.sharifirad@gmail.com (J.S.-R.)

Received: 6 January 2020; Accepted: 4 March 2020; Published: 10 March 2020

Abstract: Cardiovascular diseases (CVD) compromises a group of heart and blood vessels disorders with high impact on human health and wellbeing. Curcumin (CUR) have demonstrated beneficial effects on these group of diseases that represent a global burden with a prevalence that continues increasing progressively. Pre- and clinical studies have demonstrated the CUR effects in CVD through its anti-hypercholesterolemic and anti-atherosclerotic effects and its protective properties against cardiac ischemia and reperfusion. However, the CUR therapeutic limitation is its bioavailability. New CUR nanomedicine formulations are developed to solve this problem. The present article aims to discuss different studies and approaches looking into the promising role of nanotechnology-based drug delivery systems to deliver CUR and its derivatives in CVD treatment, with an emphasis on their formulation properties, experimental evidence, bioactivity, as well as challenges and opportunities in developing these systems.

Keywords: curcumin; cardiovascular disease; nanomedicine; nanocurcumin; liposome; nanoformulation

1. Introduction

Curcumin (1,7-bis[4-hydroxy-3- methoxyphenyl]-1,6-heptadiene-3,5-dione) is an active natural yellow colored polyphenol component that is found in *Curcuma longa* L. rhizomes (Figure 1). It is the main curcuminoid of turmeric (*C. longa*), a member of the Zingiberaceae family. It is widely used and sold as a food flavoring, herbal supplement, food coloring agent and even cosmetics ingredient with a history of usage that goes back to 1900 B.C. [1,2]. Formerly isolated in an impure form in 1815, Milobedeska and Lampe, in 1910, identified the chemical structure and chemically synthesized the compound [3–5]. Curcumin (CUR) commercial products have other CUR derivatives such as demethoxycurcumin and bisdemethoxycurcumin that has sometimes been studied instead of or beside CUR [6]. CUR is a bis-α,β-unsaturated β-diketone that shows keto-enol tautomerism. The enol form is predominant in alkaline medium while the keto form prevails in acidic and neutral pH [7]. This molecule has a unique chemical structure, anti-inflammatory, and antioxidant effects; it has been investigated and used in diverse fields, such as food, pharmaceutical, and textile industries [8].

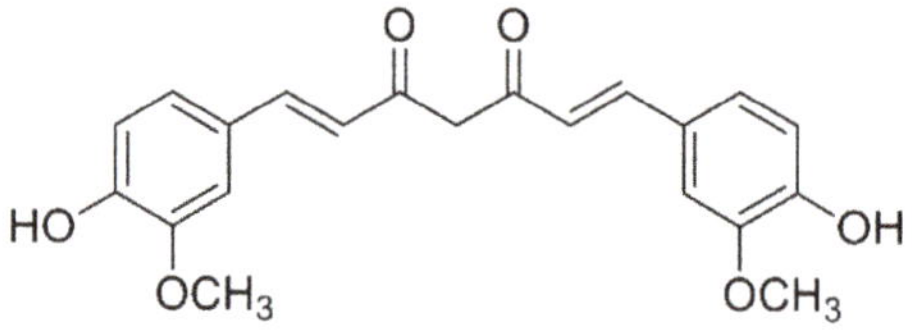

Figure 1. The chemical structure of curcumin.

Due to CUR chemical characteristics, it is considered to be a potent anti-inflammatory phytochemical that can interact with different inflammatory pathways that generated wide range pre-clinical and clinical therapeutic potentials for CUR [9,10]. In the past decade, a growing interest was noticed in CUR-based therapies in prophylaxis and treatment for different diseases, including CVD (atherosclerosis, diabetic cardiomyopathy, arrhythmia, hypertrophic cardiomyopathy, and heart failure) [11–19], cancer (colon cancer, breast cancer, and multiple myeloma) [20–27], neurodegenerative diseases (Parkinson's, Alzheimer's disease, and multiple sclerosis) [8,28–30], autoimmune diseases (osteoarthritis and rheumatoid arthritis) [31,32], psychological disorders [33–37], diabetes [38–40], pulmonary diseases [41–43], gastrointestinal disorders (gastric ulcers, indigestion, and dyspepsia) [44–48], ophthalmic disorders [49–51], and skin disorders [52–54].

A raising number of pre- and clinical studies have investigated CUR effects in CVD that is mainly put down to its antihyperlipidemic and anti-atherosclerotic properties [18]. In clinical trials, CUR was used in different doses ranging from 20–4000 mg with different effects on CV biochemical parameters [18]. CUR has protective properties against CVD through improving patients' lipid profile, and it could be used alone or as a dietary adjunctive to conventional CV drugs [55]. CUR significantly increases beneficial serum parameters, such as apolipoprotein A (Apo A) and HDL, on the other hand, it reduces low-density lipoprotein (LDL), total cholesterol (TC), Apo B, plasma fibrinogen (PF), serum Cu/Zn, serum lipid peroxides (SLP), TC/HDL ratio, non-HDL, lipoprotein A (Lp(A)), serum pro-oxidant-antioxidant balance (PAB), and triglycerides (TG) [18].

CUR has been studied as a chemopreventive agent in atherosclerosis which is a chronic CVD that leads to the thick artery wall, it is shown that this effect is due to the reduction of SLP and TC serum levels, and the increase in HDL cholesterol [56]. Different studies have reported an improved lipid profile in patients with an acute coronary syndrome which is a situation that happens when the blood supply to the myocardium is blocked [10]. In some pre-clinical studies, CUR has shown efficacy and activity in heart failure treatment. This effect is attributable to inhibition of cardiomyocyte fibrosis, improvement in ventricular hypertrophy, and related-gene expression [57]. Other CUR cardio-protective potentials are used in myocardial ischemia/reperfusion injury, diabetic cardiomyopathy, arrhythmia, hypertrophic cardiomyopathy, and doxorubicin-related cardiotoxicity. The mechanisms suggested for these effects are attenuating apoptosis, oxidative stress, and inflammation [58].

Despite having enormous potential benefits, CUR has poor bioavailability that is attributed to its poor absorption, rapid metabolism, and high rate of systemic elimination from the body [59]. One of the major obstacles to deliver CUR is the poor solubility in aqueous media (estimated to be 3.21 mg/L at 25 °C, 0.4 μg/mL at the pH 7.4, and 11 ng/mL in aqueous buffer at pH 5), thus, 60%–70% of the orally administered drug is not absorbed and is excreted in feces [60–62]. On the other hand, CUR is soluble in ethanol, methanol, acetonitrile, chloroform, ethyl acetate, and dimethyl sulfoxide (DMSO) [63,64]. CUR has hydrophobic properties with an estimated octanol-water partition coefficient (log Kow) of 3.29 providing the molecule with good permeability capabilities in passing cellular membranes, however, these lipophilic properties diminish the oral absorption of CUR, thus, in biopharmaceutical classification system (BCS) it is considered to be a class II drug (low solubility and high permeability) [64–66]. Other barriers related to the stability of this molecule are high degradation rate and instability in body fluids because of rapid hydrolyzation at physiological pH. This molecule shows more stability in an acidic environment (pH range of 1.2–6.0) than alkaline media. The products that could found when CUR is degraded in hydrolytic conditions are diferuloylmethane, trans-6-(4′-hydroxy-3′-methoxyphenyl)-2,4-dioxo-5-hexenal, vanillin, ferulic acid, and ferulic aldehyde [67]. CUR instability is extended to light, exhibiting decomposition under UV/visible light exposure in both solid state and solution. The instability is considered to be a drawback for scale-up purposes in industrial point of view because of the minimized expected shelf-life [68]. CUR is rapidly metabolized through reduction or conjugation (sulfation or glucuronidation). Afterward, it extensively undergoes through systemic clearance from the body [69]. On the other hand, CUR is primarily eliminated in the bile, as hexahydrocurcumin glucuronides and tetrahydrocurcumin in intraperitoneally/intravenously administrations [7,70,71]. Pan, Huang and Lin [61] conducted a study on CUR tissue biodistribution after intraperitoneal administration in mice have also revealed low bioavailability of CUR vis this route. As a result, these studies show that despite the administration used route, CUR exhibits suboptimal blood concentrations and poor tissue biodistribution [72].

Nanomedicine is bridging the gap between pharmaceutical limitations and the therapeutic potentials of natural phytochemicals by improving the compound's targeting, pharmacokinetics, efficacy, and cellular uptake [73–80]. Many studies have focused on CUR nanotechnology mediated drug delivery formulations in optimization the therapeutics uses of CUR for various diseases, such as cancer therapy [81–90], neurodegenerative disorders [91,92], wound healing [93], diabetes [94,95], and inflammatory diseases [96]. A wide variety of nanomedicine-based drug delivery systems are used to deliver CUR such as liposomes, polymeric nanoparticles, dendrimers, solid lipid nanoparticles, dendrosomes, nanogels, micelles, niosomes, cyclodextrin inclusion complexes, silver and gold nanoparticles, carbon nanotubes, nanoemulsions, nanosuspensions, exosomes, nanocrystals, and mesoporous silica nanoparticles. These promising platforms are also used for delivering CUR in tissue engineering [97]. This approach has emerged to face major drug delivery issues such as biodistribution limitations, rapid elimination, undesirable degradation/biotransformation, short half-life, and instability. Additionally, among different features provided by nanomedicine formulations are improving the solubility of hydrophobic drugs in water, the potentials of overcoming physiological barriers, increased permeability, offering the possibility of designing controlled release systems, and enhancing the circulation lifetime and pharmacokinetics [98–103]. One of the essential benefits that nano-mediated drug delivery could offer is the enhancement bioactivity and bioavailability through surface modifications, reduction of particle size, and entrapping CUR in within nanocarriers [104]. In the oral route, the bioavailability is enhanced by nanocarriers after improving solubility, protecting the drug from degradation in the gastrointestinal environment, and enhancing permeation in the small intestine; leading to an increase of drug levels in the blood stream [105]. Other emerging goals of nanocarriers is to achieve co-delivery of CUR with other drugs as an adjunct combinations therapy as an effective strategy to combat multi drug resistance [83,88]. Nanocarriers are also used to decrease the nonspecific drug uptake to undesirable tissues that leads to decreased toxicity [106,107]. Moreover, enhanced permeation and retention effect is one of the most important advantages of these systems which results in improving the circulation and accumulation of the loaded drug at the targeted sites, this means higher drug concentrations at the site of action which could help in minimizing the overall used dose and reduce adverse drug reactions [103]. Thus, leading to provision of agents and approaches specifically designed to improve CVD diagnosis and treatment [108,109].

In this present article, we aim to review and underline different studies and approaches looking into the promising role of nanotechnology-based drug delivery systems to deliver CUR and its derivatives in CVD treatment with emphasis on their formulation properties, experimental evidence, general bioactivity, and discussing the challenges and opportunities in developing these systems.

2. General Bioactivity of Curcumin in Cardiovascular Diseases

Studies showed very high cardioprotective potential of CUR including anticoagulant, anti-hypercholesterolemic and anti-atherosclerotic activity, as well as activities related to lowering the consequences of cardiac ischemia and reperfusion injury and regeneration of myocardium. Modes of action includes many molecular targets, including histone acetyltransferase (HAT-p300, involved in in the hypertrophy of cardiomyocytes), nuclear factor erythroid 2 (NFE2)-related factor 2 (NrF2, a major transcription factor involved in cellular redox homeostasis), NF-κB (nuclear factor kappa B, transcription factor upregulated in inflammatory/carcinogenic conditions), angiotensin II type receptor (AT1R, involved in cardiac hypertrophy), toll like receptor 4 (TLR4) and some other molecular targets such as SIRT3 and TGFβ/Smad-mediated signaling pathways.

2.1. *In Vivo Studies*

2.1.1. Anti-Hypercholesterolemic Effect

Obesity is known as the main risk factor for CVD, whereas CUR presents a potent agent in its prevention through various mechanisms. This compound inhibits adipogenesis in 3T3-L1 adipocytes, angiogenesis and thus obesity, which was demonstrated in the study of Ejaz, et al. [110] on mice. This study demonstrated increased oxidation, decreased fatty acid esterification, reduced angiogenesis in an adipose tissue as well as reduced lipid metabolism in adipocytes, resulted in reduced total serum cholesterol.

Studies on rats fed with high fat diet (HFD) demonstrated that administration of CUR significantly reduced increase in body weight as well as levels of total lipids, TC and TG in comparison to the control group. Together with this, CUR intake reduced the high inflammatory response (tumor necrosis factor alpha and C-reactive protein, CRP) noticed in the control group, and alleviated total leucocytes, monocytes and lymphocytes, accompanied by decreased nitric oxide (NO) level in serum, aorta and cardiac tissue of the HFD-group [111].

Administration of CUR for 18 weeks lead to reduced early atherosclerotic lesions, lipid infiltration, intercellular adhesion molecule 1 (ICAM-1) and vascular cell adhesion molecule 1 (VCAM-1) localization together with decreased levels of plasma cholesterol, TG, LDL, Apo B levels as well as cholesteryl ester transfer protein (CETP) activity. In contrast to the above markers, plasma HDL and liver Apo A-I expression were increased. This study demonstrated anti-atherogenic efficacy of CUR comparable to those of lovastatin [112].

2.1.2. Anti-Atherosclerotic Effect

Since CVD presents a condition highly induced by inflammatory response, CUR is a treatment of choice in their prevention due to high anti-inflammatory efficiency. Many studies have confirmed the efficacy of CUR in reducing the risk factors for atherosclerosis and CVD. For instance, a turmeric hydroalcoholic extract revealed to be protective against subcellular membranes lipoperoxidation [113], and damage of thoracic and abdominal aorta [114]. Similar findings were stated on LDL oxidation susceptibility and plasma lipid levels (cholesterol, phospholipid, and TG) [115]. However, mentioned studies used hydroalcoholic extracts of turmeric, while studies with pure CUR in this sense developed somewhat later. Olszanecki, et al. [116] administered CUR at a dose of only 0.3 mg/kg daily for four months to ApoE^{-}/$^{-}$ mice fed with HFD. The results pointed to efficiency of CUR intake in inhibition of atherosclerosis progression, but lack of impact to lipid levels (cholesterol and TG) or body weight in treated animals. The atheroprotective effect of dietary CUR (0.2% (w/w) for four months) in a mouse model of atherosclerosis was also studied together with its molecular and cellular targets at the vascular level [117]. It was found that CUR supplementation reduced atherosclerotic lesions up to 26%, together with decreased leukocyte adhesion and transendothelial migration via NF-κB-dependent pathways. The mentioned molecular mechanisms were related to increased expression of NF-κB protein inhibitor and decreased NF-κB/DNA binding and NF-κB transcriptional activity following tumor necrosis factor (TNF)-α induction, which were detected upon CUR exposure. In another study, CUR significantly ameliorated oxidized low-density lipoprotein (oxLDL)-induced cholesterol accumulation in macrophages and decreased the protein expression of scavenger receptor class A (SR-A) but increased that of ATP-binding cassette transporter (ABC) A1 [118]. Since CUR intake affected the expression of SR-A, ABCA1, ABCG1, and SR-BI in aortas and prevented atherosclerosis in apoE^{-}/$^{-}$ mice, it was proposed that inhibition of SR-A-mediated oxLDL uptake and promotion of ABCA1-dependent cholesterol efflux represent two crucial events in cholesterol accumulation suppression by CUR in macrophage foam cells transformation [118]. Similar reduction of oxLDL uptake has been reported in the study on LDLR^{-}/$^{-}$ mice after CUR administration at doses of 500–1500 mg/kg for 16 weeks [16], where inhibition of the fatty acid binding proteins aP2, together with decreased expression of cluster of differentiation 36 were detected in treated animals. In ApoE^{-}/$^{-}$ mice as model organisms, CUR (0.1% (w/w) for four months) was found to have another molecular target, toll-like receptor 4 (TLR4), whose downregulation leads to reduction in pro-inflammatory mediators and decreased atherogenesis [119]. Treatment of asthmatic ApoE^{-}/$^{-}$ mice with CUR (200 mg/kg/day, 8 weeks) demonstrated that CUR ameliorated the aggravation of atherosclerotic lesions and stabilized plaque by modulating the balance of T helper cell (Th)2 / regulatory T cells (Tregs) (Th2/Tregs) [120]. CUR intake markedly helped to normalize the elevated Th2 and Th17 cell numbers as well as Tregs in the spleen, while mRNA expression levels of M1 macrophage-related inflammatory factors (interleukin (IL)-6, IL-1β, and inducible nitric oxide synthase (iNOS)) also decreased in treated animals.

CUR significantly affects vascular smooth muscle cells (VSMC), where it was found that it presents a potent inhibitor of platelet-derived growth factor (PDGF)-stimulated vascular cell functions, including migration, proliferation, collagen synthesis, and actin-cytoskeleton reorganization [121]. Also, CUR attenuated PDGF signal transduction and inhibited the binding of this growth factor to its receptors. The same study reported efficacy of CUR in attenuating neointima development in a rat arterial balloon-injury model [121]. Additionally, CUR inhibited oxLDL-induced cholesterol accumulation on rat VSMCs [122]. Other studies reported various effects of CUR to VSMCs, including inhibition of their proliferation [123], migration [124] and causing of the cytostatic effect at doses of only 5 μM [125]. These studies found that CUR stimulates the expression of caveolin-1 [122,123] and other molecular mechanisms such as blocking of NF-κB translocation and inhibition of matrix metalloproteinase (MMP-9) [124], or causing a cell cycle arrest by protein carbonylation, oxidative DNA damage and changes in the nucleolar activity, accompanied by elevated levels of p53 and p21 [125].

Parodi, et al. [126] demonstrated that orally administered CUR reduced proinflammatory cytokine expression in aortic wall, and decreased destruction of medial elastic fibers. In porcine coronary artery, CUR blocked endothelial disfunction induced by homocysteine [127], which was detected as inhibited epithelial nitric oxide synthase expression and superoxide anion production, as well as blocked vasorelaxation. Improvements of endothelial function by pretreatment with CUR were confirmed in human umbilical vein endothelial cells, where reduced permeability and monocyte adhesion were detected [117,128]. In the same model cells, CUR blocked NF-κB activation induced by TNF-α and reduced ROS, adhesion of monocytes, phosphorylation of c-Jun N-terminal kinase p38, and STAT3 [129]. Similar effect was reported for EA.hy926 endothelial cells where CUR reduced ROS levels and NADH activation [130]. In this study, when human microvascular endothelial cells (exposed to resistin) were treated with CUR, expression of P-selectin and fractalkine, intracellular ROS level and NADPH activation were reduced, as well as monocytes adhesion to HEC. Additionally, reduced oxidative damage has been found and related to JAK2/STAT3 pathway and suppressed apoptosis, which limited the reperfusion injury in myocardium when CUR was orally administered for 20 days [131]. Another study, performed on human microvascular endothelial cells, demonstrated protective effect of CUR against PM2.5-induced oxLDL-mediated vascular inflammation, where it reduced enhanced ROS, VCAM-1 and ICAM-1 expression levels [132].

CUR was also found to enhance the permeability of coronary artery via inhibition of several related protein expression, including MMP-9, CD40L, TNF-α, and CRP [133].

2.1.3. Cardiac Ischemia and Reperfusion

Heart ischemia can be reduced by CUR, which is confirmed by many scientific studies. In an in vivo model of thrombosis, CUR administration 30 min prior the ligation prevented ischemia-induced rise of malondialdehyde (MDA) contents and lactate dehydrogenase (LDH) release and also reduced decrease in heart rate and blood pressure following ischemia [134]. Assessing of oxidative stress-related biochemical parameters in rat myocardium following ischemia showed decreased levels of xanthine oxidase, superoxide anion, lipid peroxides (LPs) and myeloperoxidase and increased levels of SOD, CAT, GPx, and GST activities [135]. Postoperative elevation of plasma inflammatory cytokines IL-8, IL-10, cardiac troponin 1 and TNF-α was found in CUR-treated groups, related to NF-κB inhibition [136]. Beneficial effects of CUR (10 μM, 3 h prior stimulation) on cardiomyocytes were demonstrated to be related to toll-like receptor 2 and monocyte chemoattractant protein (MCP)-1 inhibition [137]. In the same study, cardiac ischemia/reperfusion model performed on rats fed with or without CUR (300 mg/kg/day; 7 days before and 14 days after I/R surgery) showed unchanged TLR2 in the infarct zone, decreased macrophage infiltration (CD68) and fibrosis, as well as recovered connexin 43 in the CUR-treated group. Preserving effect of CUR (applied only in the reperfusion period) on cardiac function after ischemia and reperfusion has also been confirmed in the study of Wang, et al. [138]. In the mentioned study, CUR reduced degradation of extracellular matrix and inhibited synthesis of collagen via TGFβ/Smad-mediated signaling pathway, which resulted with reduced extent of collagen-rich scar and increased mass of viable and functional myocardium [138]. In the study of Wang, et al. [139], effect of CUR (150 mg/kg/day, administered for 5 days prior ischemia) to early growth response (EGR-1), responsible for triggering inflammation-induced tissue injury after ischemia and reperfusion, has been investigated in rats subjected to 30-min ischemia and 180-min reperfusion. It was found that CUR significantly reduced expression of EGR-1 mRNA and protein, decreased inflammatory markers TNF-α, IL-6, p-selectin and ICAM-1, and reduced infarct size. Beneficial effects of CUR were demonstrated as reduced infarct size (2.5-fold), found in rats fed with CUR (10, 20, or 30 mg/kg/day) for 20 days and subjected to myocardial injuries by ligation of the coronary artery for 60 min [131]. Silent information regulator 3 (SIRT3) is a NAD-dependent histone deacetylase and has cardioprotective effects. Wang, et al. [140] investigated the role of SIRT3 signaling pathway in protective effects of CUR and found improved cardiac function and decreased infarct size via downregulation of the proapoptotic protein Bax and AcSOD2 and activation of SIRT3.

Another very significant target for CVD prevention by CUR is its potential to prevent heart failure caused by hypertrophy of cardiomyocytes, which is a result of prolonged pressure or volume overload. It has been confirmed that CUR inhibits hypertrophic responses in cultured neonatal rat cardiomyocytes and that it prevents the deterioration of left ventricular (LV) systolic function, myocardial infarction and hypertensive heart disease [141], as well as diabetes-induced cardiac hypertrophy [142]. CUR is known to be a specific inhibitor of p300) [143], which regulates hypertrophy-responsive transcriptional factors and therefore presents a therapeutic agent for maladaptive hypertrophy of cardiomyocytes. This was demonstrated in several animal models of heart failure [141,142,144,145]. In combination with enalapril,

CUR applied orally (50 mg/kg per day for 6 weeks) to rats after myocardial infarction enhanced LV fractional shortening (FS) and reduced cardiomyocyte diameter in the non-infarct area, as well as perivascular fibrosis [146]. Changes in gene expression (total of 179 genes), improved heart function, reduced infarct size and abnormalities in the activities of LDH and creatine kinase-MB (CK-MB) were detected in the group treated with CUR for only three days (75 mg/kg daily) [147]. The same authors proposed cytokine-cytokine receptor interaction, extracellular matrix-receptor interaction, focal adhesions and colorectal cancer pathway as those involved in the cardioprotective effects of CUR.

2.2. Clinical Studies

Many clinical trials confirmed beneficial effects of CUR in the prevention and treatment of various CV conditions. Cholesterol-lowering effect of CUR consumption has been demonstrated in many studies, where healthy subjects [12,14,56] or participants with hypercholesterolemia [15,148] consumed CUR for defined period of time (per os), ranging from 7 days to 6 months. It was found that when healthy subjects consumed CUR in doses from 80–4000 mg/day, positive effect on blood lipid profiles were observed and included decrease in SLP, lowering in TC [12,14,56] and LDL cholesterol, increase in HDL and Apo B [56,148]. In addition to enhanced lipid profile, DiSilvestro, et al. [14] found lowering of TC, plasma sICAM readings, plasma ALT activities and β-amyloid proteins by CUR treatment; the results for the same subjects demonstrated an increase of salivary radical scavenging capacities, plasma CAT activities, myeloperoxidase as well as plasma NO.

CUR was also found to be beneficial in the clinical trials performed on patients suffering from obesity [149–151], metabolic syndrome [152–154] or acute coronary disease [11]. When obese individuals consumed capsules of CUR (500 mg C3 Complex (curcuminoids formula + 5 mg bioperine)) for 30 days, serum TG were decreased, as well as LDL, TC/LDL ratio, and PAB in serum [14,149,150], together with increased Zn/Cu and a reduction in Cu/Zn ratio in serum [151]. Improved lipid status was also recorded in patients suffering from metabolic syndrome, where intake of CUR extract capsules (12 weeks) or C3 Complex (8 weeks) resulted with elevated HDL concentrations and reduced LDL, TG, TC/HDL ratio, non-HDL, TC, TG, and Lp(A) [152,153]. When healthy subjects positive for metabolic syndrome consumed either black seeds, either turmeric or their combination, it was found that turmeric alone improved body mass index, waist circumference and body fat percentage (BF%) after 4 weeks and reduced LDL and CRP following 8 weeks of consummation. In combination with black seeds, reduced BF%, TC, TG, LDL, CRP, and raised HDL were recorded in the serum of the participants [154]. Similar positive effects were found in clinical trials (3 studies: 1) $n = 75$; 2) $n = 240$ and 3) $n = 70$) on hypocholesterolemic patients, those with type II diabetes and acute coronary syndrome [11,13,15].

3. Nanomedicine: Nanoformulation and Cardiovascular Effects

Therapeutic application of most of the drugs reduces their viability and potential due to use of conventional phytochemical methods [107]. More than 40% of new drugs entities has shown slow absorption rate due to poor water solubility [155,156]. As a consequence of this, most of the newly-discovered drugs have low bioavailability and inefficacy in terms of its actions. A major challenge lies in improving the poor absorption of conventional drugs by finding perfect formulation without altering the physicochemical properties of drugs and targeted delivery. Nanoformulation is a unique drug package where a drug is encapsulated with nanoparticle to tackle the challenges of poor absorption, low bioavailability and inefficacy site specific delivery of drugs. In recent years, the uses of nanoformulated drugs are prominently increasing to enhance the therapeutic value of drugs [157]. These nanoformulated drugs possess certain features like quantum size effects, targeted size delivery, target specific, high surface to mass ratio, high solubility, and absorption [158].

Nanomedicine is a new area which is growing very fast in combination with nanotechnology and pharmaceutical sciences [159–161]. Nanoparticle possesses different characters including pharmacokinetic, efficacy, safety, and target specificity. This impart character is being exploited by the pharmaceutical researcher to include in drug formulation [159–162]. Some nanomedicines are under clinical trials for wide application and indications [160]. However, many challenges like better characterization, issue related to toxicity, regulatory guidelines, cost-effective and health care warnings are faced by the nanopharmaceuticals.

3.1. Nanoformulations Characteristics

Nanoformulation size ranges from 10–100 nm in diameter [163]. Drugs are attached to the nanocarrier. Nanoformulation has certain properties while formulating nanodrugs. The nanoformulation must facilitate the drugs to timely reach site of action from the site of administrations. The site of administration may be through oral or injection as fluid. The formulation should also protect the drugs from detrimental effects of bodily environmental factors (pH, enzymes, temperature). It is being reported that preparation techniques of nanodrugs plays a great role in maintaining the desired characters for delivering the drugs at targeted area [164,165]. Nanoformulation may have nanospheres or nanocapsules types depend on method of preparation. In nanocapsules, drugs are embedded inside the cavity of polymer matrix, whereas drug is uniformly dispersed in nanospheres. Nanocapsules have larger size, higher degree of polymerization than nanosphere. In freeze drying technology, nanospheres can be easily lyophilized than nanocapsules due to its structure.

3.2. Nanoformulation Techniques

The preparation of nanoparticles with CUR is a well-established method by several authors taking advantage of the liposolubility of the drug to incorporate into the internal phase of emulsions. The solubility of approximately 6 μg/mL guarantees high encapsulation efficiency in most cases. The use of organic solvents such as acetone and ethyl acetate for the internal phase of emulsions allows rapid solubility of the drug and subsequent solvent removal [91]. The method most frequently reported in the literature for the elaboration of nanoparticles with CUR is nanoprecipitation [166]. Briefly, the drug and the nanoparticle polymer are solubilized in an organic solvent at room temperature with moderate magnetic stirring, then the stabilizer is solubilized in water in a concentration range that can range from 0.5% to 5% w/v. Subsequently, the organic phase is poured into the aqueous phase, the change in solubility of the polymer and the drug results in the formation of the nanoparticles by the presence of the stabilizer and magnetic stirring [167]. Finally, the system is subjected to reduced pressure to remove the solvent, subsequent steps include purification of the formulation usually by centrifugation and then conditioning by lyophilization.

The most commonly used polymer is poly (lactic-co-glycolic acid) (PLGA), an excipient employed in the medical area for a long time and approved by the U.S. Food and Drug Administration (FDA). This polymer is biodegradable and its by-products enter the Krebs cycle [91]. Although the by-products slightly acidify the environment where it is degraded, there are few studies that indicate severe complications from this involvement. The biodegradation time, or in other words, the control of the release time, can be manipulated by the proportion of lactic:glycolic monomers. Even today it is possible to acquire several derivatizations by the main commercial suppliers that allow a higher vectorization.

Moreover, for CV effects the option of PLGA-polyethylene glycol (PEG) is an attractive alternative due to the increase in the hydrophilicity of the nanoparticle corona, decrease in protein adsorption, increase in circulation time, and therefore, the possibility of reaching heart. The stabilizers most commonly employed in the nanoprecipitation technique for the formulation of nanoparticles with CUR include Tween 80, polyvinyl alcohol (PVA), and poloxamer 407 and 188. In general, PVA offers high stability with zeta potential values, usually greater than –20 mV and allows adequate reproducibility, while Tween 80 and poloxamers can offer a type of biological interaction that improves the therapeutic effect of the formulation. The choice of stabilizer usually consists of a balance of stability/therapeutic effect.

Certainly, the spontaneous shock of solubility when the organic phase is poured into the aqueous phase can cause a decrease in the reproducibility of the particle size, polydispersity index (PDI) and the efficiency of drug loading in the nanoparticles. However, it is a practical and fast method, even the most feasible for its industrial escalation. Today, it is possible to find in the pharmaceutical industries the appropriate instrumentation to produce PLGA nanoparticles in batches with an average capacity of 10 L or more.

An alternative to increase the reproducibility of CUR nanoparticles and drug loading efficiency is through the use of the emulsification-diffusion method [91,99]. This method also consists in the formation of an emulsion, but with the difference of the previous saturation of both phases. It also involves adding a quantity of water at the end. In the intermediate step of the emulsion, the addition of an additional fraction of water breaks the emulsion, the internal phase moves outward and causes precipitation of the polymer and drug due to the effect of the stabilizer and agitation [168]. The volume of the batch is greater than that obtained by nanoprecipitation and therefore the nanoparticles are in a lower concentration. The production time is longer than by nanoprecipitation and the stirring speed is greater than 1,500 rpm. In general, the same excipients can be used for both methods.

The first quality tests of CUR nanoparticles should consist of measuring the average particle size, PDI, zeta potential and morphology. These inspections will allow establishing parameters for the subsequent validation of the manufacturing method. The average reported size for CUR nanoparticles ranges from 100 to 200 nm, with a PDI value that reaches 0.05 in the best case, the zeta potential fluctuates depending on the type and concentration of stabilizer. The morphology by scanning electron microscopy or atomic force microscopy is usually spherical.

3.3. *Types of Nanoformulation*

In every year, new nanodrugs entered clinical investigation and some more are under pipelines in the very early stages. However, it is confirmed that nanodrugs are developing very fast beyond the expectation. The clinically trials nanodrugs has steadily increased since 2007 [159]. Selected nanoformulated drugs are listed in the following section.

3.3.1. Liposomes Nanoformulation

Liposome is a spherical vesicle made from lipid bilayer membrane having a designed of empty core structure. Due to their unique properties, liposomes can be used in nanodrug formulations by encapsulating with nanoparticles. Liposomes were firstly identified as simple drug delivery system in 1970s [159]. Their size is 90 to 150 nm in diameter and is capable of self-assembling the hydrophilic or hydrophobic therapies into its empty core [159,160]. Hydrophilic drugs such as ampicillin and, 5-fuoro-deoxyuridine can easily fit into the empty core region of liposomes without any modification in drug ratio. Hydrophobic drug such as Amphotericin B and Indomethacin attached to acyl hydrocarbon chain of the liposomes rather confining to the empty core [169]. Liposomes are considered as one of the most viable drug delivery vehicles due to their specific designed in membrane structure that can facilitate incorporation of different types of drugs in them [170]. Their structural designed enable them to carry biomolecules such as monoclonal antibodies and antigens as conjugated ligands on its surface. Liposome based nanodrugs has advantages of extended retention time period in bloodstream providing longer time for treatment as compared to nonliposomal drugs. They are very much effective at the site of tumor infection area as they can accumulate the drug and deliver to the targeted cell.

Liposomes can be divided into four types [171]: (1) conventional type liposomes, (2) PEG types, (3) ligan-targeted types, and (4) theranostic types. Drug loading in liposomes is not affected by the types of liposomes however it can be performed in two different ways, i.e., active (drug loaded after liposomes is formed) and passive (drug loaded during the liposome formation). Mechanical and solvent dispersion methods of passive loading are usually performed.

Liposomal nanoformulations for drug delivery have been significantly increasing in pharmacology. These formulations have benefitted from the stability, biodistribution on those drugs having bioavailability or high toxicity [172–175]. While treating liposome as alone in intravenous blood stream, it got cleared by immune system due to having short half-lives [172]. However, nanoformulation on liposome helps it to minimize the clearance as PEG attachment protects it from easily accessible.

3.3.2. Nanoformulation of Polymer

Polymer based nanoformulations are widely used in nanomedical research due to their unique properties such as easily synthesized, safety, and efficacy in delivery. Among the polymer, the most well-established polymer is PEG. Polymer based nanoparticle may have different size of single polymer chain (can be directly used as a therapeutic) or as a modifying agent. Polymeric nanoparticle can withstand the drug in the body for weeks and this character made it a promising carrier for numerous medications including cancer, diabetes, and vaccinations [161]. Polymer nanodrugs have following benefits over the conventional polymers: (1) Biodegradable, (2) longer retention time, (3) biocompatibility, and (4) solubility.

3.3.3. Nanocrystals

Nanocrystals are solid drug particles of sizes within a 1000 nm range. They act as drug molecules without attaching any kind of carriers on their surface [171]. Nanocrystals possess peculiar type of characters such as increase saturation solubility, increased dissolution velocity and increased glueyness on the membrane surface. These characters allowed them to be one of the most promising molecules for nanodrugs. Nanocrystals can be made in two different ways: Top-down process and bottom-up process. Top-down techniques are based on size reduction from a relatively large molecule into smaller particles. Bottom-up techniques consist of smaller molecules to form individual large molecule. Bottom-up approaches for nanocrystals are commonly called as 'precipitation methods. Bottom-up techniques includes: (1) Hot melt method, (2) solvent evaporation method, (3) hydrosol, (4) gas anti-solvent recrystallization, (5) rapid expansion of supercritical solutions, (6) and controlled crystallization during free-drying. Top-down techniques includes: (1) sono-crystallization, (2) precipitation, (3) high gravity-controlled precipitation technology, (4) multi-inlet vortex mixing techniques, and (5) limited impinging liquid jet precipitation techniques. Among all of the methods, precipitation is the most common method for production of nanocrystals. In nanosuspension nanocrystals, the dispersing medium are usually replaced by water or any aqueous media (liquid PEG and oils) [176,177].

Nanocrystals are versatile in nature, can be used to improve the pharmacokinetics or pharmacodynamics properties of organic or inorganic materials with poor solubility and bioavailability [178,179]. They possess a narrow, symmetric emission spectrum, tunable, and photochemical stability. They have optically active core region surrounded by a shell that provides a protective against the external environment, making them to less sensitive to photo-oxidation and medium changes. Nanocrystal promotes saturation solubility which can trigger on diffusion-based mass transfer across the biological membrane.

3.4. Curcumin Based Biocomposite Formulation

CUR is a natural compound having diverse properties (Figure 2) in relation to therapeutic, antineoplastic, anti-microbial, anticancer and in treating of several pathologies, neurodegenerative, inflammatory and CVD [180] and it is a good molecule that can be used as encapsulating material with other biomolecules. CUR is a promising natural photosensitizer used in photodynamic therapy [181]. CUR can be formulated with nano-emulsified materials in treating breast adenocarcinoma cell line. This biocomposite is a well-designed drug delivery system which can exploit photodynamic property as therapeutic tools in an in vitro breast cancer model, MCF-7 cells [181]. CUR-nanoemulsion composite fulfill all the requirements to be an excellent drug delivery system.

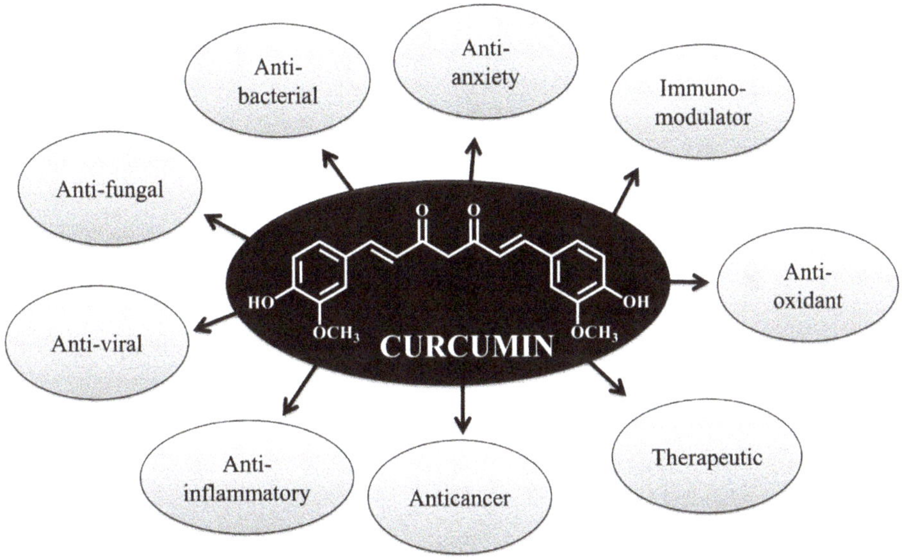

Figure 2. Different properties of curcumin.

In very interestingly, CUR can also form a composite with $CaCO_3$ based solid dispersion formulation to enhance the dissolution rate of water [182]. This formulation was carried out using ethanolic $CaCl_2$ as solution medium thereby diffusing the CO_2. The interaction between $CaCO_3$ and CUR helps 100% drug entrapment. This can be a novel solid dispersion preparation pathway for preparing oral administrated water insoluble drugs.

CUR solubilizer can be checked for its solubility by formulation with other molecules. In a series of research findings, using non-linear quantitative structure–activity relationship (QSPR model) model, CUR solubility was found to be highest in composite formation with co-crystallized with pyrogallol [183].

In another effort, for treating peptic ulcer, CUR is formulated with low density material such as polypropylene foam powder, oils and various solubilizers. This biocomposite has prolonged gastro-retention time and improve insufficient CUR release [184]. This composite is a promising carrier for drug targeted at stomach using CUR formulation.

The therapeutic potential of CUR has certain limitation in regards to poor solubility, bioavailability (Figure 3), and photostability. Onoue, et al. [185] reported to design and develop efficacious formulation of CUR with nanocrystal solid dispersion, amorphous solid dispersion, and nanoemulsion to overcome limitation of CUR formulation. These CUR-based formulations have improved physicochemical and pharmacokinetic properties.

CUR loaded nanoparticle drug delivery system plays a major role targeted delivery of drugs. Many CUR-based nanoformulations have been developed in order to ensure site specific target of cancer cells. CUR nanoparticulate is comparatively more effective than free CUR while tested against different cancer cell lines under in vitro conditions [186]. As part of the studies, this CUR-based nanocomposite showed longer half–life than free CUR while tested on mice. They have reported that, CUR nanoparticulate will have more potential as anticancer drug for treatment of malignant tumors than normal CUR treatment.

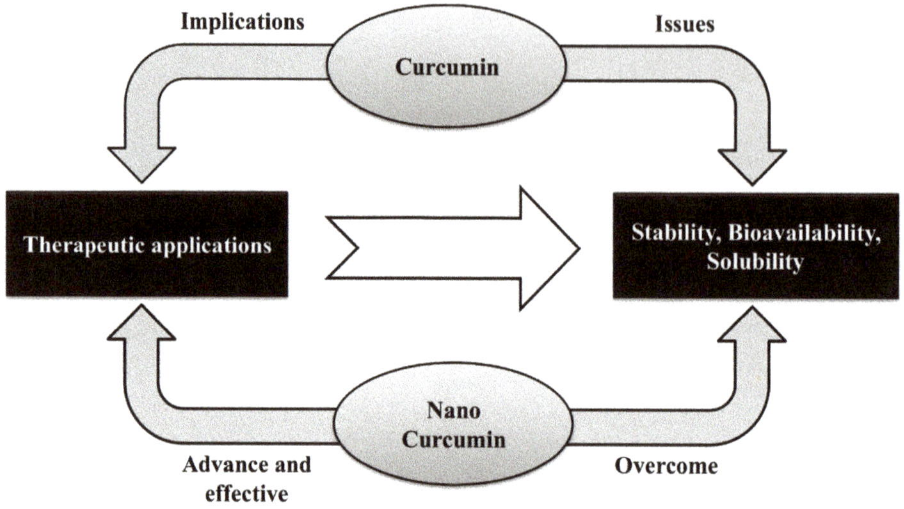

Figure 3. Curcumin and nanocurcumin.

3.5. Preparative Methods of Nanocurcumin Formulation

CUR nanoparticles are usually prepared in different ways such as (1) coacervation techniques (polymer is directly allowed to dissolve in organic solvent, e.g., ethyl acetate and CUR is suspended directly in the solution and it is allowed to homogenize. Nanoformulation is collected after centrifugation) [187], (2) nanoprecipitation (also called as solvent displacement methods, polymer and CUR is allowed to suspends together to form drug- polymeric solution and then water is added under continuous stirring which results to form precipitation. Solution is then dried by evaporation) [188], (3) spray drying technology (A CUR nano-suspension having drug concentration of 10% (w/w) is dried using mini spray dryer. The spray dried nanocrystal is directly collected after the process is over) [189], (4) single emulsion techniques (It is a conventional method in which CUR nano-suspension are dispersed in a suitable solvent followed by homogenization or ultrasonification [190], and (5) wet milling method (nano-CUR is suspended in a suitable dispersing solvent followed by ultrasonification. The obtained CUR nanoparticle is collected by centrifugation [191].

The fate of the nanoparticle depends on the type of the methods followed for its synthesis (Figure 4). Each method produces different types of nanoparticle possessing distinct physicochemical properties. In most of the cases, nanoparticle with a size of 10–200 nm is of great interest in the medicinal applications. Different shape and size ranging from spherical to other forms having positive or negative charge on the surface of nanoparticle can be administered for toxic level in cells.

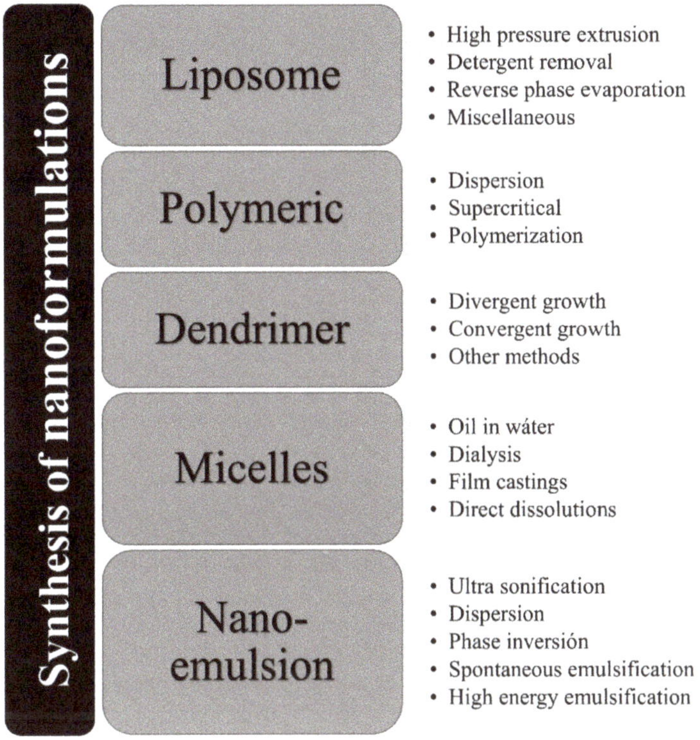

Figure 4. Different types of synthesis of nanoformulations.

3.6. Cardiovascular Effects of Curcumin-Loaded Nanoparticles

CUR possess anti-inflammatory, antioxidant, and anticancer properties. Furthermore, it has been reported that this compound may protect against myocardial injury and preserve cardiac function [8]. However, its application as treatment has been hindered due to its intrinsic characteristics, such as low bioavailability, high rate of degradation, and low solubility in aqueous medium [91,99]. For these reasons, in recent years there has been an increasing interest for the development of CUR-loaded nanoformulations to overcome its pharmacokinetic limitations, which would permit to administer the compound as therapeutic agent for CVD [96,108].

In this regard, cardioprotective effects of a CUR nanoformulation in a cell model of doxorubicin-induced cardiotoxicity were explored by Carlson, et al. [192]. These authors co-loaded CUR and resveratrol at a molar ratio of 5:1 in Pluronic® F127 micelles (Cur-Res-mP127). The size of Cur-Res-mP127 was 25.05 ± 0.539 nm with a PDI of 0.059 ± 0.018; interestingly, the encapsulation allowed 1617-fold the aqueous solubility of CUR with respect drug alone. The experimental approach showed that Cur-Res-mP127 reduced apoptosis and ROS in rat embryonic cardiomyocytes (H9C2) treated with doxorubicin hydrochloride, indicating cardioprotection.

On the other hand, increases in intracellular Ca^{2+} and ROS production mediated by L-type Ca^{2+} channel are major mediators of ischemia-reperfusion injury, a severe CVD. Thus, therapeutic efficacy of CUR encapsulated in poly (glycidyl methacrylate) nanoparticles alone (Cur-PGMA) and in combination with a peptide against the α-interacting domain of L-type Ca^{2+} channel (Cur-AID-PGMA) was evaluated in rat hearts exposed to ischemia-reperfusion [193]. Cur-AID-PGMA had an average diameter of 152 nm and a PDI of 0.062, with a CUR loading efficiency of 11.8% (w/w). Both Cur-PGMA and Cur-AID-PGMA exhibited beneficial effects against oxidative stress and myocardial injury following ischemia-reperfusion, suggesting that the formulations could possess therapeutic usefulness. In line with this, a study conducted by Ray, et al. [194] demonstrated that the encapsulation of CUR in carboxymethyl chitosan nanoparticles (Cur-CMC) increased its bioavailability, maintaining its bioactivity. In that report, the authors demonstrated that Cur-CMC produced regression of cardiac hypertrophy in a rat model. Likewise, nanoformulation allowed to observe beneficial effects at a low dose (5 mg/kg body weight) compared to free CUR (5 mg/kg body weight).

Hypertension may progress into more dangerous CVD, such as stroke and myocardial infarction. Since CUR possesses antihypertensive activity, Rachmawati, et al. [195] studied whether encapsulation of CUR in a nanoemulsion (Cur-NE) improve this activity in in vitro assays. The authors employed glyceryl monooleate as oil phase because this is more suitable in spontaneous nanoemulsification. Cur-NE had an average diameter of 42.93 ± 29.85 nm and a PDI of 0.36 ± 0.04, with a spherical morphology. Results showed that Cur-NE possesses higher inhibition rate of angiotensin converting enzyme with respect to pure CUR, suggesting an improvement of antihypertensive effect of the compound.

On the other hand, due to that LV diastolic dysfunction and myocardial apoptosis are correlated, the cardiac function can be improved by sufficient control of myocardial apoptosis [141]. Concerning this, Li, et al. [196] developed CUR-loaded polyethylene glycol methyl ether-block-poly(D,L lactide) nanoparticles (Cur-PEG-PDLLA) and evaluated their effect in cardiomyocyte apoptosis induced by palmitate exposure. Authors observed that Cur-PEG-PDLLA reduced cardiomyocyte apoptosis; besides, they reported a reduction in Bax, which plays a key role in mitochondrion-mediated apoptosis, and an increment in Bcl-2, which is an antiapoptotic protein that inhibits the oligomerization of Bax. Therefore, authors suggested that the cardioprotective effect of Cur-PEG-PDLLA could be related to the regularization of the Bcl-2/Bax ratio. Interestingly, reduction of ROS production was also observed in the cardiomyocytes treated with Cur-PEG-PDLLA. A subsequent study suggested that these effects could be mediated by activation of AMP-activated protein kinase signaling pathway and regulating the expression of downstream specific proteins [197].

In 2017, Namdari and Eatemadi [198] demonstrated the cardioprotective effect of CUR-loaded magnetic hydrogel nanocomposite (Cur-NIPAAM-MAA-NP) against doxorubicin-induced cardiac toxicity in rats. They reported that the nanoparticles were successfully synthetized with 91% of efficiency of entrapment. To evaluate the cardioprotective effect of this nanoformulation, they used H9C2 cell lines (myoblastic cells); these cells were treated with free CUR and Cur-NIPAAM-MAA-NP during 72 h. The authors analyzed the expression of three heart failure markers ANP, BNP, and b-MHC genes. The decreasing of these markers suggested that Cur-NIPAAM-MAA-NP possess cardioprotective activity.

In other study, Nabofa, et al. [199] reported the elaboration of non-toxic CUR and nisin (antimicrobial peptide) based poly lactic acid nanoparticles (CurNisNp). They evaluated the protective effect CurNisNp as pretreatment in guinea pigs with isoproterenol induced myocardial necrosis. They used two doses of CurNisNp (10 and 21 mg/kg) and demonstrated that the pretreatment with CurNisNp prevented the increment in hypertrophy index observed in guinea pigs without pretreatment (control group). The authors proposed that the ability of CUR to enhance antioxidant and reduce ROS concentration is the mechanism through the CurNisNp prevents cardiac tissue damage.

Similarly, Boarescu, et al. [200] evaluated the effects of pretreatment with CUR nanoparticles (CCNP) and with free CUR on isoproterenol induced myocardial infarction in rats. CUR and CCNP were administered in three different doses (100, 150, and 200 mg/kg) for 15 days. The authors induced the myocardial infarction in the 13th day of the study. At the end of the study, blood samples were collected, and different enzymes (CK and CK-MB and oxidative stress parameters were evaluated to analyze the cardio protective, antioxidant, and anti-inflammatory effects of the CCNP. They reported a prevention of CK-MB leakage form cardiomyocytes with all the doses of CUR and CCNP, which suggested a cardioprotective effect. In addition, rats under pretreatment did not show an increment in serum levels of TNF-α, IL-6, IL-1α, IL-1β, MCP-1, unlike the control group that presented major levels of these oxidative stress parameters after the induction of myocardial infarction.

3.7. Curcumin Nanoformulations for Cardiovascular Effects

CUR nanoformulation can improve circulation and enhance permeation retention effect of the loaded therapeutic molecule and this is one of the most important factors in drug delivery systems [201,202]. Pre-clinical and clinical trials of various therapeutic nanoformulations have been under consideration. This may include paclitaxel albumin based nanoformulations, doxorubicin liposome nanoformulation, Paclitaxel micelle based nanoformulations, siRNA based nanoformulation and docetaxel nanoformulation [203].

4. Conclusions and Perspectives

CVD are an important cause of human deaths worldwide. New alternative therapies for CVD arise from ongoing research in the whole world. Pre-clinical and clinical studies have demonstrated the effects of CUR in CVD through its anti-hypercholesterolemic and anti-atherosclerotic effects and its protective properties against cardiac ischemia and reperfusion. These effects are scientifically verified showing CUR as a potential therapeutic candidate for CVD treatment. However, in clinical trials, a wide range of doses of CUR (20–4,000 mg) have shown different effects on CV parameters. One of the challenges for the use of CUR as a therapeutic drug is to improve its bioavailability. CUR nanomedicine formulations try to solve this obstacle by improving the CUR targeting, pharmacokinetics, efficacy, and cellular uptake. CUR nanoformulations are a therapeutic alternative in a new discovery phase. Future studies need to develop new CUR nanomedicine formulations and tested it in well-designed clinical studies.

Author Contributions: All authors contributed to the manuscript. Conceptualization, J.S.-R.; validation investigation, resources, data curation, writing—all authors; review and editing, N.M., M.M., M.S.-R., W.C.C., and J.S.-R. All authors have read and agreed to the published version of the manuscript.

Acknowledgments: This work was supported by CONICYT PIA/APOYO CCTE AFB170007. N. Martins would like to thank the Portuguese Foundation for Science and Technology (FCT–Portugal) for the Strategic project ref. UID/BIM/04293/2013 and "NORTE2020—Programa Operacional Regional do Norte" (NORTE-01-0145-FEDER-000012).

Conflicts of Interest: The authors declare no conflict of interest.

References

1. Aggarwal, B.B.; Ichikawa, H.; Garodia, P.; Weerasinghe, P.; Sethi, G.; Bhatt, I.D.; Pandey, M.K.; Shishodia, S.; Nair, M.G. From traditional Ayurvedic medicine to modern medicine: Identification of therapeutic targets for suppression of inflammation and cancer. *Expert Opin. Ther. Targets* **2006**, *10*, 87–118. [CrossRef]
2. Aggarwal, B.B.; Sundaram, C.; Malani, N.; Ichikawa, H. Curcumin: The Indian solid gold. *Adv. Exp. Med. Biol.* **2007**, *595*, 1–75. [CrossRef]
3. Lampe, V.; Milobedzka, J. Studien über Curcumin. *Ber. Dtsch. Chem. Ges.* **1913**, *46*, 2235–2240. [CrossRef]
4. Gupta, S.C.; Patchva, S.; Koh, W.; Aggarwal, B.B. Discovery of curcumin, a component of golden spice, and its miraculous biological activities. *Clin. Exp. Pharmacol. Physiol.* **2012**, *39*, 283–299. [CrossRef]
5. Mehanny, M.; Hathout, R.M.; Geneidi, A.S.; Mansour, S. Exploring the use of nanocarrier systems to deliver the magical molecule; Curcumin and its derivatives. *J. Control. Release Off. J. Control. Release Soc.* **2016**, *225*, 1–30. [CrossRef]
6. Ahmad, N.; Umar, S.; Ashafaq, M.; Akhtar, M.; Iqbal, Z.; Samim, M.; Ahmad, F.J. A comparative study of PNIPAM nanoparticles of curcumin, demethoxycurcumin, and bisdemethoxycurcumin and their effects on oxidative stress markers in experimental stroke. *Protoplasma* **2013**, *250*, 1327–1338. [CrossRef]
7. Sharma, R.A.; Gescher, A.J.; Steward, W.P. Curcumin: The story so far. *Eur. J. Cancer* **2005**, *41*, 1955–1968. [CrossRef]

8. Aggarwal, B.B.; Harikumar, K.B. Potential therapeutic effects of curcumin, the anti-inflammatory agent, against neurodegenerative, cardiovascular, pulmonary, metabolic, autoimmune and neoplastic diseases. *Int. J. Biochem. Cell Biol.* **2009**, *41*, 40–59. [CrossRef]
9. Anand, P.; Sundaram, C.; Jhurani, S.; Kunnumakkara, A.B.; Aggarwal, B.B. Curcumin and cancer: An "old-age" disease with an "age-old" solution. *Cancer Lett.* **2008**, *267*, 133–164. [CrossRef]
10. Gupta, S.C.; Patchva, S.; Aggarwal, B.B. Therapeutic roles of curcumin: Lessons learned from clinical trials. *AAPS J.* **2013**, *15*, 195–218. [CrossRef]
11. Alwi, I.; Santoso, T.; Suyono, S.; Sutrisna, B.; Suyatna, F.D.; Kresno, S.B.; Ernie, S. The effect of curcumin on lipid level in patients with acute coronary syndrome. *Acta Med. Indones.* **2008**, *40*, 201–210.
12. Baum, L.; Cheung, S.K.; Mok, V.C.; Lam, L.C.; Leung, V.P.; Hui, E.; Ng, C.C.; Chow, M.; Ho, P.C.; Lam, S.; et al. Curcumin effects on blood lipid profile in a 6-month human study. *Pharmacol. Res.* **2007**, *56*, 509–514. [CrossRef]
13. Chuengsamarn, S.; Rattanamongkolgul, S.; Phonrat, B.; Tungtrongchitr, R.; Jirawatnotai, S. Reduction of atherogenic risk in patients with type 2 diabetes by curcuminoid extract: A randomized controlled trial. *J. Nutr. Biochem.* **2014**, *25*, 144–150. [CrossRef]
14. DiSilvestro, R.A.; Joseph, E.; Zhao, S.; Bomser, J. Diverse effects of a low dose supplement of lipidated curcumin in healthy middle aged people. *Nutr. J.* **2012**, *11*, 79. [CrossRef]
15. Ferguson, J.J.A.; Stojanovski, E.; MacDonald-Wicks, L.; Garg, M.L. Curcumin potentiates cholesterol-lowering effects of phytosterols in hypercholesterolaemic individuals. A randomised controlled trial. *Metab. Clin. Exp.* **2018**, *82*, 22–35. [CrossRef]
16. Hasan, S.T.; Zingg, J.M.; Kwan, P.; Noble, T.; Smith, D.; Meydani, M. Curcumin modulation of high fat diet-induced atherosclerosis and steatohepatosis in LDL receptor deficient mice. *Atherosclerosis* **2014**, *232*, 40–51. [CrossRef]
17. Sahebkar, A. Dual effect of curcumin in preventing atherosclerosis: The potential role of pro-oxidant-antioxidant mechanisms. *Nat. Prod. Res.* **2015**, *29*, 491–492. [CrossRef]
18. Salehi, B.; Stojanovic-Radic, Z.; Matejic, J.; Sharifi-Rad, M.; Anil Kumar, N.V.; Martins, N.; Sharifi-Rad, J. The therapeutic potential of curcumin: A review of clinical trials. *Eur. J. Med. Chem.* **2019**, *163*, 527–545. [CrossRef]
19. Zingg, J.M.; Hasan, S.T.; Meydani, M. Molecular mechanisms of hypolipidemic effects of curcumin. *BioFactors* **2013**, *39*, 101–121. [CrossRef]
20. Bayet-Robert, M.; Kwiatkowski, F.; Leheurteur, M.; Gachon, F.; Planchat, E.; Abrial, C.; Mouret-Reynier, M.A.; Durando, X.; Barthomeuf, C.; Chollet, P. Phase I dose escalation trial of docetaxel plus curcumin in patients with advanced and metastatic breast cancer. *Cancer Biol. Ther.* **2010**, *9*, 8–14. [CrossRef]
21. Carroll, R.E.; Benya, R.V.; Turgeon, D.K.; Vareed, S.; Neuman, M.; Rodriguez, L.; Kakarala, M.; Carpenter, P.M.; McLaren, C.; Meyskens, F.L., Jr.; et al. Phase IIa clinical trial of curcumin for the prevention of colorectal neoplasia. *Cancer Prev. Res.* **2011**, *4*, 354–364. [CrossRef]
22. Cheng, A.L.; Hsu, C.H.; Lin, J.K.; Hsu, M.M.; Ho, Y.F.; Shen, T.S.; Ko, J.Y.; Lin, J.T.; Lin, B.R.; Ming-Shiang, W.; et al. Phase I clinical trial of curcumin, a chemopreventive agent, in patients with high-risk or pre-malignant lesions. *Anticancer Res.* **2001**, *21*, 2895–2900.
23. Dhillon, N.; Aggarwal, B.B.; Newman, R.A.; Wolff, R.A.; Kunnumakkara, A.B.; Abbruzzese, J.L.; Ng, C.S.; Badmaev, V.; Kurzrock, R. Phase II trial of curcumin in patients with advanced pancreatic cancer. *Clin. Cancer Res. Off. J. Am. Assoc. Cancer Res.* **2008**, *14*, 4491–4499. [CrossRef]
24. Epelbaum, R.; Schaffer, M.; Vizel, B.; Badmaev, V.; Bar-Sela, G. Curcumin and gemcitabine in patients with advanced pancreatic cancer. *Nutr. Cancer* **2010**, *62*, 1137–1141. [CrossRef]
25. He, Z.Y.; Shi, C.B.; Wen, H.; Li, F.L.; Wang, B.L.; Wang, J. Upregulation of p53 expression in patients with colorectal cancer by administration of curcumin. *Cancer Investig.* **2011**, *29*, 208–213. [CrossRef]
26. Kanai, M.; Yoshimura, K.; Asada, M.; Imaizumi, A.; Suzuki, C.; Matsumoto, S.; Nishimura, T.; Mori, Y.; Masui, T.; Kawaguchi, Y.; et al. A phase I/II study of gemcitabine-based chemotherapy plus curcumin for patients with gemcitabine-resistant pancreatic cancer. *Cancer Chemother. Pharmacol.* **2011**, *68*, 157–164. [CrossRef]

27. Kim, S.G.; Veena, M.S.; Basak, S.K.; Han, E.; Tajima, T.; Gjertson, D.W.; Starr, J.; Eidelman, O.; Pollard, H.B.; Srivastava, M.; et al. Curcumin treatment suppresses IKKbeta kinase activity of salivary cells of patients with head and neck cancer: A pilot study. *Clin. Cancer Res. Off. J. Am. Assoc. Cancer Res.* **2011**, *17*, 5953–5961. [CrossRef]
28. Baum, L.; Lam, C.W.; Cheung, S.K.; Kwok, T.; Lui, V.; Tsoh, J.; Lam, L.; Leung, V.; Hui, E.; Ng, C.; et al. Six-month randomized, placebo-controlled, double-blind, pilot clinical trial of curcumin in patients with Alzheimer disease. *J. Clin. Psychopharmacol.* **2008**, *28*, 110–113. [CrossRef]
29. Ringman, J.M.; Frautschy, S.A.; Teng, E.; Begum, A.N.; Bardens, J.; Beigi, M.; Gylys, K.H.; Badmaev, V.; Heath, D.D.; Apostolova, L.G.; et al. Oral curcumin for Alzheimer's disease: Tolerability and efficacy in a 24-week randomized, double blind, placebo-controlled study. *Alzheimer Res. Ther.* **2012**, *4*, 43. [CrossRef]
30. Kim, D.S.; Kim, J.Y.; Han, Y. Curcuminoids in neurodegenerative diseases. *Recent Pat. CNS Drug Discov.* **2012**, *7*, 184–204. [CrossRef]
31. Arora, R.; Kuhad, A.; Kaur, I.P.; Chopra, K. Curcumin loaded solid lipid nanoparticles ameliorate adjuvant-induced arthritis in rats. *Eur. J. Pain* **2015**, *19*, 940–952. [CrossRef] [PubMed]
32. Chandran, B.; Goel, A. A randomized, pilot study to assess the efficacy and safety of curcumin in patients with active rheumatoid arthritis. *Phytother. Res. PTR* **2012**, *26*, 1719–1725. [CrossRef]
33. Bhutani, M.K.; Bishnoi, M.; Kulkarni, S.K. Anti-depressant like effect of curcumin and its combination with piperine in unpredictable chronic stress-induced behavioral, biochemical and neurochemical changes. *Pharmacol. Biochem. Behav.* **2009**, *92*, 39–43. [CrossRef] [PubMed]
34. Cox, K.H.; Pipingas, A.; Scholey, A.B. Investigation of the effects of solid lipid curcumin on cognition and mood in a healthy older population. *J. Psychopharmacol.* **2015**, *29*, 642–651. [CrossRef]
35. Esmaily, H.; Sahebkar, A.; Iranshahi, M.; Ganjali, S.; Mohammadi, A.; Ferns, G.; Ghayour-Mobarhan, M. An investigation of the effects of curcumin on anxiety and depression in obese individuals: A randomized controlled trial. *Chin. J. Integr. Med.* **2015**, *21*, 332–338. [CrossRef]
36. Jiang, H.; Wang, Z.; Wang, Y.; Xie, K.; Zhang, Q.; Luan, Q.; Chen, W.; Liu, D. Antidepressant-like effects of curcumin in chronic mild stress of rats: Involvement of its anti-inflammatory action. *Prog. Neuro Psychopharmacol. Biol. Psychiatry* **2013**, *47*, 33–39. [CrossRef]
37. Lopresti, A.L.; Maes, M.; Meddens, M.J.; Maker, G.L.; Arnoldussen, E.; Drummond, P.D. Curcumin and major depression: A randomised, double-blind, placebo-controlled trial investigating the potential of peripheral biomarkers to predict treatment response and antidepressant mechanisms of change. *Eur. Neuropsychopharmacol. J. Eur. Coll. Neuropsychopharmacol.* **2015**, *25*, 38–50. [CrossRef]
38. Chuengsamarn, S.; Rattanamongkolgul, S.; Luechapudiporn, R.; Phisalaphong, C.; Jirawatnotai, S. Curcumin extract for prevention of type 2 diabetes. *Diabetes Care* **2012**, *35*, 2121–2127. [CrossRef]
39. Nabavi, S.F.; Thiagarajan, R.; Rastrelli, L.; Daglia, M.; Sobarzo-Sanchez, E.; Alinezhad, H.; Nabavi, S.M. Curcumin: A natural product for diabetes and its complications. *Curr. Top. Med. Chem.* **2015**, *15*, 2445–2455. [CrossRef]
40. Rivera-Mancia, S.; Lozada-Garcia, M.C.; Pedraza-Chaverri, J. Experimental evidence for curcumin and its analogs for management of diabetes mellitus and its associated complications. *Eur. J. Pharmacol.* **2015**, *756*, 30–37. [CrossRef]
41. Biswas, S.; Hwang, J.W.; Kirkham, P.A.; Rahman, I. Pharmacological and dietary antioxidant therapies for chronic obstructive pulmonary disease. *Curr. Med. Chem.* **2013**, *20*, 1496–1530. [CrossRef] [PubMed]
42. Moghaddam, S.J.; Barta, P.; Mirabolfathinejad, S.G.; Ammar-Aouchiche, Z.; Garza, N.T.; Vo, T.T.; Newman, R.A.; Aggarwal, B.B.; Evans, C.M.; Tuvim, M.J.; et al. Curcumin inhibits COPD-like airway inflammation and lung cancer progression in mice. *Carcinogenesis* **2009**, *30*, 1949–1956. [CrossRef] [PubMed]
43. Suzuki, M.; Betsuyaku, T.; Ito, Y.; Nagai, K.; Odajima, N.; Moriyama, C.; Nasuhara, Y.; Nishimura, M. Curcumin attenuates elastase- and cigarette smoke-induced pulmonary emphysema in mice. *Am. J. Physiol. Lung Cell. Mol. Physiol.* **2009**, *296*, L614–L623. [CrossRef]
44. Bundy, R.; Walker, A.F.; Middleton, R.W.; Booth, J. Turmeric extract may improve irritable bowel syndrome symptomology in otherwise healthy adults: A pilot study. *J. Altern. Complemen. Med.* **2004**, *10*, 1015–1018. [CrossRef]
45. Kerdsakundee, N.; Mahattanadul, S.; Wiwattanapatapee, R. Development and evaluation of gastroretentive raft forming systems incorporating curcumin-Eudragit(R) EPO solid dispersions for gastric ulcer treatment. *Eur. J. Pharm. Biopharm. Off. J. Arb. Pharm. Verfahr. e.V* **2015**, *94*, 513–520. [CrossRef]

46. Morsy, M.A.; El-Moselhy, M.A. Mechanisms of the protective effects of curcumin against indomethacin-induced gastric ulcer in rats. *Pharmacology* **2013**, *91*, 267–274. [CrossRef]
47. Pari, L.; Tewas, D.; Eckel, J. Role of curcumin in health and disease. *Arch. Physiol. Biochem.* **2008**, *114*, 127–149. [CrossRef]
48. Yadav, S.K.; Sah, A.K.; Jha, R.K.; Sah, P.; Shah, D.K. Turmeric (curcumin) remedies gastroprotective action. *Pharmacogn. Rev.* **2013**, *7*, 42–46. [CrossRef]
49. Allegri, P.; Mastromarino, A.; Neri, P. Management of chronic anterior uveitis relapses: Efficacy of oral phospholipidic curcumin treatment. Long-term follow-up. *Clin. Ophthalmol.* **2010**, *4*, 1201–1206. [CrossRef]
50. Biswas, N.R.; Gupta, S.K.; Das, G.K.; Kumar, N.; Mongre, P.K.; Haldar, D.; Beri, S. Evaluation of Ophthacare eye drops–a herbal formulation in the management of various ophthalmic disorders. *Phytother. Res. PTR* **2001**, *15*, 618–620. [CrossRef]
51. Lal, B.; Kapoor, A.K.; Asthana, O.P.; Agrawal, P.K.; Prasad, R.; Kumar, P.; Srimal, R.C. Efficacy of curcumin in the management of chronic anterior uveitis. *Phytother. Res. PTR* **1999**, *13*, 318–322. [CrossRef]
52. Bahraini, P.; Rajabi, M.; Mansouri, P.; Sarafian, G.; Chalangari, R.; Azizian, Z. Turmeric tonic as a treatment in scalp psoriasis: A randomized placebo-control clinical trial. *J. Cosmet. Dermatol.* **2018**, *17*, 461–466. [CrossRef]
53. Kurd, S.K.; Smith, N.; VanVoorhees, A.; Troxel, A.B.; Badmaev, V.; Seykora, J.T.; Gelfand, J.M. Oral curcumin in the treatment of moderate to severe psoriasis vulgaris: A prospective clinical trial. *J. Am. Acad. Dermatol.* **2008**, *58*, 625–631. [CrossRef]
54. Ryan, J.L.; Heckler, C.E.; Ling, M.; Katz, A.; Williams, J.P.; Pentland, A.P.; Morrow, G.R. Curcumin for radiation dermatitis: A randomized, double-blind, placebo-controlled clinical trial of thirty breast cancer patients. *Radiat. Res.* **2013**, *180*, 34–43. [CrossRef]
55. Qin, S.; Huang, L.; Gong, J.; Shen, S.; Huang, J.; Ren, H.; Hu, H. Efficacy and safety of turmeric and curcumin in lowering blood lipid levels in patients with cardiovascular risk factors: A meta-analysis of randomized controlled trials. *Nutr. J.* **2017**, *16*, 68. [CrossRef]
56. Soni, K.B.; Kuttan, R. Effect of oral curcumin administration on serum peroxides and cholesterol levels in human volunteers. *Indian J. Physiol. Pharmacol.* **1992**, *36*, 273–275.
57. Saeidinia, A.; Keihanian, F.; Butler, A.E.; Bagheri, R.K.; Atkin, S.L.; Sahebkar, A. Curcumin in heart failure: A choice for complementary therapy? *Pharmacol. Res.* **2018**, *131*, 112–119. [CrossRef]
58. Jiang, S.; Han, J.; Li, T.; Xin, Z.; Ma, Z.; Di, W.; Hu, W.; Gong, B.; Di, S.; Wang, D.; et al. Curcumin as a potential protective compound against cardiac diseases. *Pharmacol. Res.* **2017**, *119*, 373–383. [CrossRef]
59. Liu, W.; Zhai, Y.; Heng, X.; Che, F.Y.; Chen, W.; Sun, D.; Zhai, G. Oral bioavailability of curcumin: Problems and advancements. *J. Drug Target.* **2016**, *24*, 694–702. [CrossRef]
60. Anand, P.; Kunnumakkara, A.B.; Newman, R.A.; Aggarwal, B.B. Bioavailability of curcumin: Problems and promises. *Mol. Pharm.* **2007**, *4*, 807–818. [CrossRef]
61. Pan, M.H.; Huang, T.M.; Lin, J.K. Biotransformation of curcumin through reduction and glucuronidation in mice. *Drug Metab. Dispos. Biol. Fate Chem.* **1999**, *27*, 486–494.
62. Tonnesen, H.H.; Masson, M.; Loftsson, T. Studies of curcumin and curcuminoids. XXVII. Cyclodextrin complexation: Solubility, chemical and photochemical stability. *Int. J. Pharm.* **2002**, *244*, 127–135. [CrossRef]
63. Priyadarsini, K.I. The chemistry of curcumin: From extraction to therapeutic agent. *Molecules* **2014**, *19*, 20091–20112. [CrossRef]
64. Williams, M. *An Encyclopedia of Chemicals, Drugs, and Biologicals*, 15th ed.; O'Neil, M.J., Ed.; Royal Society of Chemistry: Cambridge, UK, 2013; 2708p. ISBN 9781849736701; $150 with 1-year free access to The Merck Index Online. *Drug Dev. Res.* **2013**, *74*, 339. [CrossRef]
65. Fujisawa, S.; Atsumi, T.; Ishihara, M.; Kadoma, Y. Cytotoxicity, ROS-generation activity and radical-scavenging activity of curcumin and related compounds. *Anticancer Res.* **2004**, *24*, 563–569.
66. Kasim, N.A.; Whitehouse, M.; Ramachandran, C.; Bermejo, M.; Lennernas, H.; Hussain, A.S.; Junginger, H.E.; Stavchansky, S.A.; Midha, K.K.; Shah, V.P.; et al. Molecular properties of WHO essential drugs and provisional biopharmaceutical classification. *Mol. Pharm.* **2004**, *1*, 85–96. [CrossRef]
67. Shen, L.; Ji, H.F. The pharmacology of curcumin: Is it the degradation products? *Trends Mol. Med.* **2012**, *18*, 138–144. [CrossRef]
68. Aggarwal, B.B.; Surh, Y.-J.; Shishodia, S. *The Molecular Targets and Therapeutic Uses of Curcumin in Health and Disease*; Springer: Boston, MA, USA, 2007; Volume 595.

69. Marczylo, T.H.; Verschoyle, R.D.; Cooke, D.N.; Morazzoni, P.; Steward, W.P.; Gescher, A.J. Comparison of systemic availability of curcumin with that of curcumin formulated with phosphatidylcholine. *Cancer Chemother. Pharmacol.* **2007**, *60*, 171–177. [CrossRef]
70. Holder, G.M.; Plummer, J.L.; Ryan, A.J. The metabolism and excretion of curcumin (1,7-bis-(4-hydroxy-3-methoxyphenyl)-1,6-heptadiene-3,5-dione) in the rat. *Xenobiotica Fate Foreign Compd. Biol. Syst.* **1978**, *8*, 761–768. [CrossRef]
71. Ravindranath, V.; Chandrasekhara, N. Metabolism of curcumn-studies with [3H]curcumin. *Toxicology* **1981**, *22*, 337–344. [CrossRef]
72. Ma, Z.; Haddadi, A.; Molavi, O.; Lavasanifar, A.; Lai, R.; Samuel, J. Micelles of poly(ethylene oxide)-b-poly(epsilon-caprolactone) as vehicles for the solubilization, stabilization, and controlled delivery of curcumin. *J. Biomed. Mater. Res. Part A* **2008**, *86*, 300–310. [CrossRef]
73. Bonferoni, M.C.; Rossi, S.; Sandri, G.; Ferrari, F. Nanoparticle formulations to enhance tumor targeting of poorly soluble polyphenols with potential anticancer properties. *Semin. Cancer Biol.* **2017**, *46*, 205–214. [CrossRef]
74. Lagoa, R.; Silva, J.; Rodrigues, J.R.; Bishayee, A. Advances in phytochemical delivery systems for improved anticancer activity. *Biotechnol. Adv.* **2019**. [CrossRef]
75. Li, C.; Zhang, J.; Zu, Y.J.; Nie, S.F.; Cao, J.; Wang, Q.; Nie, S.P.; Deng, Z.Y.; Xie, M.Y.; Wang, S. Biocompatible and biodegradable nanoparticles for enhancement of anti-cancer activities of phytochemicals. *Chin. J. Nat. Med.* **2015**, *13*, 641–652. [CrossRef]
76. Pistollato, F.; Bremer-Hoffmann, S.; Basso, G.; Cano, S.S.; Elio, I.; Vergara, M.M.; Giampieri, F.; Battino, M. Targeting Glioblastoma with the Use of Phytocompounds and Nanoparticles. *Target. Oncol.* **2016**, *11*, 1–16. [CrossRef]
77. Rahimi, H.R.; Nedaeinia, R.; Sepehri Shamloo, A.; Nikdoust, S.; Kazemi Oskuee, R. Novel delivery system for natural products: Nano-curcumin formulations. *Avicenna J. Phytomed.* **2016**, *6*, 383–398.
78. Siddiqui, I.A.; Sanna, V. Impact of nanotechnology on the delivery of natural products for cancer prevention and therapy. *Mol. Nutr. Food Res.* **2016**, *60*, 1330–1341. [CrossRef]
79. Wang, S.; Su, R.; Nie, S.; Sun, M.; Zhang, J.; Wu, D.; Moustaid-Moussa, N. Application of nanotechnology in improving bioavailability and bioactivity of diet-derived phytochemicals. *J. Nutr. Biochem.* **2014**, *25*, 363–376. [CrossRef]
80. Davatgaran-Taghipour, Y.; Masoomzadeh, S.; Farzaei, M.H.; Bahramsoltani, R.; Karimi-Soureh, Z.; Rahimi, R.; Abdollahi, M. Polyphenol nanoformulations for cancer therapy: Experimental evidence and clinical perspective. *Int. J. Nanomed.* **2017**, *12*, 2689–2702. [CrossRef]
81. Ahmad, M.Z.; Alkahtani, S.A.; Akhter, S.; Ahmad, F.J.; Ahmad, J.; Akhtar, M.S.; Mohsin, N.; Abdel-Wahab, B.A. Progress in nanotechnology-based drug carrier in designing of curcumin nanomedicines for cancer therapy: Current state-of-the-art. *J. Drug Target.* **2016**, *24*, 273–293. [CrossRef]
82. Bansal, S.S.; Goel, M.; Aqil, F.; Vadhanam, M.V.; Gupta, R.C. Advanced drug delivery systems of curcumin for cancer chemoprevention. *Cancer Prev. Res.* **2011**, *4*, 1158–1171. [CrossRef]
83. Batra, H.; Pawar, S.; Bahl, D. Curcumin in combination with anti-cancer drugs: A nanomedicine review. *Pharmacol. Res.* **2019**, *139*, 91–105. [CrossRef]
84. Lee, W.H.; Loo, C.Y.; Young, P.M.; Traini, D.; Mason, R.S.; Rohanizadeh, R. Recent advances in curcumin nanoformulation for cancer therapy. *Expert Opin. Drug Deliv.* **2014**, *11*, 1183–1201. [CrossRef]
85. Nair, A.; Amalraj, A.; Jacob, J.; Kunnumakkara, A.B.; Gopi, S. Non-Curcuminoids from Turmeric and Their Potential in Cancer Therapy and Anticancer Drug Delivery Formulations. *Biomolecules* **2019**, *9*, 13. [CrossRef]
86. Shindikar, A.; Singh, A.; Nobre, M.; Kirolikar, S. Curcumin and Resveratrol as Promising Natural Remedies with Nanomedicine Approach for the Effective Treatment of Triple Negative Breast Cancer. *J. Oncol.* **2016**, *2016*, 9750785. [CrossRef]
87. Subramani, P.A.; Panati, K.; Narala, V.R. Curcumin Nanotechnologies and Its Anticancer Activity. *Nutr. Cancer* **2017**, *69*, 381–393. [CrossRef]
88. Tajbakhsh, A.; Hasanzadeh, M.; Rezaee, M.; Khedri, M.; Khazaei, M.; ShahidSales, S.; Ferns, G.A.; Hassanian, S.M.; Avan, A. Therapeutic potential of novel formulated forms of curcumin in the treatment of breast cancer by the targeting of cellular and physiological dysregulated pathways. *J. Cell. Physiol.* **2018**, *233*, 2183–2192. [CrossRef]

89. Wong, K.E.; Ngai, S.C.; Chan, K.G.; Lee, L.H.; Goh, B.H.; Chuah, L.H. Curcumin Nanoformulations for Colorectal Cancer: A Review. *Front. Pharmacol.* **2019**, *10*, 152. [CrossRef]
90. Yallapu, M.M.; Jaggi, M.; Chauhan, S.C. Curcumin nanoformulations: A future nanomedicine for cancer. *Drug Discov. Today* **2012**, *17*, 71–80. [CrossRef]
91. Del Prado-Audelo, M.L.; Caballero-Floran, I.H.; Meza-Toledo, J.A.; Mendoza-Munoz, N.; Gonzalez-Torres, M.; Floran, B.; Cortes, H.; Leyva-Gomez, G. Formulations of Curcumin Nanoparticles for Brain Diseases. *Biomolecules* **2019**, *9*, 56. [CrossRef]
92. Rakotoarisoa, M.; Angelova, A. Amphiphilic Nanocarrier Systems for Curcumin Delivery in Neurodegenerative Disorders. *Medicines* **2018**, *5*, 126. [CrossRef]
93. Hussain, Z.; Thu, H.E.; Ng, S.F.; Khan, S.; Katas, H. Nanoencapsulation, an efficient and promising approach to maximize wound healing efficacy of curcumin: A review of new trends and state-of-the-art. *Colloids Surf. B Biointerfaces* **2017**, *150*, 223–241. [CrossRef]
94. Mahmood, K.; Zia, K.M.; Zuber, M.; Salman, M.; Anjum, M.N. Recent developments in curcumin and curcumin based polymeric materials for biomedical applications: A review. *Int. J. Biol. Macromol.* **2015**, *81*, 877–890. [CrossRef]
95. Maradana, M.R.; Thomas, R.; O'Sullivan, B.J. Targeted delivery of curcumin for treating type 2 diabetes. *Mol. Nutr. Food Res.* **2013**, *57*, 1550–1556. [CrossRef]
96. Yallapu, M.M.; Nagesh, P.K.; Jaggi, M.; Chauhan, S.C. Therapeutic Applications of Curcumin Nanoformulations. *AAPS J.* **2015**, *17*, 1341–1356. [CrossRef]
97. Ahangari, N.; Kargozar, S.; Ghayour-Mobarhan, M.; Baino, F.; Pasdar, A.; Sahebkar, A.; Ferns, G.A.A.; Kim, H.W.; Mozafari, M. Curcumin in tissue engineering: A traditional remedy for modern medicine. *BioFactors* **2019**, *45*, 135–151. [CrossRef]
98. Bhatia, S. Nanoparticles Types, Classification, Characterization, Fabrication Methods and Drug Delivery Applications. In *Natural Polymer Drug Delivery Systems: Nanoparticles, Plants, and Algae*; Bhatia, S., Ed.; Springer International Publishing: Cham, Switzerland, 2016; pp. 33–93. [CrossRef]
99. Del Prado-Audelo, M.L.; Magaña, J.J.; Mejía-Contreras, B.A.; Borbolla-Jiménez, F.V.; Giraldo-Gomez, D.M.; Piña-Barba, M.C.; Quintanar-Guerrero, D.; Leyva-Gómez, G. In vitro cell uptake evaluation of curcumin-loaded PCL/F68 nanoparticles for potential application in neuronal diseases. *J. Drug Deliv. Sci. Technol.* **2019**, *52*, 905–914. [CrossRef]
100. Fonseca-Santos, B.; Gremiao, M.P.; Chorilli, M. Nanotechnology-based drug delivery systems for the treatment of Alzheimer's disease. *Int. J. Nanomed.* **2015**, *10*, 4981–5003. [CrossRef]
101. Ghalandarlaki, N.; Alizadeh, A.M.; Ashkani-Esfahani, S. Nanotechnology-applied curcumin for different diseases therapy. *BioMed Res. Int.* **2014**, *2014*, 394264. [CrossRef]
102. Naksuriya, O.; Okonogi, S.; Schiffelers, R.M.; Hennink, W.E. Curcumin nanoformulations: A review of pharmaceutical properties and preclinical studies and clinical data related to cancer treatment. *Biomaterials* **2014**, *35*, 3365–3383. [CrossRef]
103. Sun, M.; Su, X.; Ding, B.; He, X.; Liu, X.; Yu, A.; Lou, H.; Zhai, G. Advances in nanotechnology-based delivery systems for curcumin. *Nanomedicine* **2012**, *7*, 1085–1100. [CrossRef]
104. Gera, M.; Sharma, N.; Ghosh, M.; Huynh, D.L.; Lee, S.J.; Min, T.; Kwon, T.; Jeong, D.K. Nanoformulations of curcumin: An emerging paradigm for improved remedial application. *Oncotarget* **2017**, *8*, 66680–66698. [CrossRef]
105. Hu, B.; Liu, X.; Zhang, C.; Zeng, X. Food macromolecule based nanodelivery systems for enhancing the bioavailability of polyphenols. *J. Food Drug Anal.* **2017**, *25*, 3–15. [CrossRef]
106. Gharpure, K.M.; Wu, S.Y.; Li, C.; Lopez-Berestein, G.; Sood, A.K. Nanotechnology: Future of Oncotherapy. *Clin. Cancer Res.* **2015**, *21*, 3121–3130. [CrossRef]
107. Shakeri, A.; Sahebkar, A. Opinion Paper: Nanotechnology: A Successful Approach to Improve Oral Bioavailability of Phytochemicals. *Recent Pat. Drug Deliv. Formul.* **2016**, *10*, 4–6. [CrossRef]
108. Martin Gimenez, V.M.; Kassuha, D.E.; Manucha, W. Nanomedicine applied to cardiovascular diseases: Latest developments. *Ther. Adv. Cardiovasc. Dis.* **2017**, *11*, 133–142. [CrossRef]
109. McCarthy, J.R. Nanomedicine and Cardiovascular Disease. *Curr. Cardiovasc. Imaging Rep.* **2010**, *3*, 42–49. [CrossRef]
110. Ejaz, A.; Wu, D.; Kwan, P.; Meydani, M. Curcumin inhibits adipogenesis in 3T3-L1 adipocytes and angiogenesis and obesity in C57/BL mice. *J. Nutr.* **2009**, *139*, 919–925. [CrossRef]

111. El-Habibi, E.-S.M.; El-Wakf, A.M.; Mogall, A. Efficacy of Curcumin in Reducing Risk of Cardiovascular Disease in High Fat Diet-Fed Rats. *J. Bioanal. Biomed.* **2013**, *5*, 66–70. [CrossRef]
112. Shin, S.K.; Ha, T.Y.; McGregor, R.A.; Choi, M.S. Long-term curcumin administration protects against atherosclerosis via hepatic regulation of lipoprotein cholesterol metabolism. *Mol. Nutr. Food Res.* **2011**, *55*, 1829–1840. [CrossRef]
113. Quiles, J.L.; Aguilera, C.; Mesa, M.D.; Ramirez-Tortosa, M.C.; Baro, L.; Gil, A. An ethanolic-aqueous extract of Curcuma longa decreases the susceptibility of liver microsomes and mitochondria to lipid peroxidation in atherosclerotic rabbits. *BioFactors* **1998**, *8*, 51–57. [CrossRef]
114. Quiles, J.L.; Mesa, M.D.; Ramirez-Tortosa, C.L.; Aguilera, C.M.; Battino, M.; Gil, A.; Ramirez-Tortosa, M.C. Curcuma longa extract supplementation reduces oxidative stress and attenuates aortic fatty streak development in rabbits. *Arterioscler. Thromb. Vasc. Biol.* **2002**, *22*, 1225–1231. [CrossRef]
115. Ramirez-Tortosa, M.C.; Mesa, M.D.; Aguilera, M.C.; Quiles, J.L.; Baro, L.; Ramirez-Tortosa, C.L.; Martinez-Victoria, E.; Gil, A. Oral administration of a turmeric extract inhibits LDL oxidation and has hypocholesterolemic effects in rabbits with experimental atherosclerosis. *Atherosclerosis* **1999**, *147*, 371–378. [CrossRef]
116. Olszanecki, R.; Jawien, J.; Gajda, M.; Mateuszuk, L.; Gebska, A.; Korabiowska, M.; Chlopicki, S.; Korbut, R. Effect of curcumin on atherosclerosis in apoE/LDLR-double knockout mice. *J. Physiol. Pharmacol. Off. J. Pol. Physiol. Soc.* **2005**, *56*, 627–635.
117. Coban, D.; Milenkovic, D.; Chanet, A.; Khallou-Laschet, J.; Sabbe, L.; Palagani, A.; Vanden Berghe, W.; Mazur, A.; Morand, C. Dietary curcumin inhibits atherosclerosis by affecting the expression of genes involved in leukocyte adhesion and transendothelial migration. *Mol. Nutr. Food Res.* **2012**, *56*, 1270–1281. [CrossRef]
118. Zhao, J.F.; Ching, L.C.; Huang, Y.C.; Chen, C.Y.; Chiang, A.N.; Kou, Y.R.; Shyue, S.K.; Lee, T.S. Molecular mechanism of curcumin on the suppression of cholesterol accumulation in macrophage foam cells and atherosclerosis. *Mol. Nutr. Food Res.* **2012**, *56*, 691–701. [CrossRef]
119. Zhang, S.; Zou, J.; Li, P.; Zheng, X.; Feng, D. Curcumin Protects against Atherosclerosis in Apolipoprotein E-Knockout Mice by Inhibiting Toll-like Receptor 4 Expression. *J. Agric. Food Chem.* **2018**, *66*, 449–456. [CrossRef]
120. Gao, S.; Zhang, W.; Zhao, Q.; Zhou, J.; Wu, Y.; Liu, Y.; Yuan, Z.; Wang, L. Curcumin ameliorates atherosclerosis in apolipoprotein E deficient asthmatic mice by regulating the balance of Th2/Treg cells. *Phytomed. Int. J. Phytother. Phytopharm.* **2019**, *52*, 129–135. [CrossRef]
121. Yang, X.; Thomas, D.P.; Zhang, X.; Culver, B.W.; Alexander, B.M.; Murdoch, W.J.; Rao, M.N.; Tulis, D.A.; Ren, J.; Sreejayan, N. Curcumin inhibits platelet-derived growth factor-stimulated vascular smooth muscle cell function and injury-induced neointima formation. *Arterioscler. Thromb. Vasc. Biol.* **2006**, *26*, 85–90. [CrossRef]
122. Yuan, H.Y.; Kuang, S.Y.; Zheng, X.; Ling, H.Y.; Yang, Y.B.; Yan, P.K.; Li, K.; Liao, D.F. Curcumin inhibits cellular cholesterol accumulation by regulating SREBP-1/caveolin-1 signaling pathway in vascular smooth muscle cells. *Acta Pharmacol. Sin.* **2008**, *29*, 555–563. [CrossRef]
123. Qin, L.; Yang, Y.B.; Tuo, Q.H.; Zhu, B.Y.; Chen, L.X.; Zhang, L.; Liao, D.F. Effects and underlying mechanisms of curcumin on the proliferation of vascular smooth muscle cells induced by Chol: MbetaCD. *Biochem. Biophys. Res. Commun.* **2009**, *379*, 277–282. [CrossRef] [PubMed]
124. Yu, Y.M.; Lin, H.C. Curcumin prevents human aortic smooth muscle cells migration by inhibiting of MMP-9 expression. *Nutr. Metab. Cardiovasc. Dis. NMCD* **2010**, *20*, 125–132. [CrossRef] [PubMed]
125. Lewinska, A.; Wnuk, M.; Grabowska, W.; Zabek, T.; Semik, E.; Sikora, E.; Bielak-Zmijewska, A. Curcumin induces oxidation-dependent cell cycle arrest mediated by SIRT7 inhibition of rDNA transcription in human aortic smooth muscle cells. *Toxicol. Lett.* **2015**, *233*, 227–238. [CrossRef] [PubMed]
126. Parodi, F.E.; Mao, D.; Ennis, T.L.; Pagano, M.B.; Thompson, R.W. Oral administration of diferuloylmethane (curcumin) suppresses proinflammatory cytokines and destructive connective tissue remodeling in experimental abdominal aortic aneurysms. *Ann. Vasc. Surg.* **2006**, *20*, 360–368. [CrossRef] [PubMed]
127. Ramaswami, G.; Chai, H.; Yao, Q.; Lin, P.H.; Lumsden, A.B.; Chen, C. Curcumin blocks homocysteine-induced endothelial dysfunction in porcine coronary arteries. *J. Vasc. Surg.* **2004**, *40*, 1216–1222. [CrossRef] [PubMed]
128. Monfoulet, L.E.; Mercier, S.; Bayle, D.; Tamaian, R.; Barber-Chamoux, N.; Morand, C.; Milenkovic, D. Curcumin modulates endothelial permeability and monocyte transendothelial migration by affecting endothelial cell dynamics. *Free Radic. Biol. Med.* **2017**, *112*, 109–120. [CrossRef] [PubMed]

129. Kim, Y.S.; Ahn, Y.; Hong, M.H.; Joo, S.Y.; Kim, K.H.; Sohn, I.S.; Park, H.W.; Hong, Y.J.; Kim, J.H.; Kim, W.; et al. Curcumin attenuates inflammatory responses of TNF-alpha-stimulated human endothelial cells. *J. Cardiovasc. Pharmacol.* **2007**, *50*, 41–49. [CrossRef]
130. Pirvulescu, M.M.; Gan, A.M.; Stan, D.; Simion, V.; Calin, M.; Butoi, E.; Tirgoviste, C.I.; Manduteanu, I. Curcumin and a Morus alba extract reduce pro-inflammatory effects of resistin in human endothelial cells. *Phytother. Res. PTR* **2011**, *25*, 1737–1742. [CrossRef]
131. Liu, H.; Wang, C.; Qiao, Z.; Xu, Y. Protective effect of curcumin against myocardium injury in ischemia reperfusion rats. *Pharm. Biol.* **2017**, *55*, 1144–1148. [CrossRef]
132. Shi, J.; Deng, H.; Zhang, M. Curcumin pretreatment protects against PM2.5induced oxidized lowdensity lipoproteinmediated oxidative stress and inflammation in human microvascular endothelial cells. *Mol. Med. Rep.* **2017**, *16*, 2588–2594. [CrossRef]
133. Li, X.; Lu, Y.; Sun, Y.; Zhang, Q. Effect of curcumin on permeability of coronary artery and expression of related proteins in rat coronary atherosclerosis heart disease model. *Int. J. Clin. Exp. Pathol.* **2015**, *8*, 7247–7253. [PubMed]
134. Srivastava, R.; Dikshit, M.; Srimal, R.C.; Dhawan, B.N. Anti-thrombotic effect of curcumin. *Thromb. Res.* **1985**, *40*, 413–417. [CrossRef]
135. Manikandan, P.; Sumitra, M.; Aishwarya, S.; Manohar, B.M.; Lokanadam, B.; Puvanakrishnan, R. Curcumin modulates free radical quenching in myocardial ischaemia in rats. *Int. J. Biochem. Cell Biol.* **2004**, *36*, 1967–1980. [CrossRef] [PubMed]
136. Yeh, C.H.; Chen, T.P.; Wu, Y.C.; Lin, Y.M.; Jing Lin, P. Inhibition of NFkappaB activation with curcumin attenuates plasma inflammatory cytokines surge and cardiomyocytic apoptosis following cardiac ischemia/reperfusion. *J. Surg. Res.* **2005**, *125*, 109–116. [CrossRef]
137. Kim, Y.S.; Kwon, J.S.; Cho, Y.K.; Jeong, M.H.; Cho, J.G.; Park, J.C.; Kang, J.C.; Ahn, Y. Curcumin reduces the cardiac ischemia-reperfusion injury: Involvement of the toll-like receptor 2 in cardiomyocytes. *J. Nutr. Biochem.* **2012**, *23*, 1514–1523. [CrossRef]
138. Wang, N.P.; Wang, Z.F.; Tootle, S.; Philip, T.; Zhao, Z.Q. Curcumin promotes cardiac repair and ameliorates cardiac dysfunction following myocardial infarction. *Br. J. Pharmacol.* **2012**, *167*, 1550–1562. [CrossRef]
139. Wang, N.P.; Pang, X.F.; Zhang, L.H.; Tootle, S.; Harmouche, S.; Zhao, Z.Q. Attenuation of inflammatory response and reduction in infarct size by postconditioning are associated with downregulation of early growth response 1 during reperfusion in rat heart. *Shock* **2014**, *41*, 346–354. [CrossRef]
140. Wang, R.; Zhang, J.Y.; Zhang, M.; Zhai, M.G.; Di, S.Y.; Han, Q.H.; Jia, Y.P.; Sun, M.; Liang, H.L. Curcumin attenuates IR-induced myocardial injury by activating SIRT3. *Eur. Rev. Med Pharmacol. Sci.* **2018**, *22*, 1150–1160. [CrossRef]
141. Morimoto, T.; Sunagawa, Y.; Kawamura, T.; Takaya, T.; Wada, H.; Nagasawa, A.; Komeda, M.; Fujita, M.; Shimatsu, A.; Kita, T.; et al. The dietary compound curcumin inhibits p300 histone acetyltransferase activity and prevents heart failure in rats. *J. Clin. Investig.* **2008**, *118*, 868–878. [CrossRef]
142. Feng, B.; Chen, S.; Chiu, J.; George, B.; Chakrabarti, S. Regulation of cardiomyocyte hypertrophy in diabetes at the transcriptional level. *Am. J. Physiol. Endocrinol. Metab.* **2008**, *294*, E1119–E1126. [CrossRef]
143. Balasubramanyam, K.; Varier, R.A.; Altaf, M.; Swaminathan, V.; Siddappa, N.B.; Ranga, U.; Kundu, T.K. Curcumin, a novel p300/CREB-binding protein-specific inhibitor of acetyltransferase, represses the acetylation of histone/nonhistone proteins and histone acetyltransferase-dependent chromatin transcription. *J. Biol. Chem.* **2004**, *279*, 51163–51171. [CrossRef] [PubMed]
144. Morimoto, T.; Sunagawa, Y.; Fujita, M.; Hasegawa, K. Novel heart failure therapy targeting transcriptional pathway in cardiomyocytes by a natural compound, curcumin. *Circ. J. Off. J. Jpn. Circ. Soc.* **2010**, *74*, 1059–1066. [CrossRef]
145. Wongcharoen, W.; Phrommintikul, A. The protective role of curcumin in cardiovascular diseases. *Int. J. Cardiol.* **2009**, *133*, 145–151. [CrossRef] [PubMed]
146. Sunagawa, Y.; Morimoto, T.; Wada, H.; Takaya, T.; Katanasaka, Y.; Kawamura, T.; Yanagi, S.; Marui, A.; Sakata, R.; Shimatsu, A.; et al. A natural p300-specific histone acetyltransferase inhibitor, curcumin, in addition to angiotensin-converting enzyme inhibitor, exerts beneficial effects on left ventricular systolic function after myocardial infarction in rats. *Circ. J. Off. J. Jpn. Circ. Soc.* **2011**, *75*, 2151–2159. [CrossRef] [PubMed]

147. Hong, D.; Zeng, X.; Xu, W.; Ma, J.; Tong, Y.; Chen, Y. Altered profiles of gene expression in curcumin-treated rats with experimentally induced myocardial infarction. *Pharmacol. Res.* **2010**, *61*, 142–148. [CrossRef]
148. Ramirez-Bosca, A.; Soler, A.; Carrion, M.A.; Diaz-Alperi, J.; Bernd, A.; Quintanilla, C.; Quintanilla Almagro, E.; Miquel, J. An hydroalcoholic extract of curcuma longa lowers the apo B/apo A ratio. Implications for atherogenesis prevention. *Mech. Ageing Dev.* **2000**, *119*, 41–47. [CrossRef]
149. Mohammadi, A.; Sahebkar, A.; Iranshahi, M.; Amini, M.; Khojasteh, R.; Ghayour-Mobarhan, M.; Ferns, G.A. Effects of supplementation with curcuminoids on dyslipidemia in obese patients: A randomized crossover trial. *Phytother. Res. PTR* **2013**, *27*, 374–379. [CrossRef]
150. Sahebkar, A.; Mohammadi, A.; Atabati, A.; Rahiman, S.; Tavallaie, S.; Iranshahi, M.; Akhlaghi, S.; Ferns, G.A.; Ghayour-Mobarhan, M. Curcuminoids modulate pro-oxidant-antioxidant balance but not the immune response to heat shock protein 27 and oxidized LDL in obese individuals. *Phytother. Res. PTR* **2013**, *27*, 1883–1888. [CrossRef]
151. Mohajer, A.; Ghayour-Mobarhan, M.; Parizadeh, S.M.R.; Tavallaie, S.; Rajabian, M.; Sahebkar, A. Effects of supplementation with curcuminoids on serum copper and zinc concentrations and superoxide dismutase enzyme activity in obese subjects. *Trace Elem. Electrolytes* **2015**, *32*, 16–21. [CrossRef]
152. Yang, Y.S.; Su, Y.F.; Yang, H.W.; Lee, Y.H.; Chou, J.I.; Ueng, K.C. Lipid-lowering effects of curcumin in patients with metabolic syndrome: A randomized, double-blind, placebo-controlled trial. *Phytother. Res. PTR* **2014**, *28*, 1770–1777. [CrossRef]
153. Panahi, Y.; Khalili, N.; Hosseini, M.S.; Abbasinazari, M.; Sahebkar, A. Lipid-modifying effects of adjunctive therapy with curcuminoids-piperine combination in patients with metabolic syndrome: Results of a randomized controlled trial. *Complementary Ther. Med.* **2014**, *22*, 851–857. [CrossRef] [PubMed]
154. Amin, F.; Islam, N.; Anila, N.; Gilani, A.H. Clinical efficacy of the co-administration of Turmeric and Black seeds (Kalongi) in metabolic syndrome-A double blind randomized controlled trial-TAK-MetS trial. *Complementary Ther. Med.* **2015**, *23*, 165–174. [CrossRef] [PubMed]
155. Savjani, K.T.; Gajjar, A.K.; Savjani, J.K. Drug solubility: Importance and enhancement techniques. *ISRN Pharm.* **2012**, *2012*, 195727. [CrossRef] [PubMed]
156. Sharma, D.; Soni, M.; Kumar, S.; Gupta, G.D. Solubility Enhancement–Eminent Role in Poorly Soluble Drugs. *Res. J. Pharm. Technol.* **2008**, *2*, 220–224.
157. Kumari, A.; Yadav, S.K.; Yadav, S.C. Biodegradable polymeric nanoparticles based drug delivery systems. *Colloids Surf. B Biointerfaces* **2010**, *75*, 1–18. [CrossRef] [PubMed]
158. De Jong, W.H.; Borm, P.J. Drug delivery and nanoparticles:applications and hazards. *Int. J. Nanomed.* **2008**, *3*, 133–149. [CrossRef]
159. Bobo, D.; Robinson, K.J.; Islam, J.; Thurecht, K.J.; Corrie, S.R. Nanoparticle-Based Medicines: A Review of FDA-Approved Materials and Clinical Trials to Date. *Pharm. Res.* **2016**, *33*, 2373–2387. [CrossRef]
160. Caster, J.M.; Patel, A.N.; Zhang, T.; Wang, A. Investigational nanomedicines in 2016: A review of nanotherapeutics currently undergoing clinical trials. *Wiley Interdiscip. Rev. Nanomed. Nanobiotechnol.* **2017**, *9*. [CrossRef]
161. Ventola, C.L. The nanomedicine revolution: Part 1: Emerging concepts. *P T A Peer Rev. J. Formul. Manag.* **2012**, *37*, 512–525.
162. Havel, H.A. Where Are the Nanodrugs? An Industry Perspective on Development of Drug Products Containing Nanomaterials. *AAPS J.* **2016**, *18*, 1351–1353. [CrossRef]
163. Soppimath, K.S.; Aminabhavi, T.M.; Kulkarni, A.R.; Rudzinski, W.E. Biodegradable polymeric nanoparticles as drug delivery devices. *J. Control. Release Off. J. Control. Release Soc.* **2001**, *70*, 1–20. [CrossRef]
164. Rao, J.P.; Geckeler, K.E. Polymer nanoparticles: Preparation techniques and size-control parameters. *Prog. Polym. Sci.* **2011**, *36*, 887–913. [CrossRef]
165. Jeevanandam, J.; Chan, Y.S.; Danquah, M.K. Nano-formulations of drugs: Recent developments, impact and challenges. *Biochimie* **2016**, *128*, 99–112. [CrossRef] [PubMed]
166. Rice, K.M.; Manne, N.D.; Kolli, M.B.; Wehner, P.S.; Dornon, L.; Arvapalli, R.; Selvaraj, V.; Kumar, A.; Blough, E.R. Curcumin nanoparticles attenuate cardiac remodeling due to pulmonary arterial hypertension. *Artif. Cells Nanomed. Biotechnol.* **2016**, *44*, 1909–1916. [CrossRef] [PubMed]
167. Barreras-Urbina, C.G.; Ramírez-Wong, B.; López-Ahumada, G.A.; Burruel-Ibarra, S.E.; Martínez-Cruz, O.; Tapia-Hernández, J.A.; Rodríguez Félix, F. Nano- and Micro-Particles by Nanoprecipitation: Possible Application in the Food and Agricultural Industries. *Int. J. Food Prop.* **2016**, *19*, 1912–1923. [CrossRef]

168. Llera-Rojas, V.G.; Hernández-Salgado, M.; Quintanar-Guerrero, D.; Leyva-Gómez, G.; Mendoza-Elvira, S.; Villalobos-García, R. Comparative study of the release profiles of ibuprofen from polymeric nanocapsules and nanospheres. *J. Mex. Chem. Soc.* **2019**, *63*. [CrossRef]
169. Mohan, A.; Narayanan, S.; Sethuraman, S.; Krishnan, U.M. Novel resveratrol and 5-fluorouracil coencapsulated in PEGylated nanoliposomes improve chemotherapeutic efficacy of combination against head and neck squamous cell carcinoma. *BioMed Res. Int.* **2014**, *2014*, 424239. [CrossRef]
170. Bozzuto, G.; Molinari, A. Liposomes as nanomedical devices. *Int. J. Nanomed.* **2015**, *10*, 975–999. [CrossRef]
171. Patra, J.K.; Das, G.; Fraceto, L.F.; Campos, E.V.R.; Rodriguez-Torres, M.D.P.; Acosta-Torres, L.S.; Diaz-Torres, L.A.; Grillo, R.; Swamy, M.K.; Sharma, S.; et al. Nano based drug delivery systems: Recent developments and future prospects. *J. Nanobiotechnol.* **2018**, *16*, 71. [CrossRef]
172. Swamy, M.K.; Sinniah, U.R. Patchouli (Pogostemon cablin Benth.): Botany, agrotechnology and biotechnological aspects. *Ind. Crop. Prod.* **2016**, *87*, 161–176. [CrossRef]
173. Mohanty, S.K.; Swamy, M.K.; Sinniah, U.R.; Anuradha, M. Leptadenia reticulata (Retz.) Wight & Arn. (Jivanti): Botanical, Agronomical, Phytochemical, Pharmacological, and Biotechnological Aspects. *Molecules* **2017**, *22*, 1019. [CrossRef]
174. Rodrigues, T.; Reker, D.; Schneider, P.; Schneider, G. Counting on natural products for drug design. *Nat. Chem.* **2016**, *8*, 531–541. [CrossRef] [PubMed]
175. Siddiqui, A.A.; Iram, F.; Siddiqui, S.; Sahu, K. Role of natural products in drug discovery process. *Int. J. Drug Dev. Res.* **2014**, *6*, 172–204.
176. Junyaprasert, V.B.; Morakul, B. Nanocrystals for enhancement of oral bioavailability of poorly water-soluble drugs. *Asian J. Pharm. Sci.* **2015**, *10*, 13–23. [CrossRef]
177. Du, J.; Li, X.; Zhao, H.; Zhou, Y.; Wang, L.; Tian, S.; Wang, Y. Nanosuspensions of poorly water-soluble drugs prepared by bottom-up technologies. *Int. J. Pharm.* **2015**, *495*, 738–749. [CrossRef]
178. Bansal, S.; Bansal, M.; Kumria, R. Nanocrystals: Current Strategies and Trends. *Int. J. Res. Pharm. Biomed. Sci.* **2012**, *3*, 407–419.
179. Gao, L.; Liu, G.; Ma, J.; Wang, X.; Zhou, L.; Li, X.; Wang, F. Application of drug nanocrystal technologies on oral drug delivery of poorly soluble drugs. *Pharm. Res.* **2013**, *30*, 307–324. [CrossRef]
180. Guan, F.; Ding, Y.; Zhang, Y.; Zhou, Y.; Li, M.; Wang, C. Curcumin Suppresses Proliferation and Migration of MDA-MB-231 Breast Cancer Cells through Autophagy-Dependent Akt Degradation. *PLoS ONE* **2016**, *11*, e0146553. [CrossRef]
181. Machado, F.C.; Adum de Matos, R.P.; Primo, F.L.; Tedesco, A.C.; Rahal, P.; Calmon, M.F. Effect of curcumin-nanoemulsion associated with photodynamic therapy in breast adenocarcinoma cell line. *Bioorg. Med. Chem.* **2019**, *27*, 1882–1890. [CrossRef]
182. Zhou, H.; Wang, W.; Hu, H.; Ni, X.; Ni, S.; Xu, Y.; Yang, L.; Xu, D. Co-precipitation of calcium carbonate and curcumin in an ethanol medium as a novel approach for curcumin dissolution enhancement. *J. Drug Deliv. Sci. Technol.* **2019**, *51*, 397–402. [CrossRef]
183. Przybyłek, M.; Recki, Ł.; Mroczyńska, K.; Jeliński, T.; Cysewski, P. Experimental and theoretical solubility advantage screening of bi-component solid curcumin formulations. *J. Drug Deliv. Sci. Technol.* **2019**, *50*, 125–135. [CrossRef]
184. Treesinchai, S.; Puttipipatkhachorn, S.; Pitaksuteepong, T.; Sungthongjeen, S. Development of curcumin floating beads with low density materials and solubilizers. *J. Drug Deliv. Sci. Technol.* **2019**, *51*, 542–551. [CrossRef]
185. Onoue, S.; Takahashi, H.; Kawabata, Y.; Seto, Y.; Hatanaka, J.; Timmermann, B.; Yamada, S. Formulation design and photochemical studies on nanocrystal solid dispersion of curcumin with improved oral bioavailability. *J. Pharm. Sci.* **2010**, *99*, 1871–1881. [CrossRef] [PubMed]
186. Mohanty, C.; Sahoo, S.K. The in vitro stability and in vivo pharmacokinetics of curcumin prepared as an aqueous nanoparticulate formulation. *Biomaterials* **2010**, *31*, 6597–6611. [CrossRef] [PubMed]
187. Chirio, D.; Gallarate, M.; Peira, E.; Battaglia, L.; Serpe, L.; Trotta, M. Formulation of curcumin-loaded solid lipid nanoparticles produced by fatty acids coacervation technique. *J. Microencapsul.* **2011**, *28*, 537–548. [CrossRef] [PubMed]
188. Chin, S.F.; Mohd Yazid, S.N.A.; Pang, S.C. Preparation and Characterization of Starch Nanoparticles for Controlled Release of Curcumin. *Int. J. Polym. Sci.* **2014**, *2014*, 8. [CrossRef]

189. Yallapu, M.M.; Gupta, B.K.; Jaggi, M.; Chauhan, S.C. Fabrication of curcumin encapsulated PLGA nanoparticles for improved therapeutic effects in metastatic cancer cells. *J. Colloid Interface Sci.* **2010**, *351*, 19–29. [CrossRef]
190. Sari, T.P.; Mann, B.; Kumar, R.; Singh, R.R.B.; Sharma, R.; Bhardwaj, M.; Athira, S. Preparation and characterization of nanoemulsion encapsulating curcumin. *Food Hydrocoll.* **2015**, *43*, 540–546. [CrossRef]
191. Giat, L.V.; Sinh, Đ.T.; Toan, T.P. High Concentration Nanocurcumin Fabrication by Wet Milling Method Curcumin with Glassball. *Int. J. Sci. Technol. Res.* **2014**, *3*, 345–348.
192. Carlson, L.J.; Cote, B.; Alani, A.W.; Rao, D.A. Polymeric micellar co-delivery of resveratrol and curcumin to mitigate in vitro doxorubicin-induced cardiotoxicity. *J. Pharm. Sci.* **2014**, *103*, 2315–2322. [CrossRef]
193. Hardy, N.; Viola, H.M.; Johnstone, V.P.A.; Clemons, T.D.; Cserne Szappanos, H.; Singh, R.; Smith, N.M.; Iyer, K.S.; Hool, L.C. Nanoparticle-mediated dual delivery of an antioxidant and a peptide against the L-Type Ca2+ channel enables simultaneous reduction of cardiac ischemia-reperfusion injury. *ACS Nano* **2015**, *9*, 279–289. [CrossRef] [PubMed]
194. Ray, A.; Rana, S.; Banerjee, D.; Mitra, A.; Datta, R.; Naskar, S.; Sarkar, S. Improved bioavailability of targeted Curcumin delivery efficiently regressed cardiac hypertrophy by modulating apoptotic load within cardiac microenvironment. *Toxicol. Appl. Pharmacol.* **2016**, *290*, 54–65. [CrossRef] [PubMed]
195. Rachmawati, H.; Soraya, I.S.; Kurniati, N.F.; Rahma, A. In Vitro Study on Antihypertensive and Antihypercholesterolemic Effects of a Curcumin Nanoemulsion. *Sci. Pharm.* **2016**, *84*, 131–140. [CrossRef] [PubMed]
196. Li, J.; Zhou, Y.; Zhang, W.; Bao, C.; Xie, Z. Relief of oxidative stress and cardiomyocyte apoptosis by using curcumin nanoparticles. *Colloids Surf. B Biointerfaces* **2017**, *153*, 174–182. [CrossRef]
197. Zhang, J.; Wang, Y.; Bao, C.; Liu, T.; Li, S.; Huang, J.; Wan, Y.; Li, J. Curcuminloaded PEGPDLLA nanoparticles for attenuating palmitateinduced oxidative stress and cardiomyocyte apoptosis through AMPK pathway. *Int. J. Mol. Med.* **2019**, *44*, 672–682. [CrossRef]
198. Namdari, M.; Eatemadi, A. Cardioprotective effects of curcumin-loaded magnetic hydrogel nanocomposite (nanocurcumin) against doxorubicin-induced cardiac toxicity in rat cardiomyocyte cell lines. *Artif. Cells Nanomed. Biotechnol.* **2017**, *45*, 731–739. [CrossRef]
199. Nabofa, W.E.E.; Alashe, O.O.; Oyeyemi, O.T.; Attah, A.F.; Oyagbemi, A.A.; Omobowale, T.O.; Adedapo, A.A.; Alada, A.R.A. Cardioprotective Effects of Curcumin-Nisin Based Poly Lactic Acid Nanoparticle on Myocardial Infarction in Guinea Pigs. *Sci. Rep.* **2018**, *8*, 16649. [CrossRef]
200. Boarescu, P.M.; Chirila, I.; Bulboaca, A.E. Effects of Curcumin Nanoparticles in Isoproterenol-Induced Myocardial Infarction. *Oxidative Med. Cell. Longev.* **2019**, *2019*, 7847142. [CrossRef]
201. Kanai, M.; Imaizumi, A.; Otsuka, Y.; Sasaki, H.; Hashiguchi, M.; Tsujiko, K.; Matsumoto, S.; Ishiguro, H.; Chiba, T. Dose-escalation and pharmacokinetic study of nanoparticle curcumin, a potential anticancer agent with improved bioavailability, in healthy human volunteers. *Cancer Chemother. Pharmacol.* **2012**, *69*, 65–70. [CrossRef]
202. Petros, R.A.; DeSimone, J.M. Strategies in the design of nanoparticles for therapeutic applications. *Nat. Rev. Drug Discov.* **2010**, *9*, 615–627. [CrossRef]
203. Gunasekaran, T.; Haile, T.; Nigusse, T.; Dhanaraju, M.D. Nanotechnology: An effective tool for enhancing bioavailability and bioactivity of phytomedicine. *Asian Pac. J. Trop. Biomed.* **2014**, *4*, S1–S7. [CrossRef] [PubMed]

Journal of
Clinical Medicine

MDPI

Review

Biphasic Dose-Response Induced by Phytochemicals: Experimental Evidence

Jadwiga Jodynis-Liebert and Małgorzata Kujawska *

Department of Toxicology, Poznan University of Medical Sciences, 30 Dojazd Str., 60-631 Poznań, Poland; liebert@ump.edu.pl

* Correspondence: kujawska@ump.edu.pl; Tel.: +48-61-847-20-81 (ext. 156)

Received: 21 January 2020; Accepted: 3 March 2020; Published: 6 March 2020

Abstract: Many phytochemicals demonstrate nonmonotonic dose/concentration-response termed biphasic dose-response and are considered to be hormetic compounds, i.e., they induce biologically opposite effects at different doses. In numerous articles the hormetic nature of phytochemicals is declared, however, no experimental evidence is provided. Our aim was to present the overview of the reports in which phytochemical-induced biphasic dose-response is experimentally proven. Hence, we included in the current review only articles in which the reversal of response between low and high doses/concentrations of phytochemicals for a single endpoint was documented. The majority of data on biphasic dose-response have been found for phytoestrogens; other reports described these types of effects for resveratrol, sulforaphane, and natural compounds from various chemical classes such as isoquinoline alkaloid berberine, polyacetylenes falcarinol and falcarindiol, prenylated pterocarpan glyceollin1, naphthoquinones plumbagin and naphazarin, and panaxatriol saponins. The prevailing part of the studies presented in the current review was performed on cell cultures. The most common endpoint tested was a proliferation of tumor and non-cancerous cells. Very few experiments demonstrating biphasic dose-response induced by phytochemicals were carried out on animal models. Data on the biphasic dose-response of various endpoints to phytochemicals may have a potential therapeutic or preventive implication.

Keywords: cancer; diet; flavonoids; food supplements; hormesis; phytoestrogens; sulforaphane; resveratrol

1. Introduction

Compelling data have shown that the consumption of phytochemicals in the form of concentrated supplements can cause adverse health effects if the doses consumed exceed the toxic threshold. However, many reports provide evidence that low doses/concentrations of these compounds have the potential for adverse effects, such as enhancement of the proliferation of tumor cells [1,2]. Various phytochemicals demonstrate nonmonotonic dose/concentration-response termed biphasic dose-response and are considered to be hormetic compounds, for example, resveratrol [2,3] curcumin [4], sulforaphane [1]. The term hormesis described the phenomenon in which a chemical is able to induce biologically opposite effects at different doses; as dose decreases, there are not only quantitative changes in measured responses but also qualitative changes with reference to control and high dose level [5]. Most commonly, there is a stimulatory effect at low doses and an inhibitory effect at high doses [6]. Calabrese et al. [6] characterized two quantitative features of the hormetic response curve: the amplitude of the stimulatory response and the width of the stimulatory dose range. The maximal stimulation of the hormetic response is most typically an increase ranging from 30–60% over control. The stimulatory dose-response is within a 5–100-fold dose range; however, the majority are 5- to 10-fold below the point of response reversal [6,7].

Biphasic, hormetic-like dose-response to various phytochemicals is claimed to be a universal phenomenon. However, a detailed critical survey of source literature does not confirm such an opinion.

We revealed that the demarked hormetic nature of some phytochemicals has not been experimentally evidenced. Moreover, the term "hormesis" is often misused and the most common default refers to the identification of hormetic properties exclusively on the basis of low dose effects which is contradictory to the classic definition of hormesis [8].

Phytochemicals are natural components of the diet, food supplements, and medicines, therefore understanding the nonmonotonic response of biological systems to these compounds should receive considerable attention.

Our aim was to present the overview of the reports in which phytochemical-induced biphasic dose-response is experimentally proven. Hence, we thoroughly analyzed every original article found in the process of our literature search and selected those in which the reversal of response between low and high doses/concentrations of phytochemicals for a single endpoint was documented.

We have excluded curcumin from this work since its hormetic properties were recently reviewed elsewhere [4]. As data on the biphasic concentration/dose-response displayed by resveratrol were extensively reviewed in 2010 [2,3], we presented here reports concerning this subject published from 2010 until 2019. We have divided our review into three sections. The first one is dedicated to phytoestrogens because the majority of reports on biphasic concentration-response induced by phytochemicals referred to this group of compounds. Resveratrol deserves a separate section because it "commonly displays hormesis" [2]. The rest of the phytochemicals were discussed in one common section because for such diverse chemicals, no logical criteria for a division into subgroups were found. We limited the area of review to pure compounds; no extracts or juices were considered.

The literature search was conducted in PubMed, Web of Science and Google Scholar databases from 1990 to 2019; the key search terms were "phytochemicals" or "hormesis" or "biphasic dose-response" or "biphasic concentration-response" or "biphasic effect."

2. Phytoestrogens

Phytoestrogens are compounds of plant origin, which chemical structure is similar to 17β-estradiol (E2). Their action is mediated by both α and β subtypes of estrogen receptors (ERs). It has been demonstrated that phytoestrogens may protect against hormone-dependent cancers, for example, breast cancer. Two major soy isoflavones, genistein, and daidzein, are used as an alternative for estrogen replacement therapy because they bind to estrogen receptors and display estrogenic effects [9].

Genistein (4",5,7-trihydroxyflavone) (GEN) exerts biphasic effects in various tumor cell lines. A number of studies have shown that genistein induces proliferation of estrogen-dependent MCF-7 cells at low concentrations, below 1 μM, and is cytostatic at higher concentrations, above 10 μM [9–19]. The magnitude of stimulation of cell growth was in a wide range: 10% [15], 20% [12,14,18], 60% [17], 100% [13], and 190% [11]. These findings were confirmed in an animal experiment with MCF-7 cells implanted s.c. in ovariectomized athymic mice. Emerging tumors were about 2-fold larger in the genistein (750 ppm in the diet) treated group as compared to those in the controls [11]. The authors of the above-cited articles concluded that the proliferative effect of GEN in MCF-7 cells is associated with the estrogen receptor pathway, while the effects of higher concentrations were independent of the ER. A similar biphasic effect of GEN on prostate cancer cells PC-3 proliferation was demonstrated. At the concentration 0.5–1 μM genistein caused a 1.5-fold increase in cell number as opposed to >3-fold decrease with 50 μM, compared to vehicle-treated cells. The authors revealed that genistein could stimulate invasion of PC-3 cells via upregulation of osteopontin (metastasis promoter) and subsequent activation of matrix metalloproteinase-9 (MMP-9). The concentration 0.5 –1 μM represents a physiologically achievable level, which might enhance the proliferative and metastatic potential of undiagnosed early-stage prostate cancer via an estrogen- and phosphatidylinositol 3 kinase (PI3K)-dependent mechanism [20]. This suggestion was supported in the experiment with transgenic adenocarcinoma mouse prostate (TRAMP-FVB) mice fed genistein at the dose equivalent to the lower concentration used in the above-mentioned in vitro experiment (250 mg/kg diet) for 8 weeks. The authors observed the progression of prostate cancer by a 16% and 70% increase in the incidence of pelvic lymph node metastases. Administration of the dose 1000 mg/kg diet resulted in a much smaller progression of prostate cancer. However, the high dose did not evoke the opposite effects; hence, this pattern of dose-response cannot be classified as biphasic [20]. The biphasic effect of GEN was also demonstrated in nontumorigenic human prostate epithelial cells, RWPE-1, which express the ERβ receptor [21]. Treatment of the cells with GEN at the concentration of 1.5–12.5 μM increased cell proliferation by 4–58%. The concentrations of 50 μM and 100 μM decreased cell proliferation by 18% and 60%, respectively. Treatment of cells with a model antiestrogen (ICI 182,780) caused inhibition of genistein-induced proliferation. These changes were paralleled by the increase in extracellular signal-regulated kinase (ERK1/2) activity by the lower concentration (about 30%) and a marked decrease (about 95%) after incubation with the higher concentration. The results suggest that GEN modulates RWPE-1 cell proliferation via an estrogen-dependent pathway involving ERK1/2 activation. The effect of GEN on proliferation was examined in benign tumor cells: human uterine leiomyoma (UtLM), and uterine smooth muscle cells (UtSMCs). A low concentration of GEN, ~3.7 μM stimulated the 2-fold proliferation of UtLM cells. Simultaneously the expression of proliferating cell nuclear antigen (PCNA) and the percentage of cells in S phase was increased. This process did not occur in UtSMCs. Higher concentrations (>37 μM) inhibited proliferation, adversely affected morphology, and induced apoptosis in both cell lines. The increased responsiveness observed in UtLM cells could be due to enhanced transactivation of the ER and up-regulation of various transcription factors, growth factor peptides and receptor tyrosine kinases, which have been previously shown to be up-regulated in response to treatment with 17βE2 in UtLM cells [22].

The biphasic effects of GEN on parameters different than the proliferation/viability of cultured cells were also demonstrated [23]. At concentrations 0.1–10 μM GEN stimulated osteogenesis in mesenchymal progenitor cells KS483, as evidenced by the increase in alkaline phosphatase (ALP) activity, nodule formation, and calcium deposition, with the maximal effect at 1 μM (3.3–4.4 fold increase). At concentrations 25 μM and higher, all these parameters were inhibited by 40–90%. Similar stimulatory and inhibitory effects of GEN on bone formation were also shown in mouse bone marrow cell culture. The biphasic effect was also observed for adipogenesis. At low concentrations, 0.1–1 μM, GEN decreased adipocyte number by 85%, while at higher concentrations (>10 μM) it stimulated adipogenesis to a 3.4-fold increase. The authors proposed the mechanism of GEN effects on both parameters. They showed that GEN in addition to its ER affinity at micromolar concentrations binds to and transactivates peroxisome proliferator-activated receptor γ (PPARγ), the transcriptional factor essential for adipogenesis, leading to a down-regulation of osteogenesis and up-regulation of adipogenesis. They pointed out that the balance between ERs and PPAR activation determines the biological effects of genistein. It is well established that ligand activation of PPAR results in inhibition of cell growth and induction of apoptosis. Hence the authors concluded that GEN inhibits the cell growth of cancer cells as evidenced elsewhere [10–12,17,18] because of its ability to activate PPAR [23].

The animal experiment supporting in vitro findings related to the proliferative activity of GEN low doses, was reported by Liu et al. [14]. Transgenic erbB-2/neu mice relevant to human breast cancer were given a diet containing a mixture of soy flavones enriched with genistein and daidzein: 211 μg/g diet and 500 μg/g diet. Tamoxifen-associated mammary tumor prevention was significantly reduced (50%) in mice fed the low-dose isoflavone enriched diet. The higher-dose isoflavone diet did not cause such an effect.

Daidzein (7,4′-dihydroxyisoflavone) (DAI) affects the proliferation of human breast cancer cells T-47D in a biphasic dose-response pattern. At concentrations ~1–79 μM DAI enhanced cell growth (the maximum effect 150% increase at ~20 μM), whereas the growth was inhibited by 54% at the concentration ~157 μM. The authors suggested that the underlying mechanism might be associated with the levels of cell cycle regulatory protein, p53 [24]. A similar pattern of dose-response was observed in another human breast cancer cell line, MCF-7 which proliferation was stimulated (30% increase) by daidzein at ~1 μM. Concentrations higher than 10 μM caused the inhibition of proliferation, 50% at ~197 μM, and 65% at ~393 μM [25]. In colon cancer cell line LoVo, treated with 0.1–50 μM of

DAI, a biphasic effect of the compound tested on proliferation was observed. Concentrations 0.1 and 1 μM stimulated the growth of cells by 10–12%. At higher concentrations (10–100 μM), cell growth was inhibited in a concentration-dependent manner by 5–30%. These concentrations caused cell cycle arrest at the G0/G1 phase, DNA fragmentation, and an increase in caspase-3 activity [26]. Dang et al. [27] investigated the effects of DAI in noncancerous cells, namely mouse bone marrow cells and mouse osteoprogenitor cells KS483, which can concurrently differentiate into osteoblasts and adipocytes. DAI stimulated osteogenesis and decreased adipogenesis at concentrations below 20 μM whereas it inhibited osteogenesis and stimulated adipogenesis at concentrations >30 μM. DAI concurrently activates ERs and PPARs, and the balance between the action of these molecules determines the effect of DAI on both parameters tested [27].

Quercetin (QER) (5,7,3,4′-flavon-3-ol) found abundantly in fruit and vegetables displays estrogenic activity and can affect cultured cells' proliferation in a biphasic manner. Low concentrations of QER, up to 1 μM, caused a marked increase in proliferation of the two human breast cancer cell lines, MCF-7 SH and MCF-7 WT, by 4.2-fold and 2.6-fold, respectively. Concentrations 10 μM and higher led to massive cell death. The authors confirmed that the stimulating effects of QER (not cytotoxic) were ER-dependent [17]. Similar results were reported for the colon carcinoma cell lines HCT-116 and HT-29. High concentrations of QER, above 30 μM and 80 μM, respectively decreased proliferation of both lines. About a 20% increase in proliferation was observed at lower concentrations: 1–30 μM for HCT-116 cells and 1–67 μM for HT-29 cells. Within the concentration range tested only a stimulating effect, up to 100%, for the MCF-7 cells was noted [28]. Incubation of human oral squamous carcinoma cell line SCC-25 with various concentrations of QER also showed a biphasic dose-response. Exposure to 1–10 μM of QER resulted in growth stimulation of cells, whereas the cytotoxic effect was observed at 100 μM of the compound tested [29].

Quercetin was also found to display biphasic concentration-response not linked to its estrogenic activity. A strong stimulatory effect (about 60%) of QER on the cyclooxygenase mediated formation of prostaglandin E2 (PGE2) in murine macrophages RAW 264.7 was observed at physiologically achievable concentrations, 10–100 nM. Higher concentrations (10–100 μM) cause a severe drop in PGE2 content [30]. The authors intended to confirm these findings in the in vivo model. They investigated the effect of QER on plasma PGE2 levels in male Sprague–Dawley rats administered increasing doses of QER, 0.05–5 mg/kg b.w. in single i.v. injection [31]. At lower doses up to 0.3 mg/kg QER stimulated the formation of PGE2 by about 5-fold. Higher doses treatment (40 mg/kg) resulted in the reduction of PGE2 levels; however, the opposite effect, i.e., inhibition of PGE2 formation (as compared to controls) was not observed. Hence, it seems that the described effects in vivo cannot be classified as biphasic ones. A biphasic effect of QER on human basophil activation was reported by Chirumbolo et al. [32]. The authors incubated basophils with the bacterial peptide fMLP and evaluated the up-regulation of two membrane markers: the tetraspan CD63 and the ectoenzyme CD203c, which are commonly used to assess basophil response to external stimuli. QER at concentration ~0.03–0.33 μM increased expression of both markers by 52% and 37%, respectively, whereas ~3–33 μM caused a reduction in expression with the maximum effect observed at the highest concentration tested, 14% and 6% of the control values. The authors suggested that the enhancing effect of low QER concentrations on the activation of basophils might be considered beneficial because of the strengthening inflammatory reaction against invading bacteria [32]. The same authors extended their studies using a similar experimental model [33]. They confirmed the above findings and additionally reported on a biphasic pattern of histamine release from basophils activated by fMLP. Low concentrations of QER 0.03–0.3 μM caused a 2-fold increase in histamine level. The highest concentration tested, 33 μM, inhibited histamine release by 75% as compared to the control. Moreover, the authors suggested the involvement of PI3K in this effect of QER. Contrary to the above-cited results, low concentrations of QER are not beneficial in the context of its potential use in the prevention of allergies [33].

QER has been found to extend lifespan in nematode *Caenorhabditis elegans* in a biphasic dose-response manner. The magnitude of response was rather small but statistically significant. Concentration

100–200 μM caused about a 10% increase in lifespan, whereas treatment with 250 μM decreased lifespan by about 7%. The authors identified several genes putatively involved in QER life-extending action. They concluded that antioxidant/prooxidant properties of QER, modulation of some genes as well as the relocation of energy contributed to the observed biphasic effect on life extension [34].

Quercetin was reported to modulate the activity of model mutagens in biphasic concentration-response mode. The compound stimulated 2-fold the mutagenic activity of AFB1 at concentration 0.06–0.12 mM and inhibited mutagenesis at a lower concentration of 0.006–0.01 mM by about 10%. The authors suggested that the lack of consistency in the observed health effects of various flavonoids might be due to the fact that these compounds or their metabolites can modulate in a different way the activity of enzymes responsible for the activation and detoxication of carcinogens [35]. The biphasic effect of quercetin on the mutagenicity of 2-amino-3, 4-dimethylimidazo [4,5-f]quinoline (MeIQ) using a *Salmonella typhimurium* test was reported by Kang et al. [36]. Mutagenicity was enhanced by quercetin by 50% and 42% at 0.1 μM and 1 μM, respectively, but suppressed by 82% and 96% at 50 μM and 100 μM. The authors claimed that this effect was due to the biphasic concentration-response of CYP1A2 activity to the compound. Its low concentrations stimulated enzyme activity by 10–15%, which resulted in the elevated production of active metabolites of MeIQ. At the highest concentration tested (100 μM) CYP1A2 activity was inhibited by 40%, leading to the decreased mutagenicity of MeIQ [36].

Biochanin A (5,7-dihydroxy-4′-methoxyisoflavone) was demonstrated to elicit biphasic dose-response of the proliferation of two cancer cell lines. Human breast carcinoma cells MCF-7 were incubated with biochanin A at concentrations ~0.35–352 μM. At concentrations less than 35 μM cell proliferation was stimulated by 23% as compared to controls; concentrations higher than 106 μM biochanin A inhibited cell growth: by 50% at ~141 μM and by 75% at ~352 μM. A similar biphasic effect was observed for DNA synthesis: concentrations of ~18 μM caused a 180% increase, whereas at ~70 μM DNA synthesis was reduced to 47% of the control value. At concentrations higher than 141 μM, no measurable DNA synthesis was found [37]. Similar findings, although limited to two doses, were reported by Ying et al. [24] who examined the effect of biochanin A on the proliferation of human breast cancer T-47D cell line. Biochanin stimulated cell growth at a concentration ~4 μM by 36% and inhibited growth at ~70 μM by 40%. The level of p53 protein was higher in cells treated with ~70 μM of the compound tested [24].

Natural prenylated flavones characterized by the presence of an isopentenyl group at C-8: **artelastin, artelastocarpin, artelastochromene, and carpelastofuran** demonstrated the biphasic effect on DNA synthesis in MCF-7 cells. At low concentrations of 0.02–2.9 μM, they stimulated DNA synthesis by 130–200% as compared to controls. Concentrations higher than 3.12 μM inhibited cell growth, and DNA synthesis was stopped at a concentration 25 μM. The compounds tested did not stimulate DNA synthesis in estrogen-independent MDA-MB-231 cells, which suggests the involvement of an estrogenic receptor in their proliferative effect [38,39].

Another prenylated flavone, **breviflavone B** also stimulated the proliferation of MCF-7 cells with peak activity at 450 nM (1.9-fold increase). Higher concentrations, 2.2–6.6 μM inhibited the growth of cells and additionally, ERα protein expression, reducing it to about 15% of the control value. This could partially explain a possible mechanism for the observed biphasic effect—proliferative action of breviflavone driven by ERα stimulation was ceased as a result of ERα protein inhibition [40].

The prenylated isoflavonoid **glabridin**, the major isoflavan in licorice root, is an agonist of human ER. Glabridin stimulated the growth of breast tumor cells T-46D over the range of concentrations 0.1–10 μM, reaching the maximum level (about 2-fold of controls) at about 10 μM. Concentrations higher than 15 μM caused abrupt inhibition of cell growth [41].

Glabrene, an isoflavene isolated from licorice root, can bind to the human ER with higher affinity than glabridin. The growth of breast tumor cells T-47D and MCF-7 was increased as a result of incubation with increasing concentrations of the compound, 100 nM-10 μM 3.5-fold, and 75% (maximum values), respectively. Concentrations higher than 15 μM inhibited cell proliferation [42].

Mammalian lignan-type phytoestrogens **enterodiol** and **enterolactone** are produced by the action of colon microbiota from plant lignans. Feng et al. [43] reported on the increase (by about 20%) in the viability of human osteoblast-like cells MG-63 incubated with these compounds at a concentration of ~33 μM. Concentrations higher than 333 μM caused a marked decrease in cell viability (about 90%). Similarly, ALP activity (a marker of osteogenic activity) was increased by 35% at concentrations ~33–333 μM and reduced by 40–60% at higher concentrations (3–33 mM). Parallel mRNA levels of osteonectin and collagen I also followed biphasic response [43].

Isoliquiritigenin (ISL) (2′,4,4′-trihydroxychalcone) isolated from licorice root is the agonist of ERα. Concentrations of ISL up to 1 μM induce MCF-7 cell proliferation by about 3-fold, whereas concentration 10 μM induced a severe drop in cell number as a consequence of cytotoxicity. The authors confirmed that the ERα–mediated mechanism is involved in ISL stimulated cell proliferation [44]. Kang et al. [45] demonstrated a biphasic effect of ISL on tissue inhibitors of matrix metalloproteinases (TIMPs), which counteract matrix metalloproteinases (MMPs)-mediated tumor invasion. The protein expression of TIMP-2 was elevated in human umbilical vein endothelial cells (HUVEC) exposed to phorbol myristate acetate. Treatment of cells with ISL at concentrations <10 μM caused a further 4-fold increase in TIMP-2 expression, whereas 25 μM ISL suppressed TIMP-2 expression to a level lower by 30% than that in controls. The authors suggested that low concentrations of ISL may increase the therapeutic efficacy of antitumor drugs [45].

Kaempferol, one of the common dietary phytoestrogens, induced the proliferation of MCF-7 breast cancer cells at concentrations lower than 1 μM (the maximum effect 4-fold increase). Concentrations higher than 1 μM caused the inhibition of cell proliferation [46].

Generally, the authors of the above-presented reports concluded that the effects of low concentrations of phytoestrogens were mediated by ERs. High concentrations of phytoestrogens may function as estrogen antagonists and inhibit cell growth by competing with estradiol on binding to the ER site [9]. However, many studies revealed that their action at higher concentrations is ER-independent and other molecular targets are involved [9].

The biphasic effect of phytoestrogens on cell proliferation is essential in view of its use as an ingredient of food supplements. There is accumulating evidence that health benefits occur when phytoestrogens are consumed in appropriate quantities. It has been reported that the plasma concentration of GEN is relatively low and less than 40 nM (the level of stimulating cell proliferation) in humans consuming diets without soy. However, it can be much higher, about 40 μM in those who consume large amounts of soy products [47]. The blood serum level of QER from the ingestion of a standard diet varies around 1 μM; the concentration found to enhance cell proliferation. Higher QER concentrations are expected following the ingestion of the QER supplement [17]. The concentration of biochanin A <35 μM which stimulated the cell proliferation in vitro, is within the reported in vivo range (~1–11 μM) in the plasma of humans consuming soy-rich diet [37].

Some authors argue that long term exposure to low levels of phytoestrogens could stimulate the progression of estrogen-dependent tumors [20,28,44]. Hence, dietary recommendations should be considered carefully in women affected by hormone-sensitive breast cancer. In the recently published article, Rietjens et al. [9] presented a comprehensive overview of the health effects of phytoestrogens. Numerous health benefits of these compounds have been reported; however, there is also evidence for their potential adverse effects, e.g., endocrine disruption. The authors claimed that a more refined quantitative risk-benefit should be made to conclude definitely on the health effects.

Data on the biphasic effects of the above-discussed phytoestrogens and suggested mechanisms are presented in Table 1 and Figure 1.

Table 1. Phytoestrogens displaying biphasic concentration-response relationship.

Compound *	Model	Concentration	Effects	Mechanism	Refs
			Effects Linked to Estrogenic Activity		
Artelastin Artelastocarpin Artelastochromen Carpelastofuran isolated from *Artocarpus elasticus*	MCF-7	0.02–2.90 μM	↑proliferation, DNA synthesis		[38,39]
		>3.12 μM	↓proliferation		
		25 μM	↓DNA synthesis		
Biochanin A	MCF-7	~4–35 μM	↑proliferation		[37]
		~106–352 μM	↓proliferation		
		~18 μM	↑DNA synthesis		
		~70 μM	↓DNA synthesis		
	T-47D	~4 μM	↑proliferation	↓p53	[24]
		~70 μM	↓proliferation	↑p53	
Breviflavone B isolated from *Epimedium brevicornum*	MCF-7	450 nM	↑proliferation		[40]
		2.2–6.6 μM	↓proliferation	↓ERα	
Daidzein	T-47D	~1–79 μM	↑proliferation	↓p53	[24]
		~157 μM	↓proliferation	↑p53	
	MCF-7	~1 μM	↑proliferation		[25]
		>10 μM	↓proliferation		
	LoVo	0.1, 1.0 μM	↑proliferation		[26]
		10–100 μM	↓proliferation	G0/G1 arrest	
				↑caspase-3	
	KS483, mouse bone marrow cells	<20 μM	↑osteogenesis ↓adipogenesis	PPARs transactivation	[27]
		>30 μM	↓osteogenesis ↑adipogenesis		
Enterodiol Enterolactone	MG-63	~33 μM	↑viability	↑*osteonectin* ↑*collagen I*	[43]
		~33–333 μM	↑ALP activity		
		>333 μM	↓viability	↓*osteonectin* ↓*collagen I*	
		~3–33 mM	↓ALP activity		
Genistein	MCF-7	<1 μM	↑proliferation	↑ER transcription	[11–15,17–19]
		>10 μM	↓proliferation		
	PC-3	500–1000 nM	↑proliferation,	↑MMP-9 activity	[20]
				↑osteopontin	
		50,000 nM	↓proliferation	↓MMP-9 activity	
	RWPE-1	1.5–12.5 μM	↑proliferation	↑ERK1/2 activity	[21]
		50 and 100 μM	↓proliferation		
	UtLM	~4 μM	↑proliferation		[22]
			↑PCNA, ↑cells in S phase		
		>37 μM	↓proliferation ↑apoptosis		
	KS483, mouse bone marrow cells	0.1–10.0 μM	↑osteogenesis ↑ALP activity		[23]
			↑nodule formation and calcium deposition		
		>25 μM	↓osteogenesis ↓ALP activity		
			↓nodule formation and calcium deposition		
	KS483, mouse bone marrow cells	0.1–1.0 μM	↓adipocytes number		[23]
		10–50 μM	↓adipocytes number		
Glabrene isolated from *Glycyrrhiza glabra*	T47-D, MCF-7	100 nM–10 μM	↑proliferation		[42]
		>15 μM	↓proliferation		
Glabridin isolated from *Glycyrrhiza glabra*	T-46D	0.1–10 μM	↑proliferation		[41]
		>15 μM	↓proliferation		
Isoliquiritigenin synthesized by authors	MCF-7	<1 μM	↑proliferation		[44]
		10 μM	↓proliferation		
Kaempherol	MCF-7	<1 μM	↑proliferation		[46]
		>1 μM	↓proliferation		

Table 1. *Cont.*

Compound *	Model	Concentration	Effects	Mechanism	Refs
Quercetin	MCF-7	<1 μM	↑proliferation		[17]
		>10 μM	↓proliferation		
	HCT-116	1–30 μM	↑proliferation		[28]
		40–100 μM	↓proliferation		
	HT-29	1–67 μM	↑proliferation		
		80–100 μM	↓proliferation		
	SCC-25	1–10 μM	↑proliferation		[29]
		>100 μM	↓proliferation		
Activity not Linked to Estrogenic Properties					
Isoliquiritigenin	HUVEC/PMA	<10 μM	↑TIMP-2	↓JNK, p38 MAPK pathway	[45]
		25 μM	↓TIMP-2		
Quercetin	RAW 264.7	10–100 nM	↑PGE2		[30]
		10–100 μM	↓PGE2		
	basophils/fMLP	~0.03–0.33 μM	↑CD63, CD203c		[32]
		~3–33 μM	↓CD63, CD203c		
	basophils/fMLP	0.03–0.3 μM	↑histamine	PI3K involvement	[33]
		33 μM	↓histamine		
	Caenorhabditis elegans	100–200 μM	↑lifespan	↑*hsp*	[34]
		250 μM	↓lifespan		
	Salmonella typhimurium/AFB1	0.006–0.01 mM	↓mutagenicity		[35]
		0.06–0.12 mM	↑mutagenicity		
	Salmonella typhimurium/MeIQ	0.1, 1 μM	↑mutagenicity, CYP1A2 activity		[36]
		50, 100 μM	↓mutagenicity, CYP1A2 activity		

* If the source of the compound was not specified it was obtained commercially; ↑ = increase, ↓ = decrease; 2-AAF—2-Acetylaminofluorene; AFB1—aflatoxin B1; ALP—alkaline phosphatase; CD203c—basophil-specific ectoenzyme E-NPP3; CD63—tetraspan transmembrane protein family; CYP1A2—Cytochrome P450 1A2; fMLP—bacterial formyl peptide N-formylmethionine-leucine-phenylalanine; HCT-116, HT-29—colon carcinoma cell line; HepG-2—human liver cancer cell line; HUVEC—human umbilical vein endothelial cell line; KS483—murine osteoprogenitor cell line; JNK—c-JUN terminal kinase; LC3-II—microtubule-associated protein 2 light chain 3; LoVo—human colon adenocarcinoma cell line; MCF-7—human breast adenocarcinoma cell line; MeIQ—2-amino-3, 4-dimethylimidazo [4,5-f]quinoline; MG-63—human osteoblast-like cells; MMP-9—matrix metallopeptidase 9; p53—tumor protein p53; PC-3—human prostatic carcinoma cell line; PCNA—proliferating cell nuclear antigen; PGE2—prostaglandin E2; PI3K—phosphoinositide-3 kinase; PMA—phorbol myristate acetate; RAW 264.7—murine macrophage cell line; p38 MAPK—p38 mitogen-activated protein kinase; SCC-25—oral squamous carcinoma cell line; T-47D—human breast cancer cell lines; TIMP-2—tissue inhibitor of metalloproteinase-2; UtLM—human uterine leiomyoma.

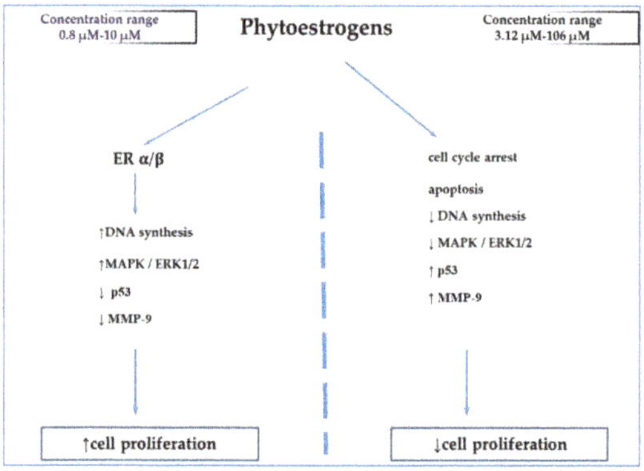

Figure 1. Suggested mechanisms of biphasic concentration-dependent effects of phytoestrogens (on the basis of references cited in the review). ↑ = increase, ↓ = decrease; ER—estrogen receptor; ERK—extracellular signal-regulated kinase protein-serine/threonine kinase; MAPK—mitogen-activated protein kinase; MMP-9—matrix metallopeptidase 9; p53—tumor protein p53.

3. Resveratrol

As mentioned above, in the current review, we presented data concerning biphasic concentration-response induced by resveratrol and published after 2010.

Biphasic concentration-response to resveratrol has been commonly demonstrated for standard parameters measured routinely in cell culture: viability and proliferation. Plauth et al. [48] found that treatment with a lower concentration of RES moderately increased the viability of several cell lines: neonatal normal human epidermal keratinocytes (NHEK) by 20% (<50 μM); neonatal normal human dermal fibroblasts (NHDF) by 15% (1–300 μM); and HepG2 cells by 15% (1–100 μM). The high concentration of RES (500 μM) markedly reduced cell viability: 75% for NHEC and NHDF, and 40% for HepG2. The authors proposed that the increased fitness of cells treated with low RES concentration is due to the enhanced expression of cellular defense genes, the process triggered by gentle oxidative stress evoked by RES [48].

At 1 μM, 10 μM and 20 μM, RES stimulated the proliferation of neural progenitor cells by 10%, 35%, and 25%, respectively. Higher concentrations, 50 μM and 100 μM decreased cell proliferation by 50% and 65%. A similar relationship was reported for proliferation markers nestin and SOX2. The levels of both molecules were increased by 10–50% in cells incubated with 1 μM, 10 μM and 20 μM. Higher concentrations tested decreased their levels by 20–50%. The authors suggested that enhanced proliferation was mediated by increased phosphorylation of extracellular signal-regulated kinases (ERKs) and p 38 kinases. Higher RES concentrations significantly reduced the activation of these molecules [49].

A similar effect of RES on cell proliferation was observed for colorectal adenocarcinoma cells HT-29. At concentrations, 1–10 μM RES increased about 2-fold a number of cells whereas at 50 μM and 100 μM, the percentage of necrotic and apoptotic cells was reduced by 76% and 90%, respectively. RES-induced cytotoxicity was associated with NADP oxidase activation and increased level of histone γH2AX, a marker of DNA damage [50].

Bovine spermatozoa viability was also affected by RES in a biphasic mode. At lower RES concentrations, 1–50 μM, an increase in this parameter by 10–75% was noted. Incubation of cells with 100 and 1000 μM resulted in inhibition of the cell viability by 50% and 65%, respectively. Superoxide anion production in spermatozoa incubated with growing concentrations of RES also displayed biphasic concentration-response mode. Low RES concentrations, 1–50 μM reduced superoxide level by 15–50%; higher concentrations, 100 and 200 μM caused a 40% and 60% increase, respectively, as compared to controls. The consistency between the effects of RES on spermatozoa viability and superoxide production once more confirmed the role of prooxidant RES action in cytotoxicity [51].

RES induced a biphasic effect on DNA synthesis in androgen-sensitive LNCaP cells. At 5 μM and 10 μM RES caused a 2–3-fold increase in DNA synthesis—due to the induction of cells' entry into S-phase, whereas at >15 μM DNA synthesis was inhibited [52]. Similar effects were observed in rat granulosa cells. RES at 10 μM stimulated thymidine incorporation by 54%, whereas concentrations of 30 and 50 μM decreased this process by 49% and 44%, respectively [53]. The authors of both reports suggested that the unique ability of RES to exert opposing action on two essential processes in cell cycle progression: induction of S phase and inhibition of DNA synthesis is responsible for the described effects.

Guo et al. [54] reported that RES biphasically modulated chromosomal instability (CIN) in human normal colon epithelial cells. At low RES concentrations (0.1–1 μM) basal levels of CIN markers micronuclei (MN) and nucleoplasmic bridge (NPB) were reduced by 17–63%; the most marked decrease was noted at 0.1 μM. The higher RES concentration, 100 μM, increased the MN value by 30% and NPB by 10%. Consistently with the above findings, cell viability was slightly increased (10%) and significantly decreased (35%) when incubated with 0.1 and 100 μM of RES. The authors suggested that the biphasic effect of RES on CIN might be attributed to the regulation of mitotic fidelity through the SAC (spindle assembly checkpoint) pathway which is a major cell-cycle regulatory network controlling chromosome segregation during mitosis [54].

Besides cell viability/proliferation and DNA synthesis, other parameters were also modulated by RES in a biphasic mode. Bosutti et al. [55] investigated the effect of RES (10–60 μM) on C12C12 myoblast and myotube plasticity. Low RES concentration (10 μM) stimulated myoblast cell cycle arrest, migration, and sprouting which were inhibited by 40–60 μM. However, only cell motility displayed biphasic concentration-response. At 10 μM cell motility was enhanced by 38% whereas the number of migrated cells was decreased by 17–70% by increasing concentrations of RES. The authors concluded that low concentrations of RES might promote in vitro muscle regeneration [55].

In a HepG2 cell culture, the high concentration of RES (100 μM) decreased the extracellular level of apolipoprotein M (apoM) by about 35% whereas moderate concentrations (1 and 10 μM) increased 2-fold its extracellular level. ApoM is a carrier and modulator of sphingosine 1-phosphate (S1P), a product of sphingosine kinase (SK), which exerts beneficial effects in cardiovascular diseases [56].

Peltz et al. [57] examined the effects of RES on cell self-renewal and differentiation of human mesenchymal stem cells (hMSCs), which could differentiate into multiple cell types. They demonstrated that at 0.1 μM RES inhibited cellular senescence by 10%, at 1 μM had no effect whereas at 5 and 10 μM the senescence rate was increased by 6% and 15%, respectively, as compared to controls. Despite their small magnitude, the changes were statistically significant. This finding was confirmed in the assay based on beta-galactosidase activity, an indicator of cellular senescence. The number of senescent cells was decreased by treatment with 0.1 and 1 μM by 30% and 50%, respectively. Higher concentrations of RES (5 μM and 10 μM) caused an increase in the number of senescent cells by 40% and 225%, respectively. These findings could be partly explained by the fact that some genes implicated in cell survival (e.g., sirtuins, birc) were upregulated by a lower concentration of RES but inhibited by higher concentrations [57].

The antigenotoxic effects of RES were investigated in HepG2 cells exposed to model mutagen 4-nitroquinoline-N-oxide (4NQO). A slight antigenotoxic effect at concentrations 10, 25, and 50 μM was observed with genotoxic inhibition rate (GIR) 12%, 26%, and 34%, respectively. For concentrations of 100 and 250 μM, the extent of DNA damage was greater than for 4NQO by 33% and 66%, respectively. The highest concentration tested significantly induced apoptosis, hence the authors suggested that the pro-apoptotic effect of RES could, in part, explain the above described biphasic concentration-response [58].

RES demonstrated the concentration-dependent biphasic effect on human natural killer (NK) cells, which play an essential role in tumor identification and surveillance. Cytotoxicity of NK cells was slightly increased by 4% and 6% (statistically significant increase) when incubated with low RES concentrations (1.56 and 3.13 μM). RES concentrations of 25 and 50 μM diminished NK cells cytotoxicity by 29% and 39%, respectively. At 3.13 μM RES was demonstrated to enhance the expression of both TNFγ (by 4.5-fold) and triggering cytotoxicity receptor NKG2D (by 6.4-fold), which might account for the enhanced cytotoxicity of NK cells [59].

A very extensive and well-documented report concerning the biphasic effects induced by RES was published by Posadino et al. [60]. The authors investigated numerous in vitro endpoints in HUVEC incubated with increasing concentrations of RES and undertook an ambitious attempt to elucidate the mechanism of the observed processes. It was found that at 1 μM RES intracellular basal level of ROS was decreased by 35% whereas higher concentrations (10 and 50 μM) enhanced the ROS level by 25% and 50%. Cell viability was slightly insignificantly (15%) increased when exposed to 1 μM of RES. Higher concentrations (10 and 50 μM) caused a significant decrease in cell viability, 40% and 60%, respectively. Consistently this pattern of results was reflected in the assay for DNA synthesis. The lowest RES concentration increased DNA synthesis by 15%; higher concentrations suppressed this parameter by 40% and 80%. The expression of antiapoptotic gene Bcl-2 in HUVECs treated with RES also followed biphasic concentration-response mode. At 1 μM RES increased Bcl-2 mRNA levels by 48%. The effects of higher RES concentration were the opposite—an expression of this gene was significantly diminished by 54% and 86%. These findings confirmed that RES at high concentration induced apoptosis in HUVECs. Similarly, the expression of two other genes playing an essential role in cell cycle progression and cell proliferation, namely c-myc and ornithine decarboxylase (ODC), displayed a biphasic response to RES. A higher RES concentration significantly decreased the mRNA levels of both genes by 30–43% whereas their expression was enhanced in cells treated with 1 μM RES by 27% and 47%. It was also demonstrated that RES biphasically modulated protein kinase C (PKC) activity in HUVECs. The lowest concentrations caused a 2.1-fold increase in PKC activity, whereas higher concentrations exerted a strong inhibitory effect by 56% and 72%, which was consistent with the biphasic effect of RES on ROS production [60]. The above findings contribute significantly to the understanding of the mechanism of RES concentration-dependent effects.

The only in vivo research concerning the biphasic effects of RES was reported by Juhasz et al. [61]. The biphasic cardioprotective effect was demonstrated in rats fed 3 doses of RES for 30 days. Their hearts were isolated and subjected to ischemia/reperfusion. The lowest dose, 2.5 mg/kg conferred maximum protection as evidenced by a 50% increase in aortic flow and left ventricular developed pressure, as well as infarct size, decreased by 40%. At 25 mg/kg cardiac function parameters were significantly reduced; at 100 mg/kg no aortic flow and no developed pressure were detected, indicating that the heart did not function. The authors suggested that this protective effect of RES was exerted through its ability to induce gentle intracellular stress, leading to the upregulation of the defense system. At high doses RES depressed cardiac function and induced apoptosis, which is in agreement with the well-known properties of RES concerning the inhibition of RNA, DNA and protein expression, chromosomal aberration and the inhibition of cell proliferation [2].

The reports presented in this section confirm the previous findings [2,3] that low concentrations of RES (1–100 μM) stimulate the proliferation of various cell lines, whereas higher concentrations (50–1000 μM) inhibit cell viability. The difference in magnitude of concentrations stimulating or inhibiting DNA synthesis was not so distinct, 1–10 μM vs. >15 μM, respectively. Much lower concentrations (0.1–1 μM) were able to protect DNA which has been shown by decreased chromosomal instability (CIN), whereas 100 μM of RES increased this parameter.

The increase in proliferation was explained by the enhanced expression of cellular defense genes resulting from mild oxidative stress as well as by activating ERKs and p38 kinases. Prooxidant properties of RES contributed to its antiproliferative action demonstrated at higher concentrations, as evidenced by NADP oxidase activation, superoxide anion generation and an increase in ROS level. Other beneficial effects of RES low concentrations presented here include a decreased stem cell senescence, antigenotoxic effect, enhanced myoblast plasticity and antiapoptotic action.

Summing up, at higher doses/concentrations, RES can act as a preventive agent with respect to carcinogenesis, the opposite effect of low concentration suggests a need for caution [2].

Data on biphasic concentration-response induced by RES are summarized in Table 2.

Table 2. Biphasic concentration/dose-response relationship induced by resveratrol.

Model	Concentration	Effects	Mechanism	Refs
NHEK	<50 μM	↑viability	↑CAT, Nrf2, KEAP1, NQO1, GCLC, GSR, G6PD, FOXO3, SIRT1, DAPK 1 (5–100 μM)	[48]
	500 μM	↓viability	↓CAT, Nrf2, KEAP1, NQO1, GCLC, GSR, G6PD, FOXO3, SIRT1, DAPK1 150 μM	
NHDF	1–300 μM	↑viability		
	500 μM	↓viability		
HepG2	1–100 μM	↑viability		
	500 μM	↓viability		
NPCs	1, 10, 20 μM	↑proliferation	↑ERK1/2, p38, p-CREB, Bcl-2, TrkA, synaptophysin, PSA-NCAM	[49]

Table 2. *Cont.*

Model	Concentration	Effects	Mechanism	Refs
	50, 100 μM	↓proliferation	↓p-ERK1/2, p-p38 MAPK	
			↑caspase-3	
HT-29	1–10 μM	↑proliferation		[50]
	50, 100 μM	↓proliferation	↑NADPH oxidase activity, ↑γH2AX, SIRT6	
Bovine spermatozoa	1–50 μM	↑viability		[51]
		↓superoxide anion production		
	100, 1000 μM	↓viability		
	100, 200 μM	↑superoxide anion production		
LNCaP	5 μM, 10 μM	↑DNA synthesis	↓p21cip1, p27kip1	[52]
			↑Cdk2 activity	
			↑cyclins A, E	
	>15 μM	↓DNA synthesis		
Rat ovarian	10 μM	↑DNA synthesis		[53]
granulosa cells	30,50 μM	↓DNA synthesis		
Normal colon epithelial cells	0.1–1 μM	↓chromosomal instability, ↑viability	↑*SAC*	[54]
	100 μM	↑chromosomal instability, ↓viability	↓*SAC*	
C12C12	10 μM	↑cell motility		[55]
	40–60 μM	↓cell motility	↓miosin Tpe1 and total ATPase activity	
HepG2	1, 10 μM	↑apoM,		[56]
	100 μM	↓apoM		
hMSCs	0.1 μM	↓cellular senescence	↑*Sirtuin1*	[57]
	5, 10 μM	↑cellular senescence	↓*Sirtuin1, Sirtuin2, Birc4, Birc5*	
			↑*Cdk2*	
HepG2/4NQO	10, 25, 50 μM	↓genotoxicity		[58]
	100, 250 μM	↑genotoxicity		
NK	1.56, 3.13 μM	↑cytotoxicity	↑*NKG2D, NKG2D*	[59]
			↑*IFN-γ, IFN-γ*	
	25, 50 μM	↓cytotoxicity		
HUVEC	1 μM	↓ROS	↑*Bcl-2, c-myc, ODC*	[60]
		↑viability, DNA synthesis	↑PKC activity	
	10, 50 μM	↑ROS	↓*Bcl-2, c-myc, ODC*	
		↓viability, DNA synthesis	↓PKC activity	
Rats	2.5 mg/kg	↑aortic flow, LVDP, ↓infarct size	↓cardiomyocyte apoptosis	[61]
	25 mg/kg	↓aortic flow, LVDP, ↑infarct size	↑cardiomyocyte apoptosis	
	100 mg/kg	no heart function	↑cardiomyocyte apoptosis	

↑ = increase, ↓ = decrease; 4NQO—4-nitroquinoline-N-oxide; γH2AX—H2A histone family member X; apoM—apolipoprotein M; Bcl-2—B-cell lymphoma 2; C2C12—mouse myoblast cell line; CAT—catalase; Cdk—cyclin-dependent kinase; CREB—cAMP-response-element-binding protein; DAPK1—death-associated protein kinase 1; ERK1/2—extracellular signaling-regulated kinase; FOXO3—forkhead box O3; G6PD—glucose-6-phosphate dehydrogenase; GCLC—glutamate-cysteine ligase catalytic subunit; GSR—glutathione reductase; HepG2—human liver cancer cell line; hMSCs—human mesenchymal stem cell line; HT-29—colon carcinoma cell line; KEAP1—Kelch-like ECH-associated protein 1; LNCaP—androgen-sensitive human prostate adenocarcinoma cell line; LVDP—left ventricular developed pressure; NHDF—neonatal normal human dermal fibroblasts; NHEK—neonatal normal human epidermal keratinocytes; NK—human natural killer cells; NPCs—neural progenitor cells; NQO1—NAD(P)H dehydrogenase [quinone] 1; Nrf2—nuclear factor erythroid 2-related factor 2; ODC—ornithine decarboxylase; $p21^{Cip1}$ cyclin-dependent kinase inhibitor 1; $p27^{Kip1}$—cyclin-dependent kinase inhibitor 1B; PSA-NCAM—polysialylated neuronal cell adhesion molecule; p38—mitogen-activated protein kinase; PKC—protein kinase C; SAC—spindle assembly checkpoint; SIRT—sirtuin; SOX2—transcription factor (sex-determining region Y-box 2), TrkA—tropomyosin receptor kinase A. Resveratrol used in cited experiments was of commercial origin.

4. Other Phytochemicals

The isothiocyanate **sulforaphane** (SFN) found in high concentrations in cruciferous vegetables has gained extensive research interest due to its anticancer and chemopreventive properties [62,63]. SFN is considered to be a hormetic molecule [1,64,65]; however, a thorough literature search revealed that very few articles are available in which a specific biphasic dose-response relationship is reported, and only these reports were selected to be presented in the current review.

Bao et al. [63] presented a study on biphasic dose-response promoted by SFN in a high number of cultured cells demonstrating that a low concentration of SFN (1–5 μM) stimulated cell growth by 20–40% as compared with controls, whereas a high concentration (10–40 μM) inhibited cell growth in some tumor cell lines: bladder cancer T24, hepatoma HepG2, and colon cancer Caco-2. A similar dose-response relationship was observed in regular cell lines, including hepatocytes HHL-5, colon epithelial CCD841 cells, and skin fibroblasts CCD-1092 SK. The migration of T24 cells also followed the biphasic dose-response manner. Incubation with 2.5 and 3.75 μM SFN increased this parameter to 128% and 133% of the corresponding controls. Concentrations higher than 5 μM decreased cell migration, which was ceased at 40 μM. A low concentration of SFN (2.5–5 μM) promoted tube formation (a marker of angiogenesis) by 18% as evidenced by 3D angiogenesis assay. Concentrations 10 and 20 μM inhibited tube formation decreasing it to 61% and 20% of the control. The authors suggested that the mechanism of cell growth stimulation by low SFN concentrations may be related to the activation of growth-promoting molecules (for example RAS, RAF, ERK, PI3K) and signal transduction pathways such as NF-kB, FOXO, Nrf2 [63].

The concentration of SFN in human plasma after consumption of cruciferous vegetables can reach 1–5 μM, the level which promotes cell growth. The authors suggested that it might explain some inconsistency of epidemiological findings regarding the association between isothiocyanates intake and cancer risk [63].

Biphasic effects of SFN were also demonstrated in human mesenchymal stem cells (MSCs). A low concentration of SFN (0.25 and 1 μM) stimulated proliferation of MSCs by 22%, whereas 20 μM caused a significant, about 60% reduction of cell growth. Similarly, the concentration of SFN up to 5 μM reduced the number of apoptotic cells with a maximum effect of 76% demonstrated by 0.25 μM. On the contrary, concentration 20 μM caused a 2.3-fold increase in the percentage of apoptotic cells. The number of senescent cells—as assessed by acid-β-galactosidase assay—was decreased by about 30% in MSCs incubated with 0.25 and 1 μM SFN. High doses of SFN (5 and 20 μM) increased senescent cell number by 62% and 4-fold, respectively. The production of cellular ROS was also affected by SFN in a biphasic manner. Low concentration (0.25 μM) reduced by 30% the production of ROS in the basal state and under stress condition. The concentration of 20 μM caused a 30% increase in ROS generation. The authors suggest that SFN should be used as an anticancer agent very carefully because the compound may impair healthy stem cells that support hematopoiesis and contribute to homeostatic maintenance [66].

A stimulating effect of a low concentration of SFN, up to 5 μM on cell proliferation was demonstrated using various cell lines: 16% increase in MCF-7 [67], 10% in HHL-5 (human hepatocytes) [68], 16% in HepG2 cells [68] as well as 30% increase in human lymphoblastoma cells [69]. At a concentration higher than 5 μM, the proliferation of every cell line was substantially inhibited as compared to controls. Misiewicz et al. [69] additionally investigated intracellular glutathione content and revealed that incubation of lymphoblastoma cells with 0.5–5 μM SFN caused a 39–340% increase in this parameter, however, the concentration 10 μM decreased the GSH level to 50% of control value.

The biphasic effect of **berberine** (BER), an isoquinoline alkaloid, on the cell growth was demonstrated in five cancer cell lines: murine melanoma cell line B16-F10, human breast cancer cells MDA-MB-231, MDA-MB-468 and MCF-7, and human colon cancer cells LS-174. At low concentrations (1.25–5.0 μM) berberine stimulated the growth of all types of cells by 12–70% as compared to controls. Higher concentrations of BER (10–80 μM) inhibited cell proliferation up to 90% [70].

Consistent with these findings, co-treatment with a low dose of BER significantly attenuated the anticancer activity of chemotherapeutic drugs: fluorouracil, camptothecin, and paclitaxel. The authors suggested that BER activates the protective stress response in cancer cells as evidenced by the up-regulation of MAPK/ERK1/2 and PI3K/AKT signaling pathways, which can partly explain the observed effects [70].

Berberine also exerted biphasic dose-response effect on the viability of another type of cells, phaeochromocytoma cell line PC-12. A low concentration of BER (0.1–1.0 μM) significantly increased the viability of PC-12 cells, maximum by 40%, whereas 2–64 μM of BER inhibited cell viability, decreasing it to 50% of the control value [71]. Additionally, on the basis of several assays, the authors suggested that BER protects against 6-hydroxydopamine (6-OHDA)-induced neurotoxicity in PC12 cells through the hormetic mechanism. Low concentrations of BER (0.25–1.0 μM) protected cells from 6-OHDA-induced cytotoxicity and apoptosis, higher concentrations (2–16 μM) did not show this effect. The authors speculated that PI3K/AKT/Bcl-2 pathway was involved in protective effect of low BER concentration. In zebrafish larvae, low doses of BER (0.3–1.3 μM) alleviated the loss of dopamine neurons caused by 6-OHDA treatment, no protective effect of a high dose of BER (20 μM) was observed. The same range of BER low doses reversed the 6-OHDA-induced reduction of larvae locomotor activity, whereas the high dose effect was very slight [71]. In all experiments referring to the neuroprotective activity of BER, no biphasic dose-response was shown since the high dose of BER did not exert an effect opposite to that observed for low doses. Thus, the objection arises whether these relationships can be considered hormetic.

The effect of the pretreatment with two polyacetylenes, **falcarinol** and **falcarindiol** on cellular stress in primary myotube cultures exposed to hydrogen peroxide was investigated. At a lower concentration of both compounds (1.6–25 μM) the formation of ROS was slightly enhanced (maximum by 10–30%). Parallelly an increase in glutathione peroxidase (GPx) mRNA expression, as well as a decreased Hsp70 and heme oxygenase1 (HO-1) mRNAs, was observed. Preincubation with higher concentrations of the compounds tested, 50 and 100 μM resulted in a substantial decrease in ROS formation (to about 10% of the control value) and GPx mRNA expression as well as the increased expression of mRNA for HSP70 and HO-1. Myoblast viability was also affected by falcarindiol in a biphasic manner. The lower concentrations of the compound (0.61–9.8 nM) increased the viability of myotubes slightly (19%). Higher concentrations (2.5–5 μM) suppressed the viability significantly, by about 96%. The authors suggested that a protective effect of both polyacetylenes was associated with the induction of antioxidant enzyme, GPx [72].

The biphasic effect of falcarinol was also demonstrated in another experiment in which the proliferation of primary bovine mammary epithelial cells was measured using the bioassay based on the incorporation of tritiated thymidine into cellular DNA. Falcarinol exerted stimulatory effects (maximum 26%) at concentration ~0.04–0.20 μM and inhibited cell growth between ~4 μM and ~41 μM with the maximum effect (90%) observed at ~41 μM [73].

Young et al. [74] reported on the biphasic effect of falcarinol on the proliferation of the human colon carcinoma cell line CaCo-2. The increase in cell proliferation was observed at the concentration range 1–10 μM, with 1 μM being the most effective (80% increase). At concentrations above 20 μM proliferation of cells decreased gradually to reach 15% of the control value. Concomitantly the expression of apoptosis indicator, caspase-3, and basal DNA strand breakage was decreased at a low concentration of falcarinol by 50% and 40%, respectively. At concentrations above 20 μM a 13-fold enhancement of caspase-3 expression, as well as a 2-fold increase in DNA strand breakage, were observed [74].

Chattopadhyay et al. [75,76] investigated the effects of two flavonoids on longevity in *Drosophila melanogaster*. **Rutin** (quercetin-3-rutinoside) was shown to extend the median lifespan in female flies at a concentration of 200 and 400 μM by 30% and 43%, respectively. The treatment of flies with higher concentrations, 600 and 800 μM resulted in a decrease in survival, by 13% and 16%. The transcript levels of genes associated with longevity were increased in flies treated with lower doses of the compound [76]. In another experiment, *D. melanogaster* was fed a diet containing **naringenin** (4′,5,7-trihydroxyflavanone) at a concentration of 50–800 μM. Concentrations 200 and 400 μM caused an increase in the lifespan of male and female flies by 13% and 23%. Administration of higher doses, 600 and 800 μM, resulted in a decrease in lifespan by 14% and 30%, respectively. A standard diet supplemented with 200 μM naringenin increased the percentage of pupae formation as well as the number of flies that eclosed after pupation, whereas the sharp decline of both endpoints was observed when the content of naringenin was 600 and 800 μM [75].

Luteolin (3′,4′,5,7-tetrahydroxyflavone) was shown to increase the viability of MCF-7 cells at concentrations 1–10 μM by about 18%. Higher concentrations of the compound, 30–1000 μM caused a decrease in cell viability to about 95% of the control value [77]. The biphasic effect of luteolin on autophagy was demonstrated in HepG2 cells. At concentrations up to 35 μM luteolin caused about a 45% increase in the level of LC3-II, a marker of autophagy. Higher concentration (~105 μM) decreased this parameter by 35%. Autophagy is an essential process for cell homeostasis, and its impairment contributes to the pathogenesis of various diseases [78]. The antimutagenic activity of some flavonoids of rooibos (*Aspalathus linearis*) displayed a biphasic dose-response relationship. *Salmonella typhimurium* mutagenicity assay was used with 2-acetamido-fluorene (2-AAF) and aflatoxin B1 (AFB1) as model mutagens. **(+) Catechin** and **rutin** displayed a co-mutagenic effect at concentrations 1.2 and 0.8 mM, respectively, and antimutagenic activity at lower concentrations (0.01–0.6 mM) in a 2-AAF assay. On the contrary, **luteolin** was co-mutagenic at the lowest concentration tested (0.006 mM) and antimutagenic at higher concentration (1.2 mM) in the same assay [35].

The rat PC12 cell line was pretreated with **Z-ligustilide**, a bioactive phthalide isolated from Rhizoma Chuanxiong. Then cells were subjected to oxygen-glucose deprivation (OGD) procedure. At a low concentration (1–25 μM) Z-ligustilide protected cells from OGD-induced apoptosis and increased cell viability by about 50%. The protective effect of the compound declined with increasing concentrations to 73% of the basal level at 50 μM. The authors suggested that low concentrations of Z-ligustilide triggered moderate ROS production in cells which stimulated the cellular defense system via activation of PI3K/AKT and Nrf2/HO-1 pathways [79]. Yi et al. [80] reported on the biphasic effects of Z-ligustilide on selected enzymes' activity in *Spodoptera litura* larvae. Low doses of the compound (0.1–0.5 mg/g diet) increased the activities of glutathione S-transferase (GST) (by 23%), cytochrome P450 (by 150%), acetylcholinesterase (by 123%) and carboxylesterase (by 50%). Doses 1 mg/g and 5 mg/g decreased the activity of these enzymes by 80–97% except for carboxylesterase. A similar biphasic dose-response relationship was observed for mRNA expression of GSTS1, CYP4S9, and CYP 4M14. The authors suggested that a low dose of Z-ligustilide stimulated Nrf2 mediated detoxification enzymes and HSP70 pathways [80].

Salvianolic acid B (a condensate of three molecules of danshennol and one molecule of caffeic acid) exhibited a biphasic effect on the total metabolic activity of a rat mesenchymal bone marrow cell culture. Low concentrations, ~4–111 μM, of the compound tested increased the metabolic activity by 40%, whereas ~223 μM caused almost complete inhibition. A similar type of effect was found with the ALP activity. Lower concentrations of salvianolic acid increased the enzyme activity by 40%. The highest concentration tested entirely suppressed ALP activity. As ALP is an indicator of early osteoblast differentiation, the authors concluded that salvianolic acid has the potential to ameliorate bone healing [81].

Glyceollin I a compound classified as prenylated pterocarpan (an induced phytoalexin isolated from soybean) demonstrated a biphasic effect on yeast life span. At low concentration (10–100 nM) glyceollin I induced a chronologic life span (CLS) extension with the maximum effect 40%, relative to the control. A concentration higher than 1.0 μM led to the reduction of CLS and toxicity [82].

Umbelliprenin, a natural sesquiterpene coumarin, affected apoptosis in Jurkat T-CLL cells in a biphasic fashion. Concentration 10 μM and 25 μM increased apoptosis by about 20%, whereas the concentration 50 and 100 μM decreased apoptosis by 50% below the level observed in control cells [83].

Nantenine, an aporphine alkaloid isolated from *Ocotea macrophylla*, affected the activity of K+ -p- nitrophenylphosphatase (K+ -p-NPPase) in synaptosomal membranes isolated from rat brain in a biphasic manner. Concentrations 50 and 0.3 mM increased the activity of the enzyme by about 20% and 40%, respectively. Concentrations higher than 0.75 mM suppressed the activity almost entirely. These findings might explain the previously observed different effects of nantenine on seizures. The authors suggested that the anticonvulsant action of nantenine is attributed to the stimulation of K+ -p-NPPase activity by low doses of alkaloid. The convulsant effect of the compound at high doses might be related to the enzyme inhibition [84].

Kafi et al. [85] demonstrated a biphasic effect of a lignan compound, **arctigenin** on the expression of antiapoptotic gene Mcl-1 in the K562 leukemia cell line. At concentrations, ~27 and ~54 μM arctigenin increased the gene expression by 75%. Concentrations 2-fold greater caused a 75% decrease in the gene expression [85].

Hunt et al. [86] reported that two naphthoquinone compounds, **plumbagin** and **naphazarin** extended the lifespan of *Caenorhabditis elegans* by 10% and 17% when nematodes were exposed to their lower concentrations (1–45 μM plumbagin and 50–500 μM naphazarin). Higher concentrations of plumbagin and naphazarin, 100 and 1000 μM, caused about 90% and only 9% reduction of a lifespan, respectively. The authors found that CNC transcription factor, SKN-1, which promotes antioxidant gene expression, mediates a beneficial effect of both compounds at low concentrations [86].

Rosmarinic acid (RA) [caffeic acid ester of 3-(3,4-dihydroxyphenyl) acetic acid] was shown to affect the lifespan in *C. elegans* in a biphasic manner. At concentrations 100–300 μM the lifespan was extended by 10% at 200 μM, whereas the treatment with concentration 600 μM resulted in a 6% decrease in lifespan. The increased expression of six hsp genes was determined in nematodes treated with RA, which suggested the involvement of stress response activation in the observed effect [34].

A similar experimental model was used to examine the biphasic effects of **epigallocatechin-3-gallate (EGCG)**. Treatment of *C. elegans* with EGCG in the concentration range of 50–300μM resulted in increased longevity (by 5–16%). Higher concentrations of EGCG (800–1000 μM) shortened lifespan by 8% and 14%, respectively. The authors suggested that the life-extending mechanism was stimulated by EGCG-induced ROS production and involved an inducible AMPK/SIRT1/FOXO-dependent redox signaling pathway [87].

The biphasic effects of **panaxatriol saponins** (PTS) isolated from *Panax notoginseng* were examined in PC-12 cells. A stimulatory effect on cell proliferation was observed at concentrations 0.03–1.0 mg/mL and peaked at 0.12 mg/mL (30% increase). The concentration of 4 mg/mL very slightly by 10% reduced cell proliferation. A similar pattern of results was gained in PC12 cells with 6-OHDA induced damage. At low concentrations (0.03–2.0 mg/mL) PTS increased cell viability by 24%. However, co-treatment with a higher concentration of PTS (4 mg/mL) resulted in further inhibition of cell growth by 16%. The authors postulated that PTS exerted neuroprotection against 6-OHDA-induced cell damage in PC-12 cells through activating the PI3K/AKT/mTOR cell proliferation pathway and AMPK/SIRT1/FOXO3 cell survival pathway. They also pointed out the potential application of PTS for the prevention and treatment of neurodegenerative diseases [88]. The biphasic effect of PTS was not confirmed in the zebrafish larvae model. Concentrations 0.01–0.1 mg/mL reversed the dopamine neuron loss induced by 6-OHDA. The higher concentration of PTS (10 mg/mL) neither exerted protection against neuron loss nor caused the opposite effect [88].

The effect of increasing concentrations of **cynarin** (1,3-O-dicaffeoylquinic acid) (CYN) found in artichoke, on cell proliferation was tested in normal human skin fibroblasts (FSF-1) and telomerase-immortalized mesenchymal stem cells (hTERT-MSC). Both cell lines showed biphasic concentration-response to CYN. Concentrations 1–50 μM caused a 10–26% increase in the number of FSF-1 cells, whereas higher concentrations (75–500 μM) decreased cell survival by 16–84%. Similarly, lower CYN concentrations, 1–10 μM, increased the survival of hTERT-MSC cells by 7–60%, and higher concentrations inhibited cell growth by 10–96%. The authors suggested that the increase in cell growth might be due, in part, to the induction of stress response by lower CYN concentrations, as evidenced by an increase in the expression of heme oxidase-1 [89].

The dose-response relationship for the carcinogenic effect of **caffeic acid** (CA) was investigated in male F344 rats fed for 4 weeks a diet containing different CA concentrations: 0.05%, 0.14%, 0.40%, and 1.64% treatment [90]. In the forestomach, a target organ of CA-induced carcinogenesis, the markers of cell proliferation, the total number of epithelial cells, and the number of S-phase cells, were increased about 2.5-fold at 0.40% and 1.64%. At 0.14% both variables were decreased by about 30%. The authors suggested that this low-dose effect could explain the well-known cancer-protective properties of caffeic acid. The lowest dietary concentration tested in the experiment was equivalent to 35 mg/kg b.w./day. This dose is much lower than that enhancing cell proliferation in the rat forestomach and lower than ingested by strong coffee drinkers. Hence, it is in the range of potential protection, assuming the extrapolation of these outcomes to humans [90].

Data on biphasic concentration/dose-dependent effects discussed in this section are collected in Table 3.

Table 3. Phytochemicals exhibiting biphasic concentration/dose-responses.

Compound *	Model	Concentration	Effect	Mechanism	Refs
Arctigenin	K-562	~27, 54 μM	↑Mcl-1mRNA		[85]
		~107 μM	↓Mcl-1mRNA		
Berberine	B16-F10,	1.25–5.00 μM	↑proliferation	↑MAPK/ERK1/2 ↑PI3K/AKT	[70]
	MDA-MB-231,	10–80 μM	↓proliferation		
	MDA-MB-468,				
	MCF-7, LS-174				
	PC-12	0.1–1.0 μM	↑viability	↑PI3K/AKT/Bcl-2	[71]
		2–64 μM	↓viability		
Caffeic acid	male F344 rats	0.14%	↓proliferation	↓epithelial cells, S-phase cells	[90]
		0.40, 1.64%	↑proliferation	↑epithelial cells, ↓S-phase cells in forestomach	
(+) Catechin, rutin	*Salmonella typhimurium*/2-AAF	0.01–0.60 mM	↓mutagenicity		[35]
		1.2, 0.8 mM	↑mutagenicity		
Cynarin	FSF-1,	1–50 μM	↑viability	↑HO-1 activity	[89]
		75–500 μM	↓viability		
	hTERT-MSC	1–00 μM	↑viability	↑HO-1 activity	[89]
		75–500 μM	↓viability		
EGCG	*Caenorhabditis elegans*	50–300 μM	↑lifespan	↑ROS; ↑AMPK/SIRT1/FOXO	[87]
		800–1000μM	↓lifespan		
Falcarinol, Falcarindiol Isolated from carrot roots	primary myotube culture/H_2O_2	1.6–25.0 μM	↑ROS production	↑*GPx*, ↓*Hsp70, HO-1*	[72]
		50, 100 μM	↓ROS production	↓*GPx*, ↑*Hsp70, HO-1*	
Falcarindiol isolated from carrot roots	primary	0.61–9.80 nM	↑viability		[72]
	myotube culture	2.5–5.0 μM	↓viability		
	pBMEC	~0.04–0.20 μM	↑proliferation		[73]
		~4–41 μM	↓proliferation		
	CaCo-2	1–10 μM	↑proliferation ↓apoptosis	↓caspase-3, DNA breakage	[74]
		>20 μM	↓proliferation ↑apoptosis	↑caspase-3, DNA breakage	

Table 3. *Cont.*

Compound *	Model	Concentration	Effect	Mechanism	Refs
Glyceollin I isolated from soybean	*Saccharomyces cerevisiae*	10–100 nM	↑CLS		[82]
		>1 μM	↓CLS		
Luteolin	MCF-7	1–10 μM	↑viability		[77]
		30–1000 μM	↓viability		
	HepG2	<35 μM	↑LC3-II		[78]
		~105 μM	↓LC3-II		
	Salmonella typhimurium/2-AAF	0.006 mM	↑mutagenicity		[35]
		1.2 mM	↓mutagenicity		
Nanteine isolated from *Ocotea macrophilla*	synaptosomal membranes	50 μM, 0.3 mM	↑K+ -p-NPPase activity		[84]
		>0.75 mM	↓K+ -p-NPPase activity		
Naringenin	*Drosophila melanogaster*	200, 400 μM	↑lifespan	↑pupae formation	[75]
		600, 800 μM	↓lifespan	↓pupae formation	
Naphazarin	*Caenorhabditis elegans*	50–500 μM	↑lifespan	↑skn-1	[86]
		1000 μM	↓lifespan		
Panaxatriol saponins isolated from *Panax notoginseng*	PC-12	0.03–1.00 mg/ml	↑proliferation		[88]
		4 mg/ml	↓proliferation		
	PC-12 /6-OHDA	0.03–2.00 mg/ml	↑viability	↑PI3K/AKT/mTOR ↑AMPK/SIRT1/FOXO3	
		4 mg/ml	↓viability		
Plumbagin	*Caenorhabditis elegans*	1–45 μM	↑lifespan	↑skn-1	[86]
		100 μM	↓lifespan		
Rosmarinic acid	*Caenorhabditis elegans*	100–300 μM	↑lifespan	↑*hsp*	[34]
		600 μM	↓lifespan		
Rutin	*Drosophila melanogaster*	200, 400 μM	↑lifespan	↑longevity associated genes	[76]
		600, 800 μM	↓lifespan		
Salvianolic acid B	BMSCs	~4–111 μM	↑metabolic activity, ALP activity		[81]
		~223 μM	↓metabolic activity, ALP activity		
Sulforaphane	T24, HepG2, Caco-2	1–5 μM	↑proliferation	↑RAS, RAF, MEK, ERK, PI3K, AKT and Nf-kB, FOXO Nrf2 pathways	[63]
		10–40 μM	↓proliferation		
	T24	2.50, 3.75 μM	↑migration		
		5–40 μM	↓migration		
	HUVEC, PVC	2.5–5.0 μM	↑angiogenesis	↑tube formation	
		10, 20 μM	↓angiogenesis	↓tube formation	
Isolated from *Brassica oleracea*	MSCs	0.25, 1.00 μM	↑proliferation		[66]
		20 μM	↓proliferation		
		<5 μM	↓apoptotic cells		
		20 μM	↑apoptotic cells		
		0.25, 1.00 μM	↓senescence cells		
		5, 20 μM	↑senescence cells		
		0.25 μM	↓ROS production		
		20 μM	↑ROS production		
Commercial source	MCF-7, HHL-5, HepG2, lymphoblastoid cells	<5 μM	↑proliferation		[67–69]
		>5 μM	↓proliferation		
	lymphoblastoid cells	0.5–5.0 μM	↑GSH		[69]
		10 μM	↓GSH		

Table 3. *Cont.*

Compound *	Model	Concentration	Effect	Mechanism	Refs
Umbelliprenin isolated from *Ferula szowitsiana*	Jurkat T-CLL	10, 25 μM	↑apoptosis		[83]
		50, 100 μM	↓apoptosis		
Z-ligustilide isolated from *Ligusticum chuanxiong*	PC-12/ OGD	1–25 μM	↑viability, ↓apoptosis	↑HO-1 and Nrf2 translocation	[79]
		50 μM	↓viability, ↑apoptosis		
	Spodoptera litura larvae	0.1–0.5 mg/g diet	↑GST, AChE, CYP, CES activities	↑*GSTS1, CYP4S9, CYP4M14*	[80]
		1, 5 mg/g diet	↓GST, AChE, CYP activity	↓*GSTS1, CYP4S9, CYP4M14*	

* If the source of the compound was not specified it was obtained commercially; ↑ = increase, ↓ = decrease; 2-AAF—2-Acetylaminofluorene; 6-OHDA—6-hydroxydopamine; AChE—acetylcholinesterase; AKT—protein kinase B; ALP—alkaline phosphatase; B16-F10—murine melanoma cell line; BMSCs—bone marrow-derived mesenchymal stem cells; CaCo-2—human colon cancer cell line; CES—carboxylesterase; CLS—chronologic life span; CYP—cytochrome P450; CYP4M14 (4S9)—cytochrome P450 4M14 (4S9); EGCG—epigallocatechin-3-gallate; FSF-1—human skin fibroblasts; GPx—glutathione peroxidase; GST—glutathione S-transferase; GSTS1—glutathione S transferase S1; HHL-5—human normal liver cell line; HO-1—heme oxygense 1; Hsp70—heat shock protein; HepG2—human liver cancer cell line; HUVEC—human umbilical vein endothelial cells; Jurkat T-CLL—Jurkat T-cell lymphocyte leukemia cells; K562—immortalized cell line derived from human leukemia; K+ -p-NPPase activity—K+ -p- nitrophenylphosphatase; LC3— microtubule-associated protein 1A/1B-light chain 3; LS-174—human colon cancer cell line; MDA-MB-231, MDA-MB-468, MCF-7MCF-7—human breast carcinoma cell lines; MSCs—mesenchymal stem cell line; OGD—oxygen-glucose deprivation; pBMEC—primary bovine mammary epithelial cells; PC-3—human prostatic carcinoma cell line; PC-12—phaeochromocytoma cell line; PI3K—phosphatidylinositol 3-kinase; PVC—pericytes; skn-1—cap'n'collar transcription factor; T24—bladder cancer cell line; hTERT-MSC—human normal telomerase-immortalized mesenchymal stem cells.

5. Comments

Apparently, there are a lot of reviews concerning biphasic dose/concentration-response to phytochemicals. However, critical analysis of their content reveals that some of them refer mainly to numerous aspects of beneficial health effects and underlying mechanisms, and no single reference related to biphasic dose-response is cited, for example [91–94]. The common feature of this kind of articles is that some phytochemicals are demarked "hormetic" solely on the basis of the induction of "adaptive stress response" or "cellular defense system" at low doses. These effects are counteracted a priori with the presumed toxicity of high doses. In our opinion, such interpretation is not justified because the opposite effects of high doses on endpoints tested were not experimentally evidenced.

The current review includes only original reports on experiments which results conform to the classic definition of biphasic hormetic like dose-response.

The majority of studies presented here were performed on cell cultures. The most common endpoint tested was a proliferation of tumor and non-cancerous cells. Therefore, the question arises: why for other endpoints this pattern of dose-response has been reported rather rarely? Is it due to the fact that such type of response is limited to simple parameters, or maybe other endpoints were not examined with respect to biphasic dose-response? This issue should be addressed in future research.

The overwhelming part of the reports presented in the current review did not contain the elucidation of the mechanism of the biphasic response to phytochemicals. Proliferative activity of low phytoestrogens concentrations was generally explained on the basis of transactivation of the estrogen receptor [9–19,21–23,29,37–40,44]. In more recent articles, some molecular aspects involving the induction of genes expression or activation by phytochemicals of various signaling pathways, for example, MAPK/ERK1/2 and PI3K/AKT were revealed [48,49,57,60,63,72,74,78,79]. In the *Caenorhabditis elegans* model, the increased expression of some genes involved in lifespan or stress response was associated with extended lifespan [34,86,87]. Examples of mechanisms involved in the cellular response to low doses of phytochemicals are presented in Figure 2.

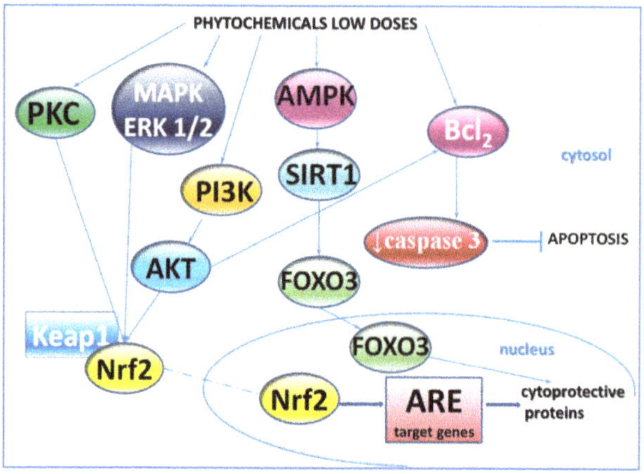

Figure 2. Examples of mechanisms involved in the cellular response to low doses of phytochemicals–on the basis of findings presented in the current review. Phytochemicals can activate kinase cascades, including PKC, MAPK/ERK1/2, PI3K/AKT, which play a critical role in the regulation of cell growth, proliferation, survival, and apoptosis. Downstream effector of these kinases is transcription factor Nrf2, which is released from the complex with keap1 and translocates to the nucleus, binds to ARE and stimulates the expression of cytoprotective proteins, e.g., antioxidant enzymes and phase-2 proteins. SIRT-1 plays a key role in the cellular response to various stressors by activating transcription factor FOXO3, which induces genes encoding cytoprotective proteins. The transcriptional activity of FOXO3 is modulated by both AMPK and SIRT-1. PI3K/AKT is the major pathway mediating cell survival and inhibiting apoptosis. Bcl-2, a pro-survival, anti-apoptotic, and cytoprotective molecule, can be activated directly by chemicals or via PI3K/AKT pathway. AKT—serine/threonine protein kinase; AMPK—AMP-activated protein kinase; ARE—antioxidant response elements; Bcl2—B-cell lymphoma 2; ERK—extracellular signal-regulated kinase protein-serine/threonine kinase; FOXO3—forkhead box O3; KEAP1—Kelch-like ECH-associated protein 1; MAPK—mitogen-activated protein kinase; Nrf2—nuclear factor erythroid 2-related factor 2; PI3K—phosphatidylinositol 3-kinase; PKC—protein kinase C; SIRT1—sirtuin1.

The current review supports the opinion of many authors that the stimulatory effects of low doses/concentrations are not always beneficial [8,95] as evidenced by the increased proliferation of tumor cells exposed to phytochemicals. On the other hand, the enhanced proliferation of neuron-like PC-12 cells induced by some phytochemicals accounts for their neuroprotective action [71,88]. Moreover, the interpretation of the impact of a stimulatory effect depends on the context of a potentially therapeutic application. Chirumbolo et al. reported that low concentrations of quercetin enhanced activation of basophils [32] and simultaneously caused an increase in histamine release [33]. The first effect was considered beneficial for the strengthening of an inflammatory reaction against invading bacteria, but the latter was harmful in the context of the potential use of quercetin in the prevention of allergy.

It is intriguing how few experiments referring to biphasic dose-response induced by phytochemicals were carried on animal models, as demonstrated in the current review. In *C. elegans* [34,86,87] and *D. melanogaster* [75,76] treated with the compounds tested, biphasic changes of lifespan were recorded. Selected enzymes' activity in *Spodoptera litura* larvae [80] and mutagenic activity tested by *Salmonella typhimurium* assay were modulated in a biphasic manner [35,36]. In transgenic mouse models [20,88] as well as in the zebrafish larvae model [71,88] solely the effects of low doses of compounds tested were demonstrated to be consistent with in vitro findings, however, no opposite effects of high doses were recorded. We found only two experiments on rodents in which regular biphasic dose-response was shown. One referred to the changes in markers of cell proliferation in the forestomach of rats fed a diet containing various amounts of caffeic acid [90], another described the cardioprotective effect of resveratrol administered to rats for 3 months [61] (Figure 3).

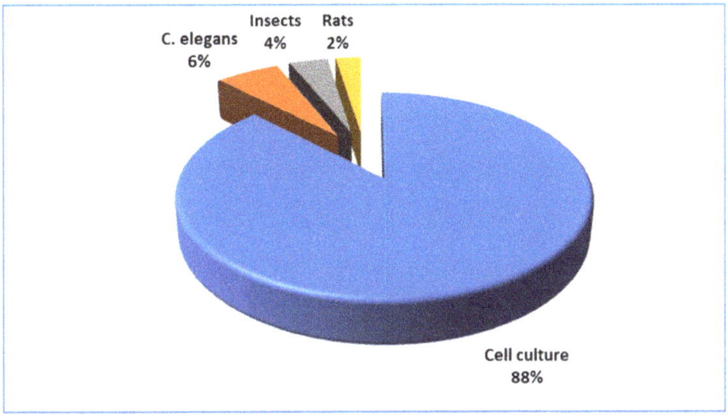

Figure 3. The percentage share of various types of experimental models applied in the reports cited in this review.

Data on the biphasic dose-response of various endpoints to phytochemicals may have a potential therapeutic or preventive implication. However, their significance is compromised by the fact that very few in vitro findings were supported by in vivo experiments. Therefore, the feasibility of extrapolating results from cell culture models to the whole organism might be questioned. The fact that low concentrations of some phytochemicals can stimulate proliferation should raise concerns with regard to carcinogenesis. However, concentrations tested in cell cultures may not be relevant to the whole organism and in various organs, different doses can evoke different effects [96]. For better extrapolation from in vitro biphasic dose-response data to in vivo conditions physiologically based pharmacokinetic models (PBPM) should be used taking into account expected plasma and tissue concentration as well as processes of biotransformation [28]. The need for caution in the assessment of pharmacological effect is supported by the report by Lutz et al. [90]. Conversely to the majority of data presented in the current review, the authors showed that high doses of caffeic acid displayed proliferative effects, whereas low doses decreased cell division in the forestomach of rats [90].

Some authors argue that biphasic dose-response is affected by a lot of factors rendering the adequate assessment of potential health benefit impossible. This type of dose-response can be differential among endpoints in a given system/model i.e., some endpoints may demonstrate positive or negative effects whereas some others may be unresponsive or clinically insignificant [97]. Moreover, low and high doses are not unequivocally defined because the low doses used in the in vitro experiments might be high doses if extrapolated to the whole organism [96].

Evidence for adverse effects of phytochemicals, depending on their concentrations/doses should provoke further mechanistic investigations to elucidate the phenomenon of their biphasic/hormetic action. Given the essential role of plant-based food in human nutrition, further preclinical and human studies aiming at establishing a safe and efficient dose of phytochemicals are required.

Author Contributions: Conceptualization, J.J.-L.; writing—original draft preparation, J.J.-L.; writing—review and editing, J.J.-L.; M.K.; graphical work, M.K. All authors have read and agreed to the published version of the manuscript.

Funding: The APC was funded by Poznan University of Medical Sciences.

Conflicts of Interest: The authors declare no conflict of interest.

Abbreviations

2-AAF	2-Acetylaminofluorene
4NQO	4-nitroquinoline-N-oxide
6-OHDA	6-Hydroxydopamine
AChE	Acetylcholinesterase
AFB1	Aflatoxin B1
AKT	Serine/threonine protein kinase
ALP	Alkaline phosphatase
apoM	Apolipoprotein M
b.w.	Bodyweight
B16-F10	Murine melanoma cell line
Bcl-2	B-cell lymphoma 2
BER	Berberine
BMSCs	Bone marrow-derived mesenchymal stem cells
C2C12	Mouse myoblast cell line
CA	Caffeic acid
CaCo-2	Human colon cancer cell line
CD203c	Basophil-specific ectoenzyme E-NPP3
CD63	Tetraspan transmembrane protein family
CES	Carboxylesterase
CIN	Chromosomal instability
CLS	Chronologic life span
CYN	Cynarin
CYP	Cytochrome P450
CYP1A2	Cytochrome P450 1A2
DAI	Daidzein
ER	Estrogen receptor
ERK	Extracellular signal-regulated kinase protein-serine/threonine kinase
fMLP	Bacterial formyl peptide N-formylmethionine-leucine-phenylalanine
FSF-1	Human skin fibroblasts
GEN	Genistein
GIR	Genotoxic inhibition rate
GPx	Glutathione peroxidase
GSH	Reduced glutathione
GSSG	Oxidized glutathione
GST	Glutathione S-transferase
HCT-116	Colon carcinoma cell lines
HepG2	Human liver cancer cell line
HHL-5	Human normal liver cell line
HO-1	Heme oxygenase-1
Hsp70	70 kDa heat shock protein
HT-29	Colon carcinoma cell lines
hTERT-MSC	Human normal telomerase-immortalized mesenchymal stem cells
HUVEC	Human umbilical vein endothelial cell line
ISL	Isoliquiritigenin
Jurkat T-CLL	Jurkat T-cell lymphocyte leukemia cells
K+ -p-NPPase activity	K+ -p- nitrophenylphosphatase
K562	Immortalized cell line derived from human leukemia
KS483	Murine osteoprogenitor cell line
LC3-II	Microtubule-associated protein 2 light chain 3
LNCaP	Androgen-sensitive human prostate adenocarcinoma cell line
LoVo	Human colon adenocarcinoma cell line

LS-174	Human colon cancer cell line
LVDP	Left ventricular developed pressure
MAPK	Mitogen-activated protein kinase
MCF-7	Human breast adenocarcinoma cell line
MDA-MB-231, MDA-MB-468, MCF-7MCF-7	Human breast carcinoma cell lines
MeIQ	2-amino-3,4-dimethylimidazo [4,5-f]quinoline
MG-63	Human osteoblast-like cells
MMPs	matrix metalloproteinases
MN	Markers micronuclei
MSCs	Mesenchymal stem cell line
NHDF	Neonatal normal human dermal fibroblasts
NHEK	Neonatal normal human epidermal keratinocytes
NK	Human natural killer cells
NPB	Nucleoplasmic bridge
NPCs	Neural progenitor cells; ODC - ornithine decarboxylase
OGD	Oxygen-glucose deprivation
pBMEC	Primary bovine mammary epithelial cells
PC-12	Phaeochromocytoma cell line
PC-3	Human prostatic carcinoma cell line
PCNA	Proliferating cell nuclear antigen
PGE2	Prostaglandin E2
PI3K	Phosphoinositide 3-kinase
PKC	Protein kinase C
PMA	Phorbol myristate acetate
PPARγ	Peroxisome proliferator-activated receptor γ
PTS	Panaxatriol saponins
PVC	Pericytes
QER	Quercetin
RA	Rosmarinic acid
RAW 264.7	Murine macrophage cell line
RES	Resveratrol
ROS	Reactive oxygen species
RWPE-1	Nontumorigenic human prostate epithelial cells
SCC-25	Oral squamous carcinoma cell line
SFN	Sulforaphane
SKN-1	Transcription factor skinhead-1
SOX2	Transcription factor (sex determining region Y-box 2
T24	Bladder cancer cell line
T-47D, T	Human breast cancer cell lines
TIMP-2	Tissue inhibitor of metalloproteinase-2
TRAMP-FVB	Transgenic adenocarcinoma of mouse prostate model
UtLM	Human uterine leiomyoma
UtSMCs	Uterine smooth muscle cells

References

1. Pal, S.; Konkimalla, V.B. Hormetic potential of sulforaphane (SFN) in switching cells' fate towards survival or death. *Mini Rev. Med. Chem.* **2016**, *16*, 980–995. [CrossRef] [PubMed]
2. Calabrese, E.J.; Mattson, M.P.; Calabrese, V. Resveratrol commonly displays hormesis: Occurrence and biomedical significance. *Hum. Exp. Toxicol.* **2010**, *29*, 980–1015. [CrossRef] [PubMed]
3. Mukherjee, S.; Dudley, J.I.; Das, D.K. Dose-dependency of resveratrol in providing health benefits. *Dose Response* **2010**, *8*, 478–500. [CrossRef] [PubMed]

4. Moghaddam, N.S.A.; Oskouie, M.N.; Butler, A.E.; Petit, P.X.; Barreto, G.E.; Sahebkar, A. Hormetic effects of curcumin: What is the evidence? *J. Cell Physiol.* **2019**, *234*, 10060–10071. [CrossRef]
5. Hayes, D.P. Nutritional hormesis. *Eur. J. Clin. Nutr.* **2007**, *61*, 147–159. [CrossRef]
6. Calabrese, E.J.; Baldwin, L.A. Defining hormesis. *Hum. Exp. Toxicol.* **2002**, *21*, 91–97. [CrossRef]
7. Calabrese, E.J.; Baldwin, L.A. A quantitatively-based methodology for the evaluation of chemical hormesis. *Hum. Ecol. Risk Assess.* **1997**, *3*, 545–554. [CrossRef]
8. Kendig, E.L.; Le, H.H.; Belcher, S.M. Defining hormesis: Evaluation of a complex concentration response phenomenon. *Int. J. Toxicol.* **2010**, *29*, 235–246. [CrossRef]
9. Rietjens, I.M.C.M.; Louisse, J.; Beekmann, K. The potential health effects of dietary phytoestrogens. *Br. J. Pharm.* **2017**, *174*, 1263–1280. [CrossRef]
10. Zava, D.T.; Duwe, G. Estrogenic and antiproliferative properties of genistein and other flavonoids in human breast cancer cells in vitro. *Nutr. Cancer* **1997**, *27*, 31–40. [CrossRef]
11. Hsieh, C.Y.; Santell, R.C.; Haslam, S.Z.; Helferich, W.G. Estrogenic effects of genistein on the growth of estrogen receptor-positive human breast cancer (MCF-7) cells in vitro and in vivo. *Cancer Res.* **1998**, *58*, 3833–3838. [PubMed]
12. Fioravanti, L.; Cappelletti, V.; Miodini, P.; Ronchi, E.; Brivio, M.; Di Fronzo, G. Genistein in the control of breast cancer cell growth: Insights into the mechanism of action in vitro. *Cancer Lett.* **1998**, *130*, 143–152. [CrossRef]
13. Le Bail, J.C.; Champavier, Y.; Chulia, A.J.; Habrioux, G. Effects of phytoestrogens on aromatase, 3beta and 17beta-hydroxysteroid dehydrogenase activities and human breast cancer cells. *Life Sci.* **2000**, *66*, 1281–1291. [CrossRef]
14. Liu, B.; Edgerton, S.; Yang, X.; Kim, A.; Ordonez-Ercan, D.; Mason, T.; Alvarez, K.; McKimmey, C.; Liu, N.; Thor, A. Low-dose dietary phytoestrogen abrogates tamoxifen-associated mammary tumor prevention. *Cancer Res.* **2005**, *65*, 879–886.
15. Limer, J.L.; Parkes, A.T.; Speirs, V. Differential response to phytoestrogens in endocrine sensitive and resistant breast cancer cells in vitro. *Int. J. Cancer* **2006**, *119*, 515–521. [CrossRef]
16. Wang, C.; Kurzer, M.S. Effects of phytoestrogens on DNA synthesis in MCF-7 cells in the presence of estradiol or growth factors. *Nutr. Cancer* **1998**, *31*, 90–100. [CrossRef]
17. Maggiolini, M.; Bonofiglio, D.; Marsico, S.; Panno, M.L.; Cenni, B.; Picard, D.; Andò, S. Estrogen receptor α mediates the proliferative but not the cytotoxic dose-dependent effects of two major phytoestrogens on human breast cancer cells. *Mol. Pharmacol.* **2001**, *60*, 595–602.
18. Miodini, P.; Fioravanti, L.; Fronzo, G.D.; Cappelletti, V. The two phyto-oestrogens genistein and quercetin exert different effects on oestrogen receptor function. *Br. J. Cancer* **1999**, *80*, 1150–1155. [CrossRef]
19. Wang, T.T.; Sathyamoorthy, N.; Phang, J.M. Molecular effects of genistein on estrogen receptor mediated pathways. *Carcinogenesis* **1996**, *17*, 271–275. [CrossRef]
20. El Touny, L.H.; Banerjee, P.P. Identification of a biphasic role for genistein in the regulation of prostate cancer growth and metastasis. *Cancer Res.* **2009**, *69*, 3695–3703. [CrossRef]
21. Wang, X.; Clubbs, E.A.; Bomser, J.A. Genistein modulates prostate epithelial cell proliferation via estrogen- and extracellular signal-regulated kinase-dependent pathways. *J. Nutr. Biochem.* **2006**, *17*, 204–210. [CrossRef] [PubMed]
22. Moore, A.; Castro, L.; Yu, L.; Zheng, X.; Di, X.; Sifre, M.; Kissling, G.; Newbold, R.; Bortner, C.; Dixon, D. Stimulatory and inhibitory effects of genistein on human uterine leiomyoma cell proliferation are influenced by the concentration. *Hum. Reprod.* **2007**, *22*, 2623–2631. [CrossRef] [PubMed]
23. Dang, Z.C.; Audinot, V.; Papapoulos, S.E.; Boutin, J.A.; Lowik, C.W. Peroxisome proliferator-activated receptor gamma (PPARgamma) as a molecular target for the soy phytoestrogen genistein. *J. Biol. Chem.* **2003**, *278*, 962–967. [CrossRef]
24. Ying, C.; Hsu, J.T.; Hung, H.C.; Lin, D.H.; Chen, L.F.; Wang, L.K. Growth and cell cycle regulation by isoflavones in human breast carcinoma cells. *Reprod. Nutr. Dev.* **2002**, *42*, 55–64. [CrossRef] [PubMed]
25. Hsu, J.T.; Jean, T.C.; Chan, M.A.; Ying, C. Differential display screening for specific gene expression induced by dietary nonsteroidal estrogen. *Mol. Reprod. Dev.* **1999**, *52*, 141–148. [CrossRef]
26. Guo, J.M.; Xiao, B.X.; Liu, D.H.; Grant, M.; Zhang, S.; Lai, Y.F.; Guo, Y.B.; Liu, Q. Biphasic effect of daidzein on cell growth of human colon cancer cells. *Food Chem. Toxicol.* **2004**, *42*, 1641–1646. [CrossRef]

27. Dang, Z.; Lowik, C.W. The balance between concurrent activation of ERs and PPARs determines daidzein-induced osteogenesis and adipogenesis. *J. Bone Min. Res.* **2004**, *19*, 853–861. [CrossRef]
28. van der Woude, H.; Gliszczynska-Swiglo, A.; Struijs, K.; Smeets, A.; Alink, G.M.; Rietjens, I.M. Biphasic modulation of cell proliferation by quercetin at concentrations physiologically relevant in humans. *Cancer Lett.* **2003**, *200*, 41–47. [CrossRef]
29. Elattar, T.M.; Virji, A.S. The inhibitory effect of curcumin, genistein, quercetin and cisplatin on the growth of oral cancer cells in vitro. *Anticancer Res.* **2000**, *20*, 1733–1738.
30. Bai, H.W.; Zhu, B.T. Strong activation of cyclooxygenase I and II catalytic activity by dietary bioflavonoids. *J. Lipid Res.* **2008**, *49*, 2557–2570. [CrossRef]
31. Bai, H.W.; Zhu, B.T. Myricetin and quercetin are naturally occurring co-substrates of cyclooxygenases in vivo. *Prostaglandins Leukot. Essent. Fat. Acids* **2010**, *82*, 45–50. [CrossRef] [PubMed]
32. Chirumbolo, S.; Conforti, A.; Ortolani, R.; Vella, A.; Marzotto, M.; Bellavite, P. Stimulus-specific regulation of CD63 and CD203c membrane expression in human basophils by the flavonoid quercetin. *Int. Immunopharmacol.* **2010**, *10*, 183–192. [CrossRef] [PubMed]
33. Chirumbolo, S.; Marzotto, M.; Conforti, A.; Vella, A.; Ortolani, R.; Bellavite, P. Bimodal action of the flavonoid quercetin on basophil function: An investigation of the putative biochemical targets. *Clin. Mol. Allergy* **2010**, *8*, 13. [CrossRef] [PubMed]
34. Pietsch, K.; Saul, N.; Chakrabarti, S.; Sturzenbaum, S.R.; Menzel, R.; Steinberg, C.E. Hormetins, antioxidants and prooxidants: Defining quercetin-, caffeic acid- and rosmarinic acid-mediated life extension in C. elegans. *Biogerontology* **2011**, *12*, 329–347. [CrossRef]
35. Snijman, P.W.; Swanevelder, S.; Joubert, E.; Green, I.R.; Gelderblom, W.C. The antimutagenic activity of the major flavonoids of rooibos (Aspalathus linearis): Some dose-response effects on mutagen activation-flavonoid interactions. *Mutat. Res.* **2007**, *631*, 111–123. [CrossRef]
36. Kang, I.H.; Kim, H.J.; Oh, H.; Park, Y.I.; Dong, M.S. Biphasic effects of the flavonoids quercetin and naringenin on the metabolic activation of 2-amino-3,5-dimethylimidazo[4,5-f]quinoline by Salmonella typhimurium TA1538 co-expressing human cytochrome P450 1A2, NADPH-cytochrome P450 reductase, and cytochrome b5. *Mutat. Res.* **2004**, *545*, 37–47.
37. Hsu, J.T.; Hung, H.C.; Chen, C.J.; Hsu, W.L.; Ying, C. Effects of the dietary phytoestrogen biochanin A on cell growth in the mammary carcinoma cell line MCF-7. *J. Nutr. Biochem.* **1999**, *10*, 510–517. [CrossRef]
38. Pedro, M.; Lourenco, C.F.; Cidade, H.; Kijjoa, A.; Pinto, M.; Nascimento, M.S. Effects of natural prenylated flavones in the phenotypical ER (+) MCF-7 and ER (-) MDA-MB-231 human breast cancer cells. *Toxicol. Lett.* **2006**, *164*, 24–36. [CrossRef]
39. Pedro, M.; Ferreira, M.M.; Cidade, H.; Kijjoa, A.; Bronze-da-Rocha, E.; Nascimento, M.S. Artelastin is a cytotoxic prenylated flavone that disturbs microtubules and interferes with DNA replication in MCF-7 human breast cancer cells. *Life Sci.* **2005**, *77*, 293–311. [CrossRef]
40. Yap, S.P.; Shen, P.; Butler, M.S.; Gong, Y.; Loy, C.J.; Yong, E.L. New estrogenic prenylflavone from Epimedium brevicornum inhibits the growth of breast cancer cells. *Planta Med.* **2005**, *71*, 114–119. [CrossRef]
41. Tamir, S.; Eizenberg, M.; Somjen, D.; Stern, N.; Shelach, R.; Kaye, A.; Vaya, J. Estrogenic and antiproliferative properties of glabridin from licorice in human breast cancer cells. *Cancer Res.* **2000**, *60*, 5704–5709. [PubMed]
42. Tamir, S.; Eizenberg, M.; Somjen, D.; Izrael, S.; Vaya, J. Estrogen-like activity of glabrene and other constituents isolated from licorice root. *J. Steroid Biochem. Mol. Biol.* **2001**, *78*, 291–298. [CrossRef]
43. Feng, J.; Shi, Z.; Ye, Z. Effects of metabolites of the lignans enterolactone and enterodiol on osteoblastic differentiation of MG-63 cells. *Biol. Pharm. Bull.* **2008**, *31*, 1067–1070. [CrossRef] [PubMed]
44. Maggiolini, M.; Statti, G.; Vivacqua, A.; Gabriele, S.; Rago, V.; Loizzo, M.; Menichini, F.; Amdo, S. Estrogenic and antiproliferative activities of isoliquiritigenin in MCF7 breast cancer cells. *J. Steroid Biochem. Mol. Biol.* **2002**, *82*, 315–322. [CrossRef]
45. Kang, S.W.; Choi, J.S.; Choi, Y.J.; Bae, J.Y.; Li, J.; Kim, D.S.; Kim, J.L.; Shin, S.Y.; Lee, Y.J.; Kwun, I.S.; et al. Licorice isoliquiritigenin dampens angiogenic activity via inhibition of MAPK-responsive signaling pathways leading to induction of matrix metalloproteinases. *J. Nutr. Biochem.* **2010**, *21*, 55–65. [CrossRef]
46. Oh, S.M.; Kim, Y.P.; Chung, K.H. Biphasic effects of kaempferol on the estrogenicity in human breast cancer cells. *Arch. Pharm. Res.* **2006**, *29*, 354–362. [CrossRef]
47. Setchell, K.D. Phytoestrogens: The biochemistry, physiology, and implications for human health of soy isoflavones. *Am. J. Clin. Nutr.* **1998**, *68*, 1333S–1346S. [CrossRef]

48. Plauth, A.; Geikowski, A.; Cichon, S.; Wowro, S.J.; Liedgens, L.; Rousseau, M.; Weidner, C.; Fuhr, L.; Kliem, M.; Jenkins, G.; et al. Hormetic shifting of redox environment by pro-oxidative resveratrol protects cells against stress. *Free Radic. Biol. Med.* **2016**, *99*, 608–622. [CrossRef]
49. Kumar, V.; Pandey, A.; Jahan, S.; Shukla, R.K.; Kumar, D.; Srivastava, A.; Singh, S.; Rajpurohit, C.S.; Yadav, S.; Khanna, V.K.; et al. Differential responses of Trans-Resveratrol on proliferation of neural progenitor cells and aged rat hippocampal neurogenesis. *Sci. Rep.* **2016**, *6*, 28142. [CrossRef]
50. San Hipólito-Luengo, Á.; Alcaide, A.; Ramos-González, M.; Cercas, E.; Vallejo, S.; Romero, A.; Talero, E.; Sánchez-Ferrer, C.F.; Motilva, V.; Peiró, C. Dual effects of resveratrol on cell death and proliferation of colon cancer cells. *Nutr. Cancer* **2017**, *69*, 1019–1027. [CrossRef]
51. Tvrdá, E.; Lukac, N.; Lukáčová, J.; Hashim, F.; Massányi, P. In vitro supplementation of resveratrol to bovine spermatozoa: Effects on motility, viability and superoxide production. *J. Microbiol. Biotechnol. Food Sci.* **2019**, *4*, 336–341. [CrossRef]
52. Kuwajerwala, N.; Cifuentes, E.; Gautam, S.; Menon, M.; Barrack, E.R.; Reddy, G.P. Resveratrol induces prostate cancer cell entry into s phase and inhibits DNA synthesis. *Cancer Res.* **2002**, *62*, 2488–2492. [PubMed]
53. Ortega, I.; Wong, D.H.; Villanueva, J.A.; Cress, A.B.; Sokalska, A.; Stanley, S.D.; Duleba, A.J. Effects of resveratrol on growth and function of rat ovarian granulosa cells. *Fertil. Steril.* **2012**, *98*, 1563–1573. [CrossRef] [PubMed]
54. Guo, X.; Ni, J.; Dai, X.; Zhou, T.; Yang, G.; Xue, J.; Wang, X. Biphasic regulation of spindle assembly checkpoint by low and high concentrations of resveratrol leads to the opposite effect on chromosomal instability. *Mutat. Res. Genet. Toxicol. Env. Mutagen.* **2018**, *825*, 19–30. [CrossRef]
55. Bosutti, A.; Degens, H. The impact of resveratrol and hydrogen peroxide on muscle cell plasticity shows a dose-dependent interaction. *Sci. Rep.* **2015**, *5*, 8093. [CrossRef]
56. Kurano, M.; Hara, M.; Nojiri, T.; Ikeda, H.; Tsukamoto, K.; Yatomi, Y. Resveratrol exerts a biphasic effect on apolipoprotein M. *Br. J. Pharm.* **2016**, *173*, 222–233. [CrossRef]
57. Peltz, L.; Gomez, J.; Marquez, M.; Alencastro, F.; Atashpanjeh, N.; Quang, T.; Bach, T.; Zhao, Y. Resveratrol exerts dosage and duration dependent effect on human mesenchymal stem cell development. *PLoS ONE* **2012**, *7*, e37162. [CrossRef]
58. Lombardi, G.; Vannini, S.; Blasi, F.; Marcotullio, M.C.; Dominici, L.; Villarini, M.; Cossignani, L.; Moretti, M. In vitro safety/protection assessment of resveratrol and pterostilbene in a human hepatoma cell line (HepG2). *Nat. Prod. Commun.* **2015**, *10*, 1403–1408.
59. Li, Q.; Huyan, T.; Ye, L.J.; Li, J.; Shi, J.L.; Huang, Q.S. Concentration-dependent biphasic effects of resveratrol on human natural killer cells in vitro. *J. Agric. Food Chem.* **2014**, *62*, 10928–10935. [CrossRef]
60. Posadino, A.M.; Giordo, R.; Cossu, A.; Nasrallah, G.K.; Shaito, A.; Abou-Saleh, H.; Eid, A.H.; Pintus, G. Flavin oxidase-induced ROS generation modulates PKC biphasic effect of resveratrol on endothelial cell survival. *Biomolecules* **2019**, *9*. [CrossRef]
61. Juhasz, B.; Mukherjee, S.; Das, D.K. Hormetic response of resveratrol against cardioprotection. *Exp. Clin. Cardiol.* **2010**, *15*, e134–e138. [PubMed]
62. Sita, G.; Hrelia, P.; Graziosi, A.; Morroni, F. Sulforaphane from cruciferous vegetables: Recent advances to improve glioblastoma treatment. *Nutrients* **2018**, *10*. [CrossRef] [PubMed]
63. Bao, Y.; Wang, W.; Zhou, Z.; Sun, C. Benefits and risks of the hormetic effects of dietary isothiocyanates on cancer prevention. *PLoS ONE* **2014**, *9*, e114764. [CrossRef] [PubMed]
64. Calabrese, V.; Cornelius, C.; Dinkova-Kostova, A.T.; Calabrese, E.J.; Mattson, M.P. Cellular stress responses, the hormesis paradigm, and vitagenes: Novel targets for therapeutic intervention in neurodegenerative disorders. *Antioxid. Redox Signal.* **2010**, *13*, 1763–1811. [CrossRef]
65. Mattson, M.P.; Cheng, A. Neurohormetic phytochemicals: Low-dose toxins that induce adaptive neuronal stress responses. *Trends Neurosci.* **2006**, *29*, 632–639. [CrossRef]
66. Zanichelli, F.; Capasso, S.; Cipollaro, M.; Pagnotta, E.; Carteni, M.; Casale, F.; Iori, R.; Galderisi, U. Dose-dependent effects of R-sulforaphane isothiocyanate on the biology of human mesenchymal stem cells, at dietary amounts, it promotes cell proliferation and reduces senescence and apoptosis, while at anti-cancer drug doses, it has a cytotoxic effect. *Age (Dordr)* **2012**, *34*, 281–293. [CrossRef]
67. Jackson, S.J.; Singletary, K.W. Sulforaphane inhibits human MCF-7 mammary cancer cell mitotic progression and tubulin polymerization. *J. Nutr.* **2004**, *134*, 2229–2236. [CrossRef]

68. Li, D.; Wang, W.; Shan, Y.; Barrera, L.N.; Howie, A.F.; Beckett, G.J.; Wu, K.; Bao, Y. Synergy between sulforaphane and selenium in the up-regulation of thioredoxin reductase and protection against hydrogen peroxide-induced cell death in human hepatocytes. *Food Chem.* **2012**, *133*, 300–307. [CrossRef]
69. Misiewicz, I.; Skupinska, K.; Kowalska, E.; Lubinski, J.; Kasprzycka-Guttman, T. Sulforaphane-mediated induction of a phase 2 detoxifying enzyme NAD(P)H:quinone reductase and apoptosis in human lymphoblastoid cells. *Acta Biochim. Pol.* **2004**, *51*, 711–721. [CrossRef]
70. Bao, J.; Huang, B.; Zou, L.; Chen, S.; Zhang, C.; Zhang, Y.; Chen, M.; Wan, J.B.; Su, H.; Wang, Y.; et al. Hormetic Effect of Berberine Attenuates the Anticancer Activity of Chemotherapeutic Agents. *PLoS ONE* **2015**, *10*, e0139298. [CrossRef]
71. Zhang, C.; Li, C.; Chen, S.; Li, Z.; Jia, X.; Wang, K.; Bao, J.; Liang, Y.; Wang, X.; Chen, M.; et al. Berberine protects against 6-OHDA-induced neurotoxicity in PC12 cells and zebrafish through hormetic mechanisms involving PI3K/AKT/Bcl-2 and Nrf2/HO-1 pathways. *Redox Biol.* **2017**, *11*, 1–11. [CrossRef] [PubMed]
72. Young, J.F.; Christensen, L.P.; Theil, P.K.; Oksbjerg, N. The polyacetylenes falcarinol and falcarindiol affect stress responses in myotube cultures in a biphasic manner. *Dose Response* **2008**, *6*, 239–251. [CrossRef] [PubMed]
73. Hansen, S.L.; Purup, S.; Christensen, L.P. Bioactivity of falcarinol and the influenceof processing and storage on its content in carrots (Daucus carota L). *J. Sci. Food Agric.* **2003**, *83*, 1010–1017. [CrossRef]
74. Young, J.F.; Duthie, S.J.; Milne, L.; Christensen, L.P.; Duthie, G.G.; Bestwick, C.S. Biphasic effect of falcarinol on caco-2 cell proliferation, DNA damage, and apoptosis. *J Agric. Food Chem.* **2007**, *55*, 618–623. [CrossRef]
75. Chattopadhyay, D.; Sen, S.; Chatterjee, R.; Roy, D.; James, J.; Thirumurugan, K. Context- and dose-dependent modulatory effects of naringenin on survival and development of Drosophila melanogaster. *Biogerontology* **2016**, *17*, 383–393. [CrossRef]
76. Chattopadhyay, D.; Chitnis, A.; Talekar, A.; Mulay, P.; Makkar, M.; James, J.; Thirumurugan, K. Hormetic efficacy of rutin to promote longevity in Drosophila melanogaster. *Biogerontology* **2017**, *18*, 397–411. [CrossRef]
77. Sato, Y.; Sasaki, N.; Saito, M.; Endo, N.; Kugawa, F.; Ueno, A. Luteolin attenuates doxorubicin-induced cytotoxicity to MCF-7 human breast cancer cells. *Biol. Pharm. Bull.* **2015**, *38*, 703–709. [CrossRef]
78. Lascala, A.; Martino, C.; Parafati, M.; Salerno, R.; Oliverio, M.; Pellegrino, D.; Mollace, V.; Janda, E. Analysis of proautophagic activities of Citrus flavonoids in liver cells reveals the superiority of a natural polyphenol mixture over pure flavones. *J. Nutr. Biochem.* **2018**, *58*, 119–130. [CrossRef]
79. Qi, H.; Han, Y.; Rong, J. Potential roles of PI3K/Akt and Nrf2-Keap1 pathways in regulating hormesis of Z-ligustilide in PC12 cells against oxygen and glucose deprivation. *Neuropharmacology* **2012**, *62*, 1659–1670. [CrossRef]
80. Yi, Y.; Dou, G.; Yu, Z.; He, H.; Wang, C.; Li, L.; Zhou, J.; Liu, D.; Shi, J.; Li, G.; et al. Z-ligustilide exerted hormetic effect on growth and detoxification enzymes of spodoptera litura larvae. *Evid. Based Complement Altern. Med.* **2018**, *2018*, 7104513. [CrossRef]
81. Liu, Y.R.; Qu, S.X.; Maitz, M.F.; Tan, R.; Weng, J. The effect of the major components of Salvia Miltiorrhiza Bunge on bone marrow cells. *J. Ethnopharmacol.* **2007**, *111*, 573–583. [CrossRef] [PubMed]
82. Liu, Y.; Wu, Z.; Feng, S.; Yang, X.; Huang, D. Hormesis of glyceollin I, an induced phytoalexin from soybean, on budding yeast chronological lifespan extension. *Molecules* **2014**, *19*, 568–580. [CrossRef] [PubMed]
83. Gholami, O. Umbelliprenin mediates its apoptotic effect by hormesis: A commentary. *Dose Response* **2017**, *15*, 1559325817710035. [CrossRef] [PubMed]
84. Ribeiro, R.A.; Rodriguez de Lores Arnaiz, G. In vitro dose dependent inverse effect of nantenine on synaptosomal membrane K+-p-NPPase activity. *Phytomedicine* **2001**, *8*, 107–111. [CrossRef]
85. Kafi, Z.; Cheshomi, H.; Gholami, O. 7-Isopenthenyloxycoumarin, arctigenin, and hesperidin modify myeloid cell leukemia type-1 (Mcl-1) gene expression by hormesis in K562 cell line. *Dose Response* **2018**, *16*, 1559325818796014. [CrossRef]
86. Hunt, P.R.; Son, T.G.; Wilson, M.A.; Yu, Q.S.; Wood, W.H.; Zhang, Y.; Becker, K.G.; Greig, N.H.; Mattson, M.P.; Camandola, S.; et al. Extension of lifespan in C. elegans by naphthoquinones that act through stress hormesis mechanisms. *PLoS ONE* **2011**, *6*, e21922. [CrossRef]
87. Xiong, L.G.; Chen, Y.J.; Tong, J.W.; Gong, Y.S.; Huang, J.A.; Liu, Z.H. Epigallocatechin-3-gallate promotes healthy lifespan through mitohormesis during early-to-mid adulthood in caenorhabditis elegans. *Redox Biol.* **2018**, *14*, 305–315. [CrossRef]

88. Zhang, C.; Li, C.; Chen, S.; Li, Z.; Ma, L.; Jia, X.; Wang, K.; Bao, J.; Liang, Y.; Chen, M.; et al. Hormetic effect of panaxatriol saponins confers neuroprotection in PC12 cells and zebrafish through PI3K/AKT/mTOR and AMPK/SIRT1/FOXO3 pathways. *Sci. Rep.* **2017**, *7*, 41082. [CrossRef]
89. Gezer, C.; Yücecan, S.; Rattan, S.I.S. Artichoke compound cynarin differentially affects the survival, growth, and stress response of normal, immortalized, and cancerous human cells. *Turk. J. Biol.* **2019**, *39*, 299–305. [CrossRef]
90. Lutz, U.; Lugli, S.; Bitsch, A.; Schlatter, J.; Lutz, W.K. Dose response for the stimulation of cell division by caffeic acid in forestomach and kidney of the male F344 rat. *Fundam. Appl. Toxicol.* **1997**, *39*, 131–137. [CrossRef]
91. Speciale, A.; Chirafisi, J.; Saija, A.; Cimino, F. Nutritional antioxidants and adaptive cell responses: An update. *Curr. Mol. Med.* **2011**, *11*, 770–789. [CrossRef] [PubMed]
92. Birringer, M. Hormetics: Dietary triggers of an adaptive stress response. *Pharm. Res.* **2011**, *28*, 2680–2694. [CrossRef] [PubMed]
93. Murugaiyah, V.; Mattson, M.P. Neurohormetic phytochemicals: An evolutionary-bioenergetic perspective. *Neurochem. Int.* **2015**, *89*, 271–280. [CrossRef] [PubMed]
94. Martel, J.; Ojcius, D.M.; Ko, Y.F.; Ke, P.Y.; Wu, C.Y.; Peng, H.H.; Young, J.D. Hormetic effects of phytochemicals on health and longevity. *Trends Endocrinol. Metab.* **2019**, *30*, 335–346. [CrossRef] [PubMed]
95. Thayer, K.A.; Melnick, R.; Burns, K.; Davis, D.; Huff, J. Fundamental flaws of hormesis for public health decisions. *Env. Health Perspect* **2005**, *113*, 1271–1276. [CrossRef] [PubMed]
96. Marques, F.Z.; Morris, B.J. Commentary on resveratrol and hormesis: Resveratrol—A hormetic marvel in waiting? *Hum. Exp. Toxicol.* **2010**, *29*, 1026–1028. [CrossRef]
97. Agathokleous, E.; Calabrese, E.J. A global environmental health perspective and optimisation of stress. *Sci. Total Env.* **2020**, *704*, 135263. [CrossRef]

Journal of
Clinical Medicine

MDPI

Review

Curcumin's Nanomedicine Formulations for Therapeutic Application in Neurological Diseases

Bahare Salehi [1], Daniela Calina [2,*], Anca Oana Docea [3], Niranjan Koirala [4], Sushant Aryal [4], Domenico Lombardo [5], Luigi Pasqua [6], Yasaman Taheri [7], Carla Marina Salgado Castillo [8], Miquel Martorell [9,10,*], Natália Martins [11,12,*], Marcello Iriti [13], Hafiz Ansar Rasul Suleria [14] and Javad Sharifi-Rad [15,*]

1 Student Research Committee, School of Medicine, Bam University of Medical Sciences, Bam 44340847, Iran; bahar.salehi007@gmail.com
2 Department of Clinical Pharmacy, University of Medicine and Pharmacy of Craiova, 200349 Craiova, Romania
3 Department of Toxicology, University of Medicine and Pharmacy of Craiova, 200349 Craiova, Romania; ancadocea@gmail.com
4 Department of Natural Products Research, Dr. Koirala Research Institute for Biotechnology and Biodiversity, Kathmandu 44600, Nepal; koirala.biochem@gmail.com (N.K.); sushantarl23@gmail.com (S.A.)
5 Italian National Research Council, Rome (CNR), 98158 Messina, Italy; lombardo@ipcf.cnr.it
6 Department of Environmental and Chemical Engineering, University of Calabria, 87036 Rende (CS), Italy; luigi.pasqua@unical.it
7 Phytochemistry Research Center, Shahid Beheshti University of Medical Sciences, Tehran 1991953381, Iran; taaheri.yasaman@gmail.com
8 Facultad de Medicina, Universidad del Azuay, 14-008 Cuenca, Ecuador; csalgado@uazuay.edu.ec
9 Department of Nutrition and Dietetics, Faculty of Pharmacy, University of Concepcion, Concepcion 4070386, Chile
10 Unidad de Desarrollo Tecnológico, Universidad de Concepción UDT, Concepcion 4070386, Chile
11 Faculty of Medicine, University of Porto, Alameda Prof. HernâniMonteiro, 4200-319 Porto, Portugal
12 Institute for Research and Innovation in Health (i3S), University of Porto, 4200-135 Porto, Portugal
13 Department of Agricultural and Environmental Sciences, Milan State University, 20133 Milan, Italy; marcello.iriti@unimi.it
14 Department of Agriculture and Food Systems, The University of Melbourne, Melbourne 3010, Australia; hafiz.suleria@unimelb.edu.au
15 Zabol Medicinal Plants Research Center, Zabol University of Medical Sciences, Zabol 61615-585, Iran
* Correspondence: calinadaniela@gmail.com (D.C.); mmartorell@udec.cl (M.M.); ncmartins@med.up.pt (N.M.); javad.sharifirad@gmail.com (J.S.-R.)

Received: 4 January 2020; Accepted: 3 February 2020; Published: 5 February 2020

Abstract: The brain is the body's control center, so when a disease affects it, the outcomes are devastating. Alzheimer's and Parkinson's disease, and multiple sclerosis are brain diseases that cause a large number of human deaths worldwide. Curcumin has demonstrated beneficial effects on brain health through several mechanisms such as antioxidant, amyloid β-binding, anti-inflammatory, tau inhibition, metal chelation, neurogenesis activity, and synaptogenesis promotion. The therapeutic limitation of curcumin is its bioavailability, and to address this problem, new nanoformulations are being developed. The present review aims to summarize the general bioactivity of curcumin in neurological disorders, how functional molecules are extracted, and the different types of nanoformulations available.

Keywords: curcumin; nanocurcumin; neurological disorders; nanocarriers; liposomes

1. Introduction

Curcumin (CUR), also known as diferuloylmethane, is a turmeric (*Curcuma longa* L. rhizomes)-derived polyphenol, with multiple applications in traditional medicine for more than 2000 years [1,2]. Its use as a food ingredient and industrial dye, in cosmetics and medicinal products formulation, and even to alleviate muscle pain and inflammation and treat various pathological conditions, such as rheumatoid arthritis, gastrointestinal and inflammatory disorders, intermittent fever, renal problems, and leukoderma are amongst to the most commonly reported applications [3]. CUR was described in 1815 by Vogel and Pelletier [4] as a mixture of resin and turmeric oil. Later, in 1842, Vogel Jr. obtained the pure form of curcumin, and 68 years later, Milobedzka and Lampe identified its structure as (1*E*,6*E*)-1,7-bis(4-hydroxy-3-methoxyphenyl)-1,6-heptadiene-3,5-dione [5]. In the past decades, CUR has received a high interest due to its anti-inflammatory, antioxidant and immunomodulatory effects [6], and its benefits in cancer [7], cardiovascular diseases [8,9], diabetes mellitus [10], autoimmune diseases [11,12], and brain or psychiatric conditions [13–15]. Regarding the latter, there is a particular focus on CUR impact in cognition [16], dementia, Alzheimer's disease (AD) [17,18], schizophrenia [14], and depression [19].

Neurological disorders are a significant cause of human deaths worldwide. Based on a World Health Organization (WHO) report in 2015, near 12% of global mortality was caused by neurological disorders. Among them, AD and other dementias represent a high percentage of the total deaths compared to others, consisting of 2.84% percent of mortality in high-income countries in 2005 [20]. Since neurological disorders such as AD mostly affect elderly individuals, the worldwide aging of the population has caused an increase in the human and economic burden. So far, no treatment to cure or reverse AD has been approved, but new studies could change this picture.

Several studies have shown that polyphenols such as CUR can modulate cellular signaling pathways involved in cognitive processes, such as cAMP-response element-binding protein (CREB) signaling and brain-derived neurotrophic factor (BDNF) activation [21,22]. This is crucial for both neurons' development and survivaland for synaptic plasticity. Polyphenols play a beneficial role in maintaining brain health [23]. They are potent antioxidants, and their presence in the diet decreases the markers of oxidative stress, which reduces the risk of neurological diseases [24]. Besides, memory, attention and concentration are enhanced by polyphenols, which may contribute to improved cerebral blood flow [25]. Adding the fact that CUR is inexpensive and has little to no side effects [26], it becomes a strong candidate for a neuroprotective agent.

However, CUR and its metabolites' application is limited due to its weak absorption, rapid metabolism, rapid systemic elimination, limited blood-brain barrier (BBB) permeability and, the most challenging factor, a low water solubility (0.4 μg/mL at normal gastric pH: 1.5–4) [27,28]. Many different formulations have been developed to resolve these issues [29,30]. In general, these innovative mechanisms improve CUR's bioavailability by increasing its chemical stability and solubility, better permeability, and tissue distribution [31,32]. Despite the challenges that need to be answered, CUR possesses numerous advantages such as excellent biological and pharmacological activity, extensive clinical trials, and low side effects that can lead to CUR formulations becoming medicine. This has inspired scientists to develop CUR nanomedicine formulations for better bioavailability, efficacy, and therapeutic index.

As might be expected, specific differences in these novel formulations can influence their efficacy, explaining why most of the clinical trials show conflicting results regarding the beneficial effects of CUR in brain diseases, especially when it comes to the treatment of AD [33]. For this reason, we must understand how existing CUR nanomedicine formulations act, including their particular benefits and disadvantages in AD and other brain conditions. This literature review aims to summarize the general bioactivity of CUR in neurological disorders, how functional molecules are extracted, and the different nanoformulation types available.

2. Chemical Properties of Curcumin

Chemically, CUR has two ferulic acid moieties connected by an additional carbon to shorten the carboxyl groups. It has seven carbon linkers and three major functional groups: an aromatic methoxy phenolic group; α,β-unsaturated β-diketo linker and keto-enol tautomerism [34]. CUR exists in tautomeric keto and enol conformations in equilibrium due to the intramolecular hydrogen atoms transfer at the β-diketone chain (Figure 1). The relative concentrations of keto-enol tautomers may vary depending on the temperature, pH, solvent polarity, and aromatic ring substitution [35]. In neutral and acidic aqueous solutions (from pH 3 to 7), the keto form dominates CUR, which is capable of transferring H-atom's crucial for antioxidant activity. However, under alkaline conditions (≥pH 8), the enolic form predominates, and the phenolic part of the molecule is a major contributor for antioxidant activity through electron donation [36]. CUR's aromatic groups provide hydrophobicity of compound, resulting in poor water solubility [37]. Typical CUR composition of commercial varieties is the combination of CUR (~77%), desmethoxycurcumin (~17%) and bisdemethoxycurcumin (~3%) known as curcuminoids [38].

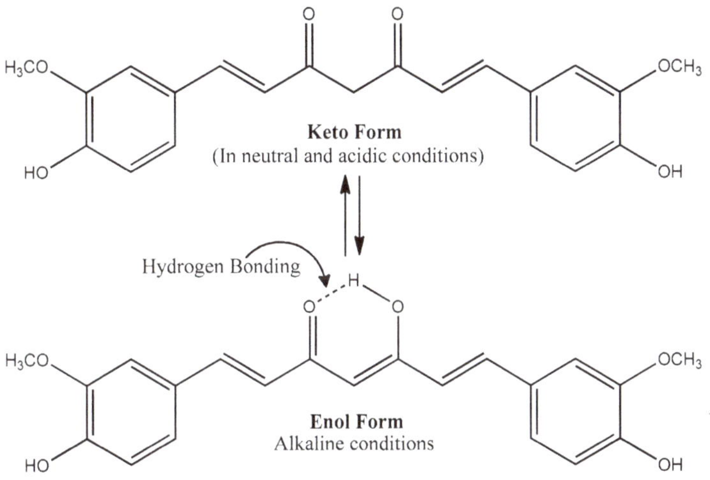

Figure 1. Chemical structure of curcumin and equilibrium between keto and enol tautomerism.

3. Curcumin and Neurological Disorders

CUR has shown promising therapeutic potential in the management of biliary disorders, LDL oxidation, blood cholesterol, anorexia, cough, diabetic wounds, thrombosis, hepatic disorders, rheumatism, sinusitis, inflammations and wounds [39]. Over the past half-decade, CUR has gained attention as a key molecule in neurological disorders, being tested both for its effectiveness and safety. Numerous preclinical studies have suggested its use in treating disorders such as AD [40,41], Parkinson disease (PD) [42,43], multiple sclerosis (MS) [44,45], migraine [46,47], epilepsy [48,49], stroke [50,51], traumatic brain injury [52,53], and spinal cord injury [54]. Various studies indicate that the antioxidant, anti-inflammatory, anti-amyloidogenic, antidepressant, antidiabetic, and antiaging properties of CUR are responsible for the neuroprotective effects as in Figure 2 [55–57].

At the molecular level, CUR reduces the reactive oxygen species (ROS) and advanced glycation products generation and accumulation, by down-regulating the nicotinamide adenine dinucleotide phosphate oxidaseexpression [58]. Moreover, CUR also inhibits the activation of glial cells, reduces the nuclear factor kappa B (NF-κB) activity and decrease the activity of proinflammatory interleukin (IL)-1β; IL-6, and IL-8 and cytokines (tumor necrosis factor-α (TNF-α)) in the neuronal system [44]. Furthermore, CUR attributes in metalloproteinase-9, inducible nitric oxide synthase (iNOS), cyclooxygenase-2

(COX-2), and 5-lipoxygenase (5-LOX) downregulation, where proteins related to antioxidant defense (hemeoxygenase-1 (HO-1) and heat shock proteins are upregulated to prevent the neuronal disorder [59,60].

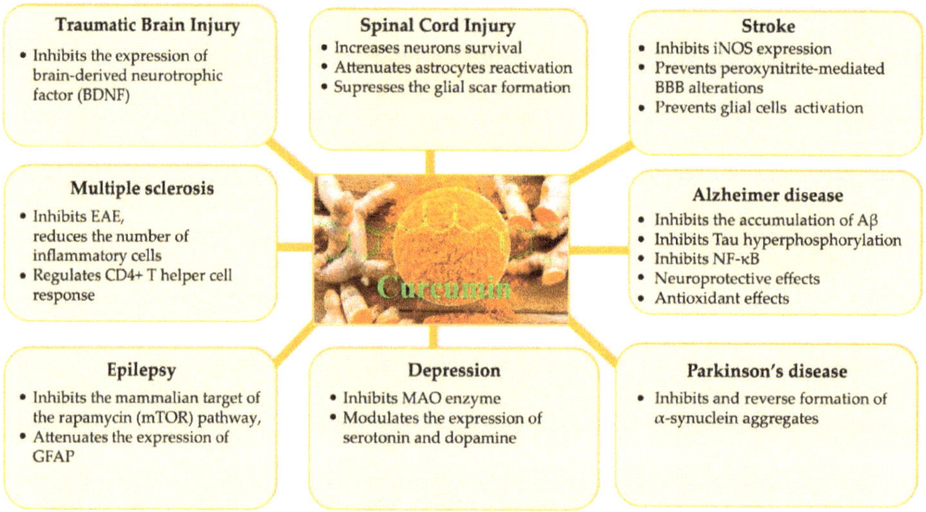

Figure 2. Potential mechanisms and applications of curcumin in neurological and psychiatric disorders [40–43,48–51,55–57]. Legend: experimental allergic encephalomyelitis (EAE), Glial fibrillary acidic protein (GFAP), inducible nitric oxide synthase (iNOS), Blood Brain Barrier (BBB).

3.1. Curcumin in Alzheimer's Disease

AD is a pathological condition determined by neurofibrillary tangle (NFT) and senile plaque (SP) aggregation, severe neuroinflammation, synaptic, and neuronal loss [61]. The loss of neurons and synapses determine atrophy of the cerebral cortex, mainly in the temporal, parietal and frontal lobe. An important pathogenic event in the development of AD is the sequential proteolysis of the transmembrane amyloid-β precursor protein (AβPP) by β-APP cleaving enzyme 1 (BACE1) and γ–secretase in Aβ peptides and its aggregation around the cells. β-amyloid peptides (Aβ) deposition is the first event that triggers NFT formation, cell death, and finally, dementia [62]. Besides Aβ plaques, the other evidence for AD is the hyper-phosphorylation tau that induces disruption of microtubules and intracellular transport. However, most of the evidence suggests that inhibition of Aβ accumulation is an ideal target for pharmacotherapy [63].

Despite the remarkable advances in the knowledge of AD pathogenesis, the typical selective neurodegeneration of the AD brains is not fully understood. Due to the lack of an early diagnosis before the onset of symptoms, approved effective disease-modifying treatments are not currently available. However, there are few clinical treatments that slow down disease progression and control symptoms [64]. Based on the old cholinergic hypothesis for the etiology AD, acetylcholinesterase (AChE) inhibitors were used to maintain the level of acetylcholine and reverse the symptoms of short-term memory loss and confusion caused by a loss in cholinergic neurons. However, none of these drugs is curative, acting mainly through reducing the degeneration of cholinergic neurons and the progression of the disease [62]. The current research focuses on the development of novel treatment, which helps to restore the degenerated neurons. CUR is a natural product extensively used in India. Indian epidemiological studies showed that the incidence of AD in this country is the lowest worldwide. The relationship between CUR consumption in India and lower AD prevalence is the basic to investigate the protective mechanisms of CUR in AD [65,66]. Multiple molecular mechanisms (Figure 3) have been scientifically verified, where CUR appears as an upcoming therapeutic candidate for AD prevention, treatment, and diagnosis [40].

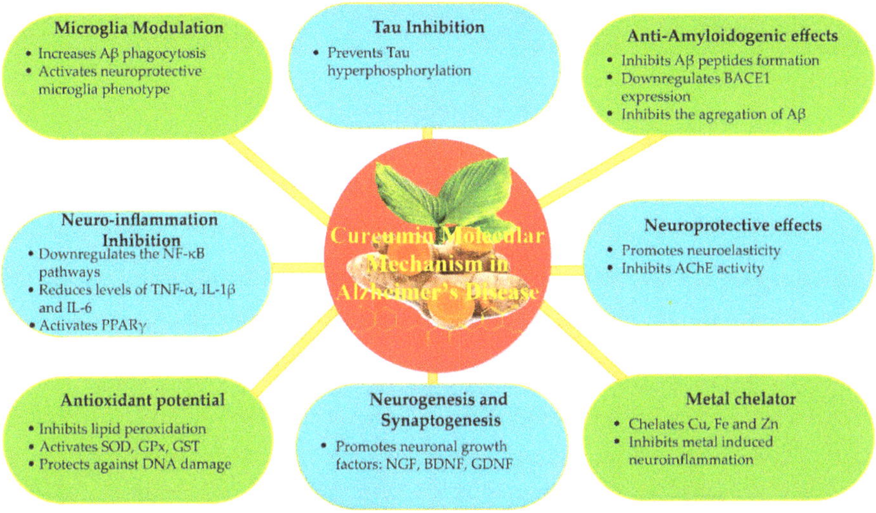

Figure 3. Multiple molecular mechanisms of curcumin to ameliorate Alzheimer's disease [40,62,65,66]. Legend: β-secretase 1 (BACE1), nuclear factor κ B (NF-κB), tumour necrosis factor α (TNF α), Interleukin I beta (IL-1β), Interleukin 6 (IL-6), Peroxisome proliferator-activated receptor γ (PPAR-γ), superoxide dismutase (SOD), glutathione peroxidase (GPx), glutathione (GSH), nerve growth factor (NGF), brain-derived neurotrophic factor (BDNF), glial cell-derived neurotrophic factor (GDNF), acetylcholine esterase (AChE).

3.1.1. Aβ Peptides Inhibition

Evidence suggests that Aβ plaques formation and accumulation is prevented by CUR. CUR's enol forms, which stain the amyloid plaques and neurofibrillary tangles (NFTs)in the brain demonstrate its binding to Aβ fibrils [67]. Zhang et al. [68] have developed aCUR fluorescence analogs with binding affinity to aggregated β-amyloid (CRANAND-2) or solubleβ-amyloid (CRANAND-58). These molecules have been increasingly detected in AD transgenic mice before plaques can be observed.

Multiple literature records have demonstrated that CUR inhibits the formation of Aβ peptides. Intragastric CUR administration to an AD mice model reduced Aβ formation by downregulating BACE1 expression, the enzyme that cleaves AβPP to Aβ [69]. Another enzymatic target for Aβ production is γ-secretase, the catalytic component of presenilin-1 (PS-1) and glycogensynthase kinase-3β (GSK-3β), which decreased when human neuroblastoma SHSY5Y cells were treated with CUR, suggesting that CUR decreased Aβ production by inhibiting GSK 3β-dependent PS-1 activation [70].

In addition to inhibiting Aβ production, CUR also inhibits the aggregation of fibrillar Aβ in vivo and in vitro and promotes disaggregation. Reinke and Gestwicki [71] examined the presence of hydrophobicity, keto or enol rings, two phenyl groups and polar hydroxyl groups on the two aromatic rings of CUR for inhibition of amyloid aggregation. The two polar hydroxyl groups present at both extremes, capable of taking part in hydrogen bonding with polar pockets of the Aβ peptide are crucial for destabilizing β-sheets and disintegratingAβ dimers.

The neuroprotective effects of CUR are not only limited in preventing the formation of Aβ fibril and its aggregations, but it also prohibits Aβ-mediated neurotoxicity. The in vitro study on human neuroblastoma SHSY5Y cells showed that CUR attenuates Aβ-membrane interactions, Aβ-induced membrane disruption, prevent intracellular calcium elevation and shift the Aβ aggregation pathway to the formation of nontoxic soluble oligomers and prefibrillar aggregates which stills requires in vivo study [72].

3.1.2. Tau Inhibition

The risk of developing Alzheimer's disease increases with age. Alzheimer's disease usually begins with memory decline and later affects other cognitive abilities. Two different types of protein deposits are involved in the brain, namely "amyloid-beta plaques" and "Tau neurofibrillary tangles" [73].

The appearance of your neurofibrillary tangles reflects the progression of the disease, they first manifest in the memory centers of the brain and then appear in other areas as the disease progresses. Tau proteins (or Tau aggregates) migrate along nerve fibers and thus contribute to the spread of the disease throughout the brain [74]. If proteins spread more quickly in the aging brain, this might explain why most people with Alzheimer's disease are older [75].

The aggregation of hyperphosphorylated tau is crucial for AD pathogenesis and scientific studies have shown that CUR prevents tau hyperphosphorylation into NFTs [76]. The tau protein is phosphorylated after by phosphatase and tensin homolog (PTEN)/protein kinase B (Akt)/GSK-3β pathway induced by the GSK-3β enzyme, Aβ peptides which are inhibited by CUR to alleviate tau-induced neurotoxicity [77].

3.1.3. Microglia Modulation and Neuro-Inflammation Inhibition

Decades of research have linked neuropathy with neuroinflammatory phenomena that can be provoked by microvascular damage, atherosclerosis, Aβ accumulation, age-related inflammatory factors and bacterial or viral infections that affect the BBB [78]. Any neurological damage/disorder can lead to microglial activation, followed by phenotypic proliferation and change [79]. In this process, Aβ diverts microglia from its neuroprotective phenotype to its neurotoxic phenotype. The neurotoxic phenotype express iNOS and major histocompatibility complex (MHC) II, activating the NF-κB pathway to produce several pro-inflammatory cytokines, such as TNF-α, IL-1β, IL-6, IL-12 and IL-23, and generate ROS and NO, which subsequently induce immune stimulation, neuroinflammation, the block of axonal remodeling and prevent neurogenesis. However, neuro- protective phenotypes mediate neuroprotection by Aβ phagocytosis and clearance, neuronal regeneration modulation, and arginase 1 (Arg1) release for tissue remodeling, wound healing and debris clearance [80].

Indeed, CUR has been proposed as a potent anti-inflammatory agent, able to reduce many neuroinflammatory mediators and modulate the activation of microglial. In an in vitro study in Aβ-activated microglia, CUR improved microglial viability and suppressed the activation and blocked extracellular signal-regulated kinase 2 (ERK1/2) and p38 kinase signaling, reducing TNF-α, IL-1β, and IL-6, mRNA and protein levels production [81]. In addition, and despite the CUR stimulatory activity on anti-inflammatory cytokines production (i.e., IL-4 and IL-10), namely in lipopolysaccharide (LPS)-activated microglia, it also has the ability to upregulates the expression of suppressors of cytokine signalling (SOCS-1), whereas reducing the phosphorylation of Janus Kinase 2 (JAK2) and Signal Transducer and Activator of Transcription-3 (STAT3). Thus, by preventing microglial inflammatory responses and inhibiting the plaque accumulation, the neuroprotective potential of CUR is enhanced, besides its direct effect on neuroinflammatory reactions by eliciting anti-inflammatory responses in microglia through JAK/STAT/SOCS signalling pathway modulation [82].

Liu et al. [83] demonstrated the ability of CUR to activate the peroxisome proliferator-activated receptor-γ (PPARγ) and amplify the PPARγ protein, which downregulates the NF-κB pathways. In addition, CUR reduced microglia and astrocytes activation, and cytokine production responsible for neuroinflammation. Besides this, when the isolated microglia of AD patients were treated with curcuminoids, Aβ phagocytosis by microglia raised by 50% compared to the control group suggesting activation of neuroprotective microglia phenotype [84]. Thus, preventing microglial inflammatory response, and inhibiting the plaque accumulation, CUR enhancement of neuroprotective.

3.1.4. Antioxidant Potential

In general, neuronal inflammation is a protective response for numerous cellular and tissue injury [85]. It represents a complex of local and general reactions of the body, which includes alternative phenomena, changes in vascular dynamics, proliferative events and finally, reparative phenomena [86]. But when the inflammation is uncontrolled, the effect initiates an excessive injury of cells and tissues, causing the destruction of healthy tissues and the occurrence of chronic inflammation. Inflammatory brain diseases, including Alzheimer's disease and Parkinson's disease, are characterized by an imbalance of redox status but also by chronic inflammation, the primary cause of injury, and cell death [87]. Reactive oxygen species (ROS) are recognized as key mediators of cell survival, proliferation, differentiation, but also apoptosis [88]. Excessive production of ROS (also known as oxidative stress) by mitochondria and NADPH oxidase is recognized as responsible for tissue injury associated with brain damage, inflammatory processes and neurodegenerative diseases, such as Alzheimer's disease [89].

Many of the well-known inflammatory proteins, including matrix metalloproteinases-9 (MMP-9), cytosolic phospholipase A2 (cPLA2), cyclooxygenase 2 (COX-2), inducible nitric oxide synthase (iNOS), and adhesion molecules, are associated with oxidative stress (ROS generation) induced by proinflammatory factors (cytokines, peptides, infectious factors, peroxides). (Figure 4) Nerve cells, especially neurons, are susceptible to the adverse effects of oxidative stress. Numerous studies have concluded, the release of various inflammatory mediators by astrocytes and microglia, in response to oxidative stress [90].

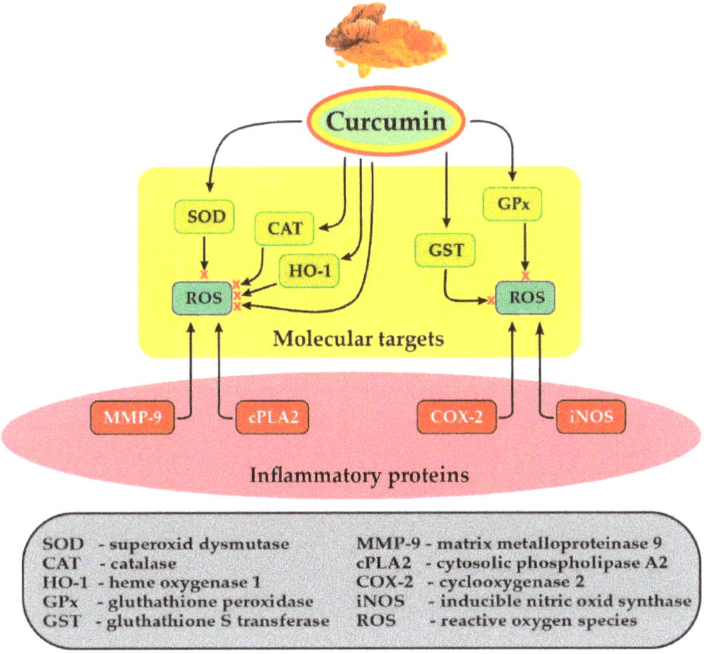

Figure 4. The molecular targets, anti-inflammatory and antioxidant mechanisms of Curcumin on the cells of the nervous tissue.

Due to the demanding metabolic rate, increased oxygen demand, lower enzymatic defense against free radicals, and composed of easily oxidized lipids, the brain is particularly vulnerable to oxidative damages. The imbalance in the redox state with ROS accumulation or a decrease in antioxidant defense is linked to the development and progression of neurodegenerative diseases [91]. In AD, an excess of ROS may be produced by mitochondrial dysfunction, aggregation of Aβ proteins, phosphorylation and polymerization of tau and/or anomalous buildup of transition metals fostering the progression of the disease [92].

CUR has shown potent antioxidant activity either by scavenging the free radicals or upregulating cytoprotective mediators. Inhibited of lipid peroxidation or reduction of ferric ions, CUR has displayed comparable antioxidant activity with standard antioxidants [93]. Moreover, CUR can also scavenge superoxide anions (O_2^-) and hydroxyl radicals (OH^-), and upregulate the expression of genes encoding for antioxidant proteins, such as catalase (CAT), heme oxygenase-1 (HO-1) and superoxide dismutase (SOD) [94,95]. In the brain, CUR can stabilize antioxidant enzymes, including SOD, glutathione peroxidase (GPx), glutathione S-transferase (GST) and protect for radical-induced DNA damages in neuronal cells [96,97].

3.1.5. Neurogenesis and Synaptogenesis Promotion

The human brain is an organ capable of amazing activity in terms of its organization as a result of learning and experience [98]. This extraordinary property called neuroplasticity manifests itself in three main hypostases: during human development from the newborn stage to old age, during learning and during recovery after a neurological injury or disease at the sensory, motor or cognitive level [99].

There are several mechanisms of neuroplasticity, including Hebb's law, synaptic plasticity, synaptogenesis, axonal growth and regeneration, growth factors, neurogenesis [100]. Synaptogenesis is a phenomenon by which neurons send new extensions that, by meeting the extensions of other neurons, form new synapses. Synaptogenesis begins *in utero* and continues after birth. It is carried out sequentially and has been followed especially at the level of neuromuscular junctions [101].

In the vicinity of a striated muscle fiber, the emergence cone (growth) of the axon begins to flatten and adhere to its surface, without any specialization being observed at the level of the two cell membranes. In an immediate next step, synaptic vesicles appear in the axonal end, and on the surface of the muscle fiber–acetylcholine receptors, distributed diffusely.

The accumulation of receptors in the area of the future postsynapse occurs under the influence of agrin, secreted by the neuron and fibroblast growth factor (FGF-β) from the extracellular environment; other molecules secreted by the neuron stimulate the activity of acetylcholine receptor-encoding genes in the juxtasynaptic nuclei [102].

The onset of synaptic activity, by generating action potential, inhibits gene activity for the same receptors in extrasynaptic nuclei. Later, there is a concentration of calcium channels in the presynaptic area, determining its intracellular growth, with a role in the organization of the cytoskeleton. Contact with the target is essential in synaptogenesis [103].

Multiple literature reports indicate the potential risk of synaptic damage and neuronal death due to declining neuronal growth factors and supporting factors, such as platelet-derived growth factor PDGF [104]. The in vivo study on animal models showed that the CUR-containing diet increases the level of neurotrophic factors and promotes neurogenesis, synaptogenesis, and improved memory functions [105]. Specifically addressing the effects of CUR on neural cells, it has revealed to have a great potential to limit histone acetylase activity and to promote neurogenesis, thus exerting a high impact on longevity and slowing down aging [106].

3.1.6. Metal Chelation

In addition to tau and Aβ, an imbalance in metal homeostasis can induce misfolded protein aggregation and promote neurological diseases such as AD. Studies have suggested that metal ions stimulate the processing of AβPP, BACE1, and mRNA and promote the misfolding of Aβ oligomers [107]. Chemically, CUR is an excellent metal chelating ligand due to the presence of OH groups and one CH_2 group [108]. CUR effectively chelate copper (Cu), iron (Fe), and zinc (Zn), making them unavailable to induce Aβ aggregation. Furthermore, CUR reduces expression of NF-κB levels induced by heavy metals in the neuroinflammation process [109].

4. Nanoformulation: Molecules, Extraction Techniques and Alzheimer's, and Brain Diseases Effects

Initially, for CUR extraction from turmeric dried roots, a liquid-solid extraction procedure needs to be used [110]. By vacuum filtration or by gravity, the insoluble material is separated from the soluble one (CUR), which is extracted into the solvent. The solution obtained can be used in its liquid form, or instead, the solvent can be evaporated to recover the extracted material in crystalline powder [110].

In a study reported by Mandal et al. [111], a better method of extraction was discovered using the extraction process with ultrasound. The researchers found that ultrasound utilization in CUR extraction was much faster, just 70 min, compared to the liquid-liquid extraction process that required many hours. In addition, this method allows for obtaining a larger amount of CUR from the turmeric root. This study highlighted that this is a method who can be used in an effective way to reduce long botanical extraction times to a few minutes, non-thermic, without using heat [111].

Thus, the shorter and better extraction methods of CUR open new windows in the research of the phytotherapeutic actions of CUR such as: cholagogue action (stimulates bile release), anticancer, inhibition of the development of cancerous tumors and metastases (breast, stomach, colon, lung, liver, skin) [112–115], anti-inflammatory action, hepatoprotective inclusive in non-alcoholic fatty liver disease [116], antiatherosclerotic, antiplatelet effects but not in cases of vitamin K coagulopathies [117], prevents AD and other neurodegenerative disorders [118,119].

However optimal therapeutic results cannot be achieved due to its poor solubility, low gastrointestinal absorption with a reduced bioavailability [120]. An important objective for the researchers was to increase the bioavailability of CUR, especially its polyphenols with a low absorption rate and an increased liver metabolism rate. This low absorption is correlated with the size of the polyphenols, as they cannot penetrate through the intestinal barrier, and with their low solubility in both water and lipids [121].

It was observed an increased affinity of CUR polyphenols for phospholipids that are both hydrophobic and hydrophilic and act as emulsifying agents, increasing bioavailability and consequently, the researchers decided to associate the two types of substances [122]. Because the most abundant phospholipid in the human tissues is phosphatidylcholine, it was chosen to use it, with the role of improving both the absorption of polyphenols in the intestine and their penetration into the cell [123,124], so the CUR phytosomes were obtained, as a special CUR formulation with a curcuminoid bioavailability of up to 29 times higher compared to the simple form of CUR [124].

The challenges of increasing CUR bioavailability have continued and culminated with the development of nanoparticles. In recent years, with the development of nanotechnologies [125], nanoformulations have made it possible to develop nano curcumins (CUR encapsulated nanoparticles). Different types of CUR nanocarriers such as liposomes, solid-lipid nanoparticles, micelles, polymer nanoparticles, and polymeric conjugates have been developed to the treatment of different disorders, among them neurodegenerative disorders.

Nanocurcumin is the result of compression of the bulky CUR molecule at less than 100 nm with higher bioavailability properties. A lot of new technological methods have been developed to design nanoparticles with CUR who have an increased bioavailability [126]. The CUR nanoparticles are effective ways of administering of some drugs due to their increased bioavailability and superior cellular absorption characteristics. Nanocurcumin can also be obtained only from filtered CUR without using the nanocarrier conjugates. CURdissolution can be achieved with ethanol and then homogenized under high pressure with water containing 0.1% citric acid [127].

Cyclodextrin-CUR inclusion complexes are composed of cyclic oligosaccharides formed from a variable number of glycopolymeric monomer units, which varies between six to eight units. These contain a lipophilic central cavity and a hydrophilic external layer [128]. Of the three different types of cyclodextrins (α, β, γ), β-cyclodextrins have been widely used, since they are easily accessible and cost-effective, improve stability, reduce bitterness, improve water solubility and bioavailability. Using solvent evaporation or pH change technologies, CUR is conjugated with β-cyclodextrins in order to obtain inclusion complexes for increasing the CUR absorption [128].

Microspheres andmicrocapsules with encapsulated CUR or dispersed in polymeric particles (camptothecin, routine, zedoaric oil) form microscopic spheres/capsules that significantly increase bioavailability and pharmacological efficacyin the target organs, especially the brain [129]. The microcapsules were formulated with a layer and the CUR was incorporated into hollow microcapsules with polyetheresis of the ectrolytic multilayer. Studies highlighted that microcapsules andmicrospheres had demonstrated a remarkable increase in CUR's stability and bioactivity [129].

Liposomal CUR (liposomes) are closed round particles, phospholipids, with CUR included into an aqueous interior, widely used as nanocarriers to increase CUR absorption and efficacy [130,131]. Strong migraine headaches experimentally induced in mice were successfully treated by the combination of sumatriptan with intravenous liposomal CUR at doses of 2 mg per 100 g body weight [47]. Recently, several changes in polymeric conjugate liposome CUR have developed to achieve better clinical outcomes in AD [132].

The CUR polymeric micelles represent another nanocarrier of CUR that significantly increases its low solubility, poorbioavailability and stability characteristics [133]. In a recent study, CUR was encapsulated in cationic micelles such as dodecyl trimethyl ammonium bromide or cetyltrimethyl-ammonium bromide with increased CUR loading capacity, increased solubility, reduced toxicity and decreased metabolic degradation [133].

CUR microemulsions are small drop dispersions (1–100 μM size) of isotropic oil and water mixtures stabilized using the interfacial films of the surfactant molecules [134]. These microemulsion systems are the pharmaceutical forms used for the administration of hydrophobic drugs. Advantages of lipid CUR microemulsion include improved CUR dissolution, thermodynamic stability and superior solubility. Tween-20 as emulsifier and triacylglycerol were used to formulate the microemulsion droplets under rapid and high-pressure homogenization procedures [134].

Solid dispersion with CUR involves dispersing it in a non-pharmacological solid nanocarrier or matrix using the solvent melting technological process [135]. Recently more nanoformulations have been designed to obtain crystalline and amorphous solid dispersions that have been shown to remarkably enhance CUR physicochemical and pharmacokinetic activities [135,136]. These include wet melting and freeze-drying.

The CUR nanogels made up of three-dimensional hydrophilic polymer networks that can absorb large amounts of water or physiological fluids internally while maintaining the internal structure of the network [137]. These nanogels are an effective CUR release formulation, high dispersibility stability, CUR release efficiency, and rapid release.without histopathological changes of nasal mucosae. CUR has the great advantage of being easily encapsulated inside of a nanogel [137].

CUR solid lipid nanoparticles (SLNs) are composed of natural lipids such as lecithins or triglycerides that remain solid at normal temperature (37 °C). Theseprotects labile compounds from chemical degradation and can improve the bioavailability of CUR with increased cellular absorption [138].

CUR polymer nanoparticles have nanometric dimensions, are highly biocompatible and circulate slightly in the blood for a more extended period of time. Some of the widely used synthetic polymeric conjugates include chitosan (CS); poly(lactic-co-glycolic acid) (PLGA) [139], polyethyleneglycol (PEG) [140] and hydrophobically modified starch. PLGA with PEG-5000 carrier stabilizer was used to design CUR nanoparticles with an efficiency of 97.5%, 81 nm diameter. Experimental studies have shown that PLGA loaded CUR nanoparticles have higher cellular absorption andincreased bioavailability [139] and easily crossing the hematoencephalic barrier with brain release of CUR with a beneficial effect in neurological diseases [141].

More recently, CUR-encapsulated exosomes have been the target of increasing attention, as they have shown to be of great interest, namely on neural therapy, besides to have a high bioavailability and safety, have ability to stimulate the immune system, and able to reach high concentrations in blood [142]. Recent experimental studies on rats have highlighted the efficacy of curcumin treatment encapsulated in exosomes, vesicles with tiny membranes in Alzheimer's disease [142]. Curcumin encapsulated in exosomes crosses the BBB and reaches the neuronal tissue where it inhibits the hyperphosphorylation of Tau proteins, thus reducing the symptoms of Alzheimer's disease. This mechanism is explained by the activation of the AKT/GSK-3β pathway [143].

Magnetic CUR nanoparticles can be used in neurodegenerative disorders under the influence of external magnetic fields [144]. CURinclusion into Fe_3O_4-CUR conjugate with oleic acid or CS on the outside results in the formation of water-dispersible fluorescence magnetic nanoparticles with increasing cellular absorption andincreased bioavailability [144]. All these nanoformulations which have the main purpose increasing of CUR's bioavailability have beenused as alternative therapies in neurodegenerative diseases such as AD [145], PD and MS [30].

4.1. Alzheimer's disease

Unfortunately, no really effective treatment is still available for AD. Therefore, prevention is first of all the most important. CUR, formulated as nanoparticles, can cross the BBB and act on brain cells, being active against various neurological diseases [146,147].The mechanisms of action of CUR in AD (Figure 5) have been proven by many studies [62].

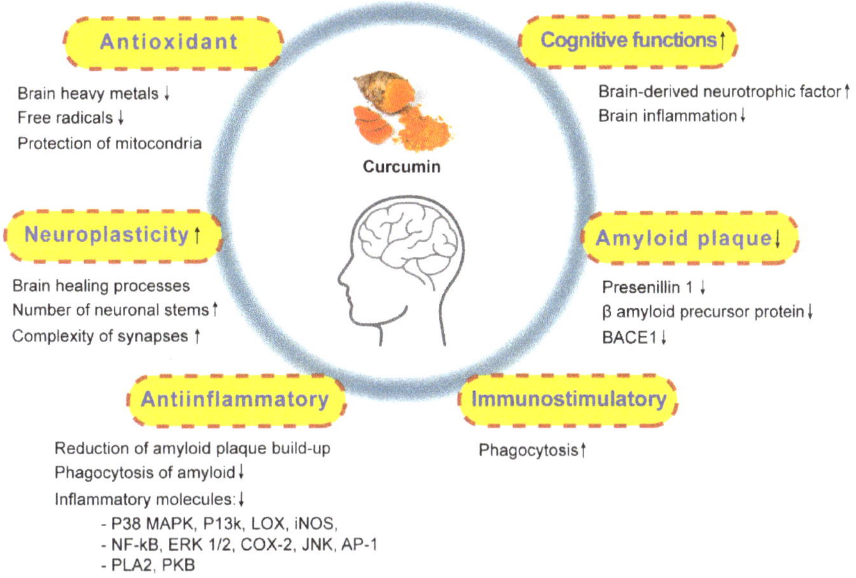

Figure 5. The mechanism of action of curcumin nanoformulations in Alzheimer's disease [142,143,146,147]. Legend: p38 mitogen-activated protein kinase (p38 MAPK), phosphatidylinositide 3-kinase (PI3K), 5-lipoxygenase (5-LOX), inducible nitric oxide synthase (iNOS), Tumor necrosis factor-alpha (TNF-α), nuclear factor-κB (NF-kB), extracellular signal-regulated kinase 1/2 (ERK1/2), cyclooxygenase 2 (COX-2), c-Jun N-terminal kinase (JNK), activator protein-1 (AP-1), phospholipase A_2 (PLA_2), protein kinase B (PKB, also named Akt), β site amyloid precursor protein cleaving enzyme 1 (β-secretase 1, BACE1).

4.1.1. The Prevention of Amyloid Plaque Accumulation

The active substance in turmeric, CUR, blocks β-amyloid plaques formation throughdifferentways [84,148]. On the one hand, CUR blocks PS-1 which contributes to plaque formation and, on the other hand, it reduces the accumulation of amyloid formations [70]. Due to their ability to reduce BACE1, there is the possibility of developing a CUR treatment for AD [149].

Bukhari et al. [150] have shown that CUR derivatives inhibit protein accumulation in the dementia-affected brain, thus reducing their neurotoxicity. A recent study demonstrated a significant decrease in amyloid plaque because free CURcan cross the BBB and attaches to neurotoxic proteins, preventing them from sticking together and forming amyloid plaques between neurons [151].

4.1.2. Antioxidant Mechanism of Curcumin in Alzheimer's

With physiologic aging, the brain accumulates metal ions (Fe, Zn and Cu) and inflammation and accumulation of amyloid plaques are triggered. It has been found that CUR derivatives inhibit the accumulation of heavy metals in AD [152]. A study conducted by Fan et al. [153] analyzed the role of different antioxidants in foods, including CUR, in AD. The result showed that due to its chelating action, CUR prevents the accumulation of heavy metals in the brain.

4.1.3. Neuroplasticity Stimulation by Curcumin Nanoparticles

The brain has a fantastic recovery capacity, called neuroplasticity [154]. CUR nanoparticles have shown that this therapy induces a regeneration process of neurons. Fan et al. demonstrated in an experimental study on mice that CUR reduces the dysfunction of neuronal plasticity structures inducedviaIL-1β/NF-κBpathway [155]. A study by Hucklenbroich et al. [156] revealed that a turmeric compound, aromatic-turmerone, can be a promising aid in regenerating neurons. It was also shown that when neuronsare exposed to aromatic-turmerone, neural stem cells grow in both number and complexity, characteristic of the healing process. This effect was seen also in vivo on a rat model that, after exposure to aromatic-turmerone, increased their stem cell production and generated healthy new brain cells [156].

4.1.4. Reducing Neuroinflammation

In AD, neuroinflammation is associated with exposure to toxic agents, infections, or amyloid plaque formation [157]. An experimental study performed by Yang et al. [158] on transgenic mice showed that CUR may bind to amyloid plaques when injected through the carotid artery.CUR caninhibit many molecules (Figure 4) involved in inflammation [159] and can cross the BBBthus reducing neuroinflammation [158]. CUR reduces inflammation from AD and prevents the formation of amyloid plaques. It also acts on the kappa-B factor, a macro protein involved in the regulation of inflammation [160] and translocation produced by IL-1β and subsequent expression of NF-κB determined by pro-inflammatory genes [161].

4.1.5. Curcumin Supports Cognitive Function and Memory

CUR protects nerve cells and increases memory skills and learning [105]. The mechanism is provided by a study of Xu et al. [162] on a rat model, according to which CUR increases the level of BDNF, a protein that supports the activity of neurons. A placebo-controlled trial conducted by Rainey-Smith et al. [163] analyzed the effect of a CUR supplement on a group of elderly people over a period of one year. Cognitive decline was found in different stages in the placebo group, but not among those who received CUR [163]. Another study conducted by Small et al. [164] showed that CUR can improve mood and memory in the case of patients with mild loss of memory related to age.

CUR is easily absorbed in people who have memory problems without dementia, emphasizing good results on microscopic plaques and nodules in the brain in patients diagnosed with AD [164].

It is not known exactly how the effects of CUR are produced, but it may be due to its possibility to decrease brain inflammation that has been correlated to AD and major depression. These actions were demonstrated in a double-blind, placebo-controlled study that included 40 volunteer patients aged 50–90 years with mild memory problems. Subjects were randomly assigned to the placebo or group treated with 90 milligrams of CUR twice a day for 18 months. 40 subjects were evaluated using standardized cognitive tests at the start of the study, and after 6-month intervals. Blood CUR concentration was controlled at the start of the study and after 18 months [164]. The results show that those who took CUR have significantly improved their memory and attention, while subjects receiving placebo did not show any improvement. In memory tests, people who took CUR improved 28% in the 18 months and increased their mood.On the other hand, their brain scans showed fewer signs of amyloid and your tonsillitis and hypothalamus than those who took a placebo. Only four people who took CUR and two of those taking placebo experienced mild side effects (abdominal pain and nausea) [164].

4.1.6. Immunostimulatory Effect

AD is also characterized by dysfunction of the immune system [165]. In the normal brain, the innate immune system is supported by astrocytes and microglial cells that clean the amyloid plaques, but this is not the case also for AD [166]. A study led by Teter et al. [167] demonstrated in mice that natural CUR derivatives restore immune function and stimulate immune cells to eliminate amyloid plaques by phagocytosis (a process by which phagocytes swallow damaged cells and other residues). In another experimental study, researchers isolated immune cells from Alzheimer's patients and treated them with curcuminoids. The ability of these cells to remove amyloid particles has increased due to CUR [168]. The results suggest that curcuminoid therapy could be applied as immunotherapy in AD.

4.2. Parkinson's Disease

The difficulty of movement is one of the main PD-associated symptoms. α-Synuclein protein leads to rigidity in locomotion [169]. It is demonstrated that the simple administration of CUR can bring a significant improvement in walking in PD patients. A recent study demonstrated that CUR manages to attenuate PD-related deficits by increasing the level of antioxidant enzymes. By reducing oxidative stress, CUR slows the loss of motor function and increases the life span [169]. Kundu et al. [170] have demonstrated on a rat model of PD that nanocarriers with CUR and piperine in the form of nanoparticles formulated with glyceryl monooleate improve their penetration into the brain by crossing the BBB. Increasing the bioavailability of CUR released from nanoparticles has reduced the synuclein fibrils by reducing their aggregation, thus decreasing dopaminergic neuronal degeneration and improving motor coordination [170].

4.3. Multiple Sclerosis (MS)

MS is a chronic autoimmune disease that affects the brain, spinal cord, and optic nerves and it is caused by demyelination of myelin plaques and inflammatory infiltrations in brain [171]. The main symptoms observed are loss of vision or double vision, loss of balance, stiffness, tiredness, difficulty in speaking and/or swallowing, intellectual deficits, changes in emotional states [171]. Unfortunately, there is no complete treatment for MS but CUR can be a good alternative therapy to relieve these symptoms, according to in vivo study conducted by Natarajan and Bright [172]. These researchers used an animal model of MS, represented by experimental allergic encephalomyelitis (EAE) autoimmune produced by injection of myelin in mice. To these EAE mice were administered parenterally 50–100 micrograms of CUR three times a week for one month. CUR-treated mice showed very few MS symptoms; and mice that did not receive CUR were paralyzed by the disease within 15 days. At the study end, CUR-treated mice (100 μg) exhibited imperceptible symptoms of the disease [172]. This effect is explained by the inhibition of IL-12, one of the main causes of myelin plaque damage [172].

In a recent experimental study on Lewis rats with induced EAE it was demonstrated that polymerized nanoparticles with CUR administered in doses of 12.5 mg/kg favor the remyelination process of neurons by repairing of myelin sheaths and reduces neuroinflammation by inhibiting the following pro-inflammatory genes: NF-ββ, IL-17, IL-1, TNF-α, and monocyte chemoattractant protein-1 (MCP-1) [173].

5. Nanocarrier Formulations for Curcumin Delivery

Despite CUR's therapeutic efficacy in neurological and brain diseases, a number of drawbacks still remain for its briader use, such as its poor bioavailability and low cellular uptake (low tissue levels) [174]. Those critical issues, that reduce its clinical application, are mainly connected to the low absorption and rapid systemic elimination (hepatic metabolism) [175]. Moreover, the high hydrophobicity and low solubility of CUR in the water at acidic (or neutral) pH cause a major limitation for their wider therapeutic use [175]. It is well known that nanocarrier-based delivery systems can enhance the drug colloidal stability as well as its ability to cross the biological barriers and to reach the targeted regions [176,177]. For this reason, the employment of the nanocarriers as delivery systems for CUR represents a promising approach for the development of nano-platforms dedicated to the treatment of neurological disorders and brain diseases [177,178].

However, the treatment of the human neurological and brain diseases requests that the delivery of CUR happens at specific target sites, by overcoming the complex microenvironment of the BBB. Within these general issues, recent progress in drug delivery approaches stimulated the development of novel nanocarriers encapsulating CUR, such as polymer nanoparticles (and micelles), lipid-based (and liposome) nanocarriers, liquid crystalline nanocarriers (LCNs) andcyclodextrins (Figure 6).

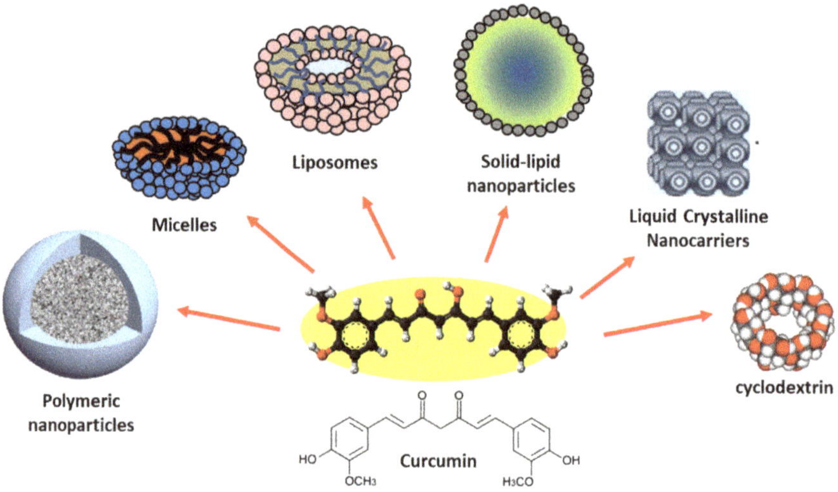

Figure 6. Main types of CUR-based nanocarrier formulations for the treatment of Alzheimer's and brain diseases.

CUR encapsulation into nanocarriers improves not only its bioavailability and solubility, but also increases its colloidal stability by protecting it from the influence of the tissue micro-environment, thus enhancing the sustained release of CUR at target sites. There are a number of key factors that govern the distribution parameters of drugs within brain tissues, including the plasma protein binding, drug–tissue interactions (and binding) in the brain region, blood (influx/efflux) flow rate at the BBB level and the rate of drug metabolism in the brain region.

Nowadays, newer formulations of nanocarriers are designed with the aim to achieve efficient transport and improved the therapeutic efficacy of CUR. In this section, we describe the main types of formulated CUR-based nanocarriers and their effectiveness in specific drug delivery processes.

5.1. Polymer-Based Nanocarriers: Polymer Nanoparticles and Micelles

Nanocarriers composed of biocompatible and biodegradable polymers nanoparticles are of high interest as drug delivery systems, given their versatility in boththerapeutic drug preparation and delivery into target tissues. Polymers employed have distinctchemical-physical characteristics, and the modification of their chemical groups has been used for functionalization and drug conjugation of many polymer-based nanocarrier platforms, increasingly employed for therapeutic drug delivery processes at the central nervous system (CNS) level [178].

Among the variety of polymer-based systems, PLGA is the most commonly-used biocompatible polymer for the treatment of neurological disorders [179]. A recent investigation analyzed different CUR-loaded PLGA nanoformulations developed with the scope to improve the kinetics of tissue distribution and BBB penetration, in a freely-moving rat model [180]. In that case, CUR exposure in the body was increased with either intravenous or oral nanoparticle administration and the relative bioavailability of CUR-loaded PLGA formulations showed a 22-fold increase over conventional CUR [180]. In another study, a sensitively prolonged retention time of CUR in the cerebral cortex (increased by 96%) and hippocampus (increased by 83%) was observed with the PLGA nanoparticle encapsulation [181]. Furthermore, neuronal uptake and neuroprotective effect of CUR-loaded PLGA nanoparticles have been recently investigated, in vitro, to the human neuroblastoma SK-N-SH cells [182]. In that case, the CUR-loaded PLGA nanoparticles were able to protect human neuroblastoma SK-N-SH cells against H_2O_2-induced oxidative damage thus evidencing a promising (nontoxic) drug delivery method to protect neurons against oxidative damage as observed in AD [182]. Moreover, CUR-encapsulated PLGA 50:50 nanoparticles (NPs-Cur 50:50) displayed higher antioxidant and anti-inflammatory activities than free CUR, and have evidenced the ability to prevent the phosphorylation of Akt and tau proteins in SK-N-SH cells induced by H_2O_2 [183].

Poly(butyl)cyanoacrylate (PBCA) nanoparticles represent another interesting polymer-based nanocarrier for CUR drug delivery [184,185]. Preparation of apolipoprotein-E3 (ApoE3) mediated PBCA nanoparticles (ApoE3-C-PBCA) containing CUR evidenced an enhanced (in vitro) apoptosis-induced anticancer activity against SH-SY5Y neuroblastoma cells [184], compared to CUR plain solution and CUR loaded PBCA nanoparticles (C-PBCA), with apoptosis being the underlying mechanism [184]. Moreover, in vitro cell culture study revealed an enhanced therapeutic efficacy of ApoE3-C-PBCA nanoparticles against β-amyloid induced cytotoxicity in SH-SY5Y neuroblastoma cells compared to CUR solution [185].

Finally, CS, a natural linear biocompatible and biodegradable polysaccharide, represents another interesting polymer for brain delivery purpose, due to its low toxicity and immunogenicity. CS polymer contains primary amine groups, which make CS-nanocarriers positively charged vehicles and efficient tools for brain therapeutic interventions [186–188]. CUR inclusion into CS nanoparticles improves its chemical stability, prevents its degradation, and facilitates the uptake of the cell membrane and the (controlled) release of CUR [186]. In a recent investigation, CUR-conjugated CS nanoparticles with diameter < 50 nm evidenced efficacy against arsenic-induced toxicity in rats [187], while CUR-loaded CS–bovine serum albumin nanoparticles showed their efficacy in the enhancement of Aβ 42 phagocytosis and modulated macrophage polarization in AD [188].

Efficient release of the encapsulated CUR and improved bioavailability can also be achieved by means of the polymer micellesnanocarriers, obtained by the self-assembly of amphiphilic polymers. In this case, the micelles hydrophobic core creates a microenvironment for the incorporation of the hydrophobic CUR, while the hydrophilic shell ensures their water solubility. Particularly interesting is the use of PEG for the hydrophilic polymer block, as it creates a local surface concentration of highly hydrated polymer brushes [189–191] that sterically inhibit the interactions with plasma proteins (or cells), thus reducing the nanocarrier uptake process by mononuclear phagocytic systems (MPS). Moreover, the surface coatings with PEG blocks have been shown to increase colloidal stability, solubility as well as to improve polymeric nanoparticle diffusion in brain tissues [191,192]. Recently, the in vivo investigation of CUR-loaded PLGA-PEG micellar nanocarriers evidenced an increase of the relevant pharmacokinetic parameters [193]. More specifically, the CUR-loaded nanocarriers could overcome the impaired BBB, efficiently diffuse through the brain parenchyma, and deliver a protective effect in the regions of injured neonatal rats'brains (with hypoxic-ischemic encephalopathy) [193]. Moreover, micelles formed by synthetic PLGA-PEG-PLGA triblock copolymers have been revealed to be able to modifyCUR pharmacokinetics and tissue distribution [194].

It is worth pointing out that the use of simple PLGA nanocarriers without further modifications presents a number of intrinsic drawbacks, connected with the short blood circulation time and the difficulty of passing through the BBB. After crossing the BBB, the polymer nanocarriers must then overcome and penetrate the brain tissues and diffuse some distance before diseased cells can be targeted. For this reason, cell-specific delivery can be promoted by the surface modifications on the polymer nanocarriers with targeting ligands or peptides. Recently a variety of approaches have been developed for the engineering of modified PLGA nanocarriers (with targeting ligands) for enhanced drug delivery to the brain and the CNS [179]. For example, in vitro investigation of CUR loaded-PLGA nanoparticles were conjugated with Tet-1 peptide for potential use in vitro in AD [195], and with glutathione that is able to modify the route of internalization (enabling them to escape the uptake through micropinocytosis) toward a safer pathway and avoiding the lysosomal degradation [196]. Furthermore, an innovative PLGA nanocarrier was designed and the results evidenced that compared to other PLGA nanoparticles, CRT peptide modified-PLGA nanoparticles (co-delivering S1 and CUR) exhibited enhanced beneficial effect in AD treatment in mice [197].

Finally, it is worth pointing that mixed polymeric micelles provide an interesting alternative approach for the formation of CUR delivery systems, due to enhanced colloidal (long-term) stability, drug-loading capacities compared with simple polymer micelles [198]. Moreover, mixed micelles can provide addition (and multiple) functionalities by the constituent copolymers to the micellar nanocarrier, thus increasing their performances in the involved drug delivery process [199]. In conclusion, polymer micelles encapsulation of CUR provides a sensitive increase in solubility and bioavailability, making this formulation very promising for the development of therapeutic tools for AD and brain disease clinical applications.

5.2. *Lipid-Based Nanocarriers*

Lipid-based nanocarriers represent a versatile nanomaterial platform to develop enhanced drug delivery systems formultiple applications in nanomedicine and biotechnology [200,201]. Synthetic or natural lipids are more biocompatible than the polymeric and inorganic nanocarriers, and they present a marked ability to penetrate the BBB even without any specific functionalization (passive targeting). Moreover, mixed lipid-based systems present enhanced colloidal stability as well as a wide range of morphological and structural properties generated by a versatile self-assembly process, as evidenced by various structural investigations [201,202]. The formation of lipid-based nanocarriers is controlled by specific soft interactions that regulate the colloidal stability of therapeutic drugs in a harsh bio-environment of diseased tissues, thus allowing better control over drug release kinetics [203]. SLNs [204], nanostructured lipid carriers (NLCs) [205] and liposomes [200], are the most important representatives of the lipid-based nanocarriers, that have been used for the treatment of brain diseases in the last decades.

5.2.1. Solid Lipid Nanoparticles and Nanostructured Lipid Carriers

Due to their inherent ability to cross theBBB, SLNs and NLCs are drug delivery systems that have been used for the active and passive targeting treatment of a variety of brain cancers and neurodegenerative diseases [206,207]. SLNs present a small spherical shape (with a radius ranging between 50 to 200 nm) with a (lipid matrix) solid core at the body (and room) temperature. They are composed of a mixture between different lipids and amphiphilic molecules (about 1–5% w/v of surfactants/cosurfactant) that stabilize the lipid core region. The glyceride derivatives (such as the monoglycerides, triglycerides, and complex glyceride mixtures), which are easily assimilated by our metabolism, are generally the most abundant component. SLNs represent an efficient drug delivery system for both lipophilic and hydrophilic therapeutic drugs. Their specific composition, made of lipids and surfactants, strongly influence their physicochemical properties such as size (and polydispersity), colloidal stability, loading and release properties of the active drugs [204]. SLNs are able to naturally cross the BBB due to their highly lipophilic nature (passive targeting). Brain uptake is performed by the paracellular pathway through the opening of the tight junctions in the brain microvasculature. Brain targeting with ApoE receptors, which is predominantly expressed in the brain, facilitated transport across the BBB (active targeting) [207].

With the aim to achieve an efficient and optimized CUR loaded nanoparticles with high drug payload, a preparation process of (small size) CUR loaded SLNs and NLCs was performed using experimental design and a multi-objective optimization approach [208]. The investigation evidenced that by the modulation of the key and control factors (such as the drug-to-lipid ratio, surfactant concentration, and homogenization rate), it is possible an experimental optimization of their effects on the nanoparticle size (and polydispersity) and loading efficiency. More specifically, the entrapment efficiency of CUR was found to be 82% (in SLNs) and 94% (in NLCs). The pharmacokinetic studies (after intravenous administration of 4 mg/kg dose of CUR in rat) evidenced that the amount of CUR available in the brain in CUR-loaded NLCs (AUC0-t = 505.76 ng/g·h), was significantly higher than the CUR-loaded SLNs (AUC0-t = 116.31 ng/g·h) and the free CUR (AUC0-t = 0.00 ng/g·h) [176]. Furthermore, CUR-loaded SLNs were investigated to assess their efficacy in the treatment of the BV-2 microglial cells against LPS-induced neuroinflammation [208]. The SLNs showed higher inhibition of NO production compared to conventional CUR in a dose-dependent manner. Moreover, the mRNA and proinflammatory cytokine levels were reduced in a dose-dependent manner in comparison to those with free CUR [208]. Finally, CUR-loaded SLNs exhibited a greater permeability than dietary CUR in vitro and showed marked effectiveness for AD therapy [209]. In that case, CUR has been shown to prevent Aβ 42-induced neuronal death by inhibiting ROS production or by blocking apoptotic death pathways and boosting cell survival pathways [209].

NLCs represent a slightly modified version of SLNs, where the structure of the solid lipid core contains imperfections in the crystal structure. This imperfect crystal, (obtained by mixing liquid/solid lipids and the addition of mono-, di- and triglycerides lipids with different chain lengths) increases the internal free space of the solid, thus resulting in a higher drug loading efficiencies [204,206]. A recent study showed that CUR-loaded NLCs significantly increase the accumulation rate of CUR in rat brain, as also its serum levels [210]. Their effects were evidenced by reduced oxidative stress parameters in hippocampal tissue and improved spatial memory. Moreover, histopathological studies revealed the CUR-loaded NLCs potential in decreasing the Aβ hallmarks in the animal model with AD. The neuroprotective potential of Cur-NLC in both pre-treatment and treatment modes also showed that loading CUR in NLCs is an effective strategy to increase CUR delivery to the brain and to reduce the Aβ-induced neurological abnormalities (and memory defects) [210]. A recent study evidenced that NLCs enhance the bioavailability and brain cancer inhibitory efficacy of CUR both in vitro and in vivo [211]. Observation of the time-dependent cellular uptake and ROS production, evidenced that CUR loaded NLC formulation not only improved the apoptotic induction effect of CUR, but markedly increased bio-availability and brain (and tumor) targeting effect, thus allowing trigger effect on the carcinoma digression [211]. Finally, both SLNs and NLCs can be produced byusing diverse formation methods, easily scaled up and without requiring the use of organic solvents, thus avoiding toxicity effects of the final product. The high-pressure homogenization technique (HPH) represents the most common technique due to its relatively low cost, and its ability for large-scale production [212].

5.2.2. Liposomes

Liposomes are a highly versatile and biocompatible drug delivery system, with the potential for carrying different types of bioactive drugs and molecules across the BBB [213,214]. They consist of uni- or multi-lamellar lipid bilayers structures composed of phospholipids, with an internal aqueous core. They exhibit various architectures that depend on the preparation methods and the involved self-assembly process. Despite their intrinsic colloidal stability, depending on the conditions of the solution and the incorporated components, liposomes may aggregate and/or fuse together, thus changing their size or surface charge expression [215,216]. For this reason, liposome surface functionalization represents a widely used strategy to avoid the evolution of an inefficient drug delivery system and the degradation of the performances to the point of action. Liposomes can incorporate both hydrophilic drugs (entrapped in the aqueous core) and lipophilic (or hydrophobic) therapeutic compounds inserted in the hydrophobic region of the lipid bilayer.

Concerning the mechanism of action with biomembranes, the positively charged nanocarriers (cationic liposomes) can facilitate cell internalization and (nonspecific) uptake by electrostatic interactions with the negative charge of the endothelial cell membrane. It is worth pointing that charge expression of (bio-)membranes may induce complex aggregation behavior and morphological transition in the presence of soft nanoparticles or drugs macromolecules within the charged complex microenvironment of the biological systems [217,218]. In any case, once in the bloodstream, most liposomes are covered around their surface by a (plasma) proteins corona (e.g., fibrinogen, immunoglobulins), leading to MPS activation and successive liposomes removal from the bloodstream [213]. This circumstance causes a reduction of the sufficient number of liposomes that can be delivered to the brain tissues and consequently requests a higher dose to reach a sensitive therapeutic efficacy. In these cases, the surface-modified (targeted) liposomes are required for effective delivery across the BBB and to stimulate a (specific) molecular interaction for an effective therapy for AD [214,218,219]. The main efficient strategy for crossing the BBB is obtained by the functionalization of the liposome surface by using biomolecular ligands that enhance the BBB transport and targeting processes for AD therapy. It has been shown that liposomes modified with transferrin [220,221] and lactoferrin [222], the most commonly employed targeted receptors, could cross and penetrate the BBB via receptor-mediated endocytosis. Moreover, the surface functionalization of liposomes with PEG (stealth liposomes) cause a drastic reduction in the formation of the so-called proteins corona thus providing a longer circulation time and improvement of their pharmacokinetic profile [192,213]. These attractive properties of liposomes stimulate a growing interest in the development of suitable nanocarrier systems for the delivery of active drugs, such as CUR, that act on the CNS. Encapsulation of CUR with liposomes areused for therapies targeting Aβ in AD, through a contrasting action against the accumulation (and deposition) of plaques of Aβ peptide in the brain, with minimum side-effects, and the enhancement of CUR solubility and its cellular uptake [218,219].

Recently, liposome nanocarriers were bifunctionalized with both a peptide derived from the ApoE receptor-binding domain (for BBB targeting) and with phosphatidic acid (for Aβ-binding). The electron microscopy experiments evidenced that the bifunctionalized liposomes are able to disaggregate and hinder the formation of Aβ assemblies in vitro.These results evidenced the versatility of bi-functional liposomes in their tasks to destabilize brain Aβ aggregate, favor peptide removal across the BBB, and its final peripheral clearance [218]. Moreover, CUR-conjugated nanoliposomes with high affinity for Aβ deposits, recently found application in diagnosis and targeted drug delivery in AD. More specifically the nanoliposomes strongly labeled Aβ deposits in the post-mortem brain tissue of AD patients and in the APPxPS1 mice. The injection of the CUR-conjugated nanoliposomes in the neocortex and hippocampus of mice evidenced the ability to specifically stain the Aβ deposits in vivo [219].

An alternative way to reach the brain tissue region consists of the exploitation of the (non-specific) interaction of liposomes with the BBB, by means of the cell-penetrating peptides (CPPs). The CPP action is based mainly on the interaction between the positively charged (peptide) amino acids with the negatively charged moieties present at the surface of the biomembranes, including the BBB [223]. For example, the presence of the amino acids arginine and lysine facilitates the formation of hydrogen bonds with the negatively charged phosphates which are present on the (bio-)membranes. CPPs that showed different properties might undergo slightly different internalization mechanisms, including (specific and non-specific) endocytosis, pore formation and energy-dependent and -independent mechanism (via caveolin- and clathrin-independent lipid rafts) [132]. Among all CPPs, the modified HIV-1 transactivating transcriptional activator (TAT) peptide (having positive charges that can interact with negative charges of the BBB) has been successfully used for specific endocytosis delivery of liposome nanoparticles into the brain [224]. It has been demonstrated that nanoliposomes double-functionalized with a CUR derivative and with a TAT peptide enhances BBB crossing in vitro, carrying a CUR-derivative to bind Aβ peptide [225]. Also, CUR derivatives containing lipid ligands can be exploited for targeted drug delivery for brain diseases. Recently, the formation of nanoliposomes with CUR, or with CUR derivatives containing lipid ligands (phosphatidic acid, cardiolipin, or GM1 ganglioside) was able to inhibit the formation of fibrillar and/or oligomeric Aβ in vitro [226]. In Figure 7, we show a sketch of the two main mechanisms of liposome activity: direct penetration and the receptor-mediated transcytosis transport processes across the BBB.

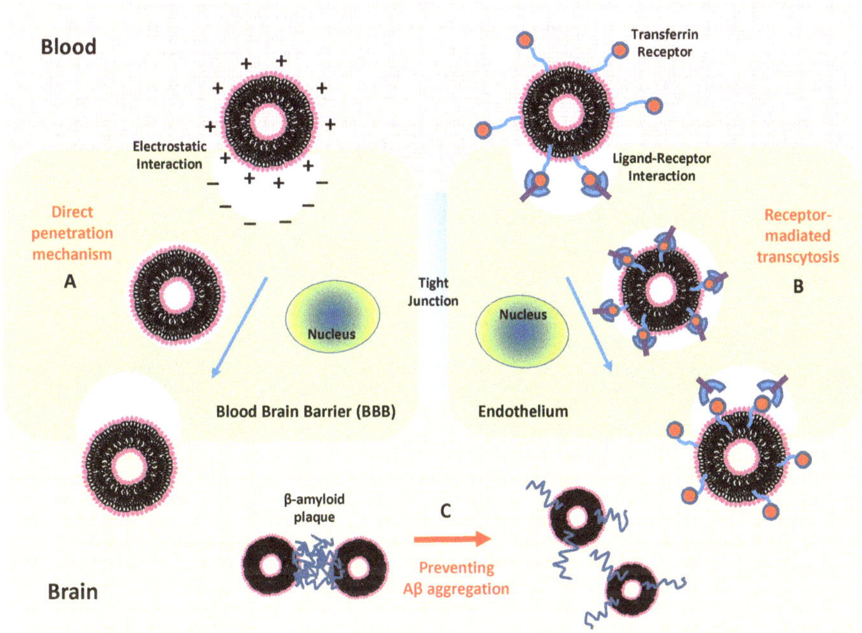

Figure 7. Transport process of liposome nanocarriers across the blood-brain barrier (BBB).In the direct penetration mechanism (**A**), liposome endocytosis is favored by the ionic interaction of positively charged liposome surface groups (due to the presence of cationic lipids, or positively charged (+++) amino acids) with the negative charge (− − −) of the endothelial cell membrane of the BBB. As an example, liposomes internalization may be favored by the negative charge exhibited by cell-penetrating peptides (e.g., CPPs TAT - transactivator of transcription of human immunodeficiency virus). Receptor-mediated transcytosis mechanism (**B**) exploits the specific interaction with receptors highly expressed at the BBB (e.g., transferrin receptor). Receptor-ligand binding interaction regulates both liposome internalization (crossing the BBB) and the delivery process of the liposome nanocarriers within the brain. Once that the liposome reaches the inside brain region, multi-functional liposomes can direct their action at the Aβ target, for AD therapy (**C**).

Finally, multifunctional liposomes obtained by the suitable combination of more functionalities, that enhance both BBB transport and target diseased tissues, seem to be an efficient approach to design advanced treatments for AD and other brain diseases. Recently, multifunctional liposomes incorporating a lipid-PEG-CUR derivative and further functionalized with a BBB transport mediator (anti-transferrin antibody) evidenced an improved intake by the BBB cellular model [130].

5.3. Liquid Crystalline Nanocarriers

LCNs are self-assembled, thermodynamically stable, liquid crystalline nanostructures (e.g., bicontinuous cubic, inverted hexagonal or sponge phases) formed upon water dispersion of lyotropic lipids (such as unsaturated monoglycerides, phospholipids, glycolipids) and other amphiphilic molecules (surfactants). These amphiphilic molecules spontaneously self-assemble into organized nanostructures (such as cubosomes and hexosomes) containing hydrophilic and hydrophobic compartments which can encapsulate hydrophilic or lipophilic guest compounds [227]. Incorporation of drugs into LCNs for delivery processes through the BBB evidenced several advantages like controlled drug release, improved drug bioavailability, reduced chemical and physiological degradation, in vivo, and reduction of side effects [228,229]. Recently, entrapment of CUR into monoolein-based liquid crystalline nanoparticle dispersion (with almost 100% encapsulation efficiency) evidenced enhancement of the colloidal stability of CUR in the nanoformulation (about 75% of the CUR survived after 45 days of storage at 40 °C), while the in vitro release of CUR was sustained (10% or less over 15 days) [230]. Moreover, the release of CUR in bulk mesophases and in inverse hexagonal (HII) liquid crystals and the radical scavenging activity of LCNPs were also recently investigated [228]. The inverse hexagonal (HII) liquid crystals mesophases were constructed by a water solution of soybean lecithin (SL) and castor oil (Coil) and characterized by polarized light microscopy (POM), small-angle X-ray scattering (SAXS) and rheology. In that case, the biphasic drug sustained-release pattern for the LCNs evidenced a relatively fast release at the initial stage and then sustained release [228].

5.4. Macrocyclic Host-Macromolecules: Curcumin Loaded Cyclodextrin Nanocarriers

An efficient, alternative way to increase the water solubility of CUR consists in the complexation of CUR with macrocyclic host-macromolecules such as cyclodextrins. These macro- molecules have an interior hydrophobic surface which can host poorly water-soluble (macro-)molecules, while the external hydrophilic region ensures its aqueous solubility and colloidal stability [231]. They were proved to create CUR complexes and to improve its solubility [232–234]. The mechanisms for brain uptake and BBB crossing seems to be connected to a direct action of cyclodextrins that extract lipids (cholesterol and phospholipids) and some proteins from cell membranes (and lipid raft regions) modifying the molecular composition and properties of the lipid bilayers [231].

Recently, the therapeutic effect of CUR-cyclodextrinnanocarriers formulation on amyloid plaques in Alzheimer's transgenic mice was demonstrated, in vivo, after intravenous and subcutaneous injection [233], and in vitro BBB model [234]. Alternatively, CUR complexation with calix(n)arenes macromolecules is also employed in brain drug delivery applications. Stable nanocarriers formed by combined methyl-β-cyclodextrin, *para*-sulphonato-calix(4)arene and *para*-sulphonato-calix(6)arene for the solubilization of CUR were recently investigated [232]. The nanocarriers, that self-assemble in a way that retains part of the CUR at the surface of the nanoparticles, showed a high affinity for the amyloid deposits, strongly labeling the SPs and also the diffuse deposits of AD brains. These nanocarriers were able to strongly label various amyloid aggregates in AD brains, thus proving their potential as trackers of AD pathology. Their biocompatibility was proved on several cell lines. Moreover, they were shown to interact with the Aβ peptide, reducing its aggregation and preventing the evolution of the disease and its toxicity [232]. We summarize in Table 1 the main characteristic and transport mechanism of the main CUR-conjugated nanocarriers.

5.5. Combining Therapeutic, Diagnostic and Stimuli-Responsive Functions: Theranostic Nanocarriers

Recently, the design of nanocarriers with combined therapeutic, diagnostic and stimuli-responsive multi-functionalities (theranosticnanocarriers) has stimulated research efforts concerning the treatment of different disease including brain disease and AD [235,236]. Different strategies can be used to engineer the surface of the nanoparticles, including the use of biomarkers, ligands, proteins and genes. Moreover, smart nanocarriers can take advantage of the specific microenvironment using (internal or external) stimuli-responsive triggers [237].

As an example, a CUR-conjugate, generation 3 PAMAM dendrimer (G3-Curc) nanocarrier proved to be a promising targeted theranosticnanocarrier for the treatment of glioblastoma brain tumors [238]. Together with the improvement of CUR water solubility and bioavailability, exvivo fluorescence imaging showed a tumor-specific distribution of G3-Curc conjugate (avoiding other major organs). While the *ex vivo* fluorescence imaging (and fluorescence microscopy) of the tumor tissue evidenced its specificity for nuclear distribution [238].

Table 1. Characteristic and the transport mechanism of the main curcumin-conjugated nanocarriers.

Nanocarrier Type	Most Investigated Components	Shape/Size	Advantages/Disadvantages	Mechanisms for Brain Uptake and BBB Crossing
Polymer Nanoparticles 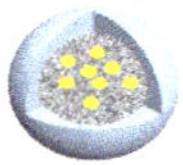	Poly(lactic-co-glycolic acid) (PLGA) is the most investigated polymer. Poly(butyl)cyanoacrylate (PBCA) and Chitosan (CS) also investigated.	Globular (10–200 nm)	Tunable physicochemical properties (through the choice of component polymers), easy preparation method, controlled pharmacokinetic, high biocompatibility, biodegradability, neurotoxic	Endocytosis and/or transcytosis through the endothelial cells, tight junctions opening. Surface conjugation with targeting ligands improve the transcytosis across the BBB [178,182,188].
Micelles 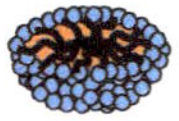	PLGA-PEG diblock and PLGA-PEG-PLGA triblock copolymers	Spherical (20–100 nm)	Negligible neurotoxic effects, improved drug bioavailability, high physicochemical and colloidal stability, sustained and controlled release/can be used only for lipophilic (hydrophobic) drug, slow drug loading capacity.	Endocytosis and/or transcytosis. Surface conjugation with targeting ligands improve the transcytosis across the BBB [198,199]
Solid Lipid Nanoparticles 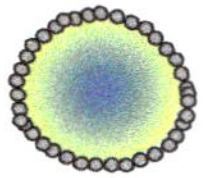	Glyceride derivatives (complex glyceride mixtures, triglycerides, monoglycerides, hard fats, stearic acid, cetyl alcohol, cholesterol butyrate, emulsifying wax. The lipid core is usually stabilized by surfactants (about 1–5% w/v) and/or cosurfactant (such as poloxamer 188 and/or Tween® 80)	Spherical (50–300)	High entrapment efficiency for hydrophobic drugs, biocompatibility, high physical stability and drug protection, controlled release, ease of formation methods (that can be easily scaled up and do not require organic solvents thus avoiding (neuro-)toxicity)/reduced hydrophilic drug entrapment efficiency, sterilization difficulties	Brain uptake by the paracellular pathway through the opening of the tight junctions in brain microvasculature, passive diffusion, and endocytosis. Active targeting with receptors (apolipoprotein E) [204,206,210]
Liposome 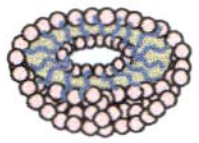	Lipids:1,2-dipalmitoyl-sn-glycero-3-phospho-choline ethyl-phosphatidyl-choline (DPPC), phosphatidylcholine (PC), sphingomyelin (SP), and lecithin (LC),Cholesterol. PEGylated 1,2-distearoyl-sn-glycero-3-phospho-ethanolamine-PEG 2000 (DSPE)	Globular/lamellar (20–200 nm)	Possibility of entrapping both hydrophilic and hydrophobic drugs, high drug protection and targeting efficiency/neurotoxicity, physicochemical instability, the tendency of fusion, rapid clearance, sterilization difficulties	Passive targeting, adsorption-mediated transcytosis, or receptor-mediated endocytosis. Active targeting. with receptors glutathione, glucose, transferrin, lactoferrin, apolipoprotein E, phosphatidic acid. Use of cell-penetrating peptides (CPPs - such as TAT, penetratin) [215,216,218,219]
Liquid Crystalline Nanocarriers 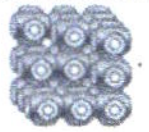	Unsaturated monoglycerides, phospholipids, glycolipids and surfactants	Bicontinuous cubic (cubosome), inverted hexagonal (hexosomes) or sponge phases (20–200 nm)	Enhancement colloidal stability, controlled andsustained (in vitro) release of curcumin, improved drug bioavailability, reduced chemical and physiological degradation (in vivo), reduction of side effects	Passive targeting, adsorption-mediated transcytosis, or receptor-mediated endocytosis. [228,229]
Cyclodextrins 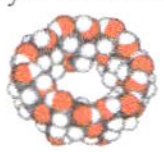	Mainly the β-cyclodextrin derivatives	Cyclic (150–500 nm)	High biocompatibility, lipophilic cavity sensitively improve curcumin solubilization, outer hydrophilic surfacefacilitate dispersion and colloidal stability of the formulation	The direct action of cyclodextrin by extracting lipids (cholesterol and phospholipids) and some proteins from cell membranes (and lipid raft region) modifying the molecular composition and properties of the lipid bilayers. [231–234].

Moreover, a novel approach of CUR-conjugated superparamagnetic iron oxide (SPION) evidenced that amyloid plaque could be visualized in (ex vivo) magnetic resonance imaging (MRI) in AD mice, while no plaque was found in non-transgenic mice [144]. Significant accumulation and co-localization of amyloid plaques with nanoparticles were observed in an immune-histochemical analysis of the mouse brains. Therefore, this formulation has great potential for non-invasive diagnosis of AD using MRI. Furthermore, anti-amyloid antibody (IgG4.1)-conjugated gadolinium/magneticnanocarriers loaded with CUR/dexamethasone drugs were proposed for early diagnosis, targeting, and as a therapeutic agent(s) of cerebrovascular amyloid (CVA) [239]. The study evidenced that the nanocarriers efficiently distribute from the blood flow to the brain vasculature and target CVA deposit, owing to the IgG4.1. Thesetheranosticnanocarriers provide then both MRI and single-photon emission computed tomography (SPECT) agents contrast, specific to the CVA in the brain. In addition, they also carry CUR/dexamethasone therapeutic agents to reduce cerebrovascular inflammation associated with cerebral amyloid angiopathy (CAA), which is believed to trigger hemorrhage in CAA patients [239].

Finally, hybrid materials composed of mesoporous silica nanoparticles (MSNPs) have been, recently proposed as a promising class of versatile drug delivery nanocarriers, as well as an efficient nanoplatform for fluorescent cell tracking and bioimage applications [240–243]. The homogenous and regular nanostructure and the good biocompatibility of MSNPs facilitate the construction of an advanced biomedical platform for the delivery of therapeutics through the encapsulation of hydrophobic drugs inside the void volumes and the delivery of covalently linked therapeutic agents functionalized at the (large external/internal) silica surface [240–243]. Recently, CUR encapsulated MSNPs showed improved solubility, in vitro release profile and significantly enhanced cell cytotoxicity compared to the pure CUR [244]. MSNPs also provide a promising strategy to target cancer cells reducing peripheral nervous system uptake [245,246]. Recently, using a nano-templating approach, a novel MSNPs (with a size of ~220 nm) loaded with the CUR and chrysin have been developed for nose-to-brain delivery applications [247]. In that case, confocal microscopy experiments demonstrated that, following a 2 h incubation, the nanoparticles of <500 nm were able to accumulate within cells with fluorescein isothiocynate (FITC)-loaded MSNP showing membrane-localized and cytoplasmic accumulation [247]. These results evidenced the ability of the novel MSNPs to target and deliver active drugs into the CNS and bypass the BBB through olfactory drug delivery [247]. Moreover, a pH-responsive MSNPs (MCM-41) and capped by CS polymer (CS-MCM-41) were recently synthesized for the controlled CUR release near the cancer cells acidic environment [248]. The presence of CS acted as a pH-responsive shield to increase the solubility, bioavailability and anticancer efficacy of CUR against U87MG glioblastoma cancer cell line. Cytotoxicity investigations on the U87MG glioblastoma cancer cell line evidenced, in fact, that CS-MCM-41 nanoparticles have more cytotoxicity than free CUR and CUR-loaded MSNPs (MCM-41) without CS [248].

In conclusion, the suitable combination of those multi-functional properties allows identifying, within a single theranostic nano-platform, the diseased tissue location, the nanocarrier delivery, and the biodistribution, thus allowing profitable monitoring of the progress/efficacy of the therapeutic treatment. The targeting of overexpressed receptors on brain diseased tissues and cells allows a specific release of CUR cargo in the target site [235]. Moreover, real-time monitoring of the pharmacokinetic profiles and target site accumulation may direct the proper selection of treatment and therapy. Finally, the improvement of theranostic approaches and the assessment of the therapeutic efficacy may stimulate the development of personalized medicine-based therapeutic protocols of interventions.

6. Conclusions and Future Remarks

AD and other brain diseases are an important cause of human deaths worldwide. New alternative therapies for AD and neurodegenerative diseases arise from ongoing research in the whole world. Because CUR may cross the hematoencephalic barrier, studies have shown that it leads to various improvements in the pathological process of AD. The molecular mechanisms of CUR in AD are several, including antioxidant, Aβ-binding, anti-inflammatory, tau inhibition, metal chelation, neurogenesis, and synaptogenesis promotion. These effects are scientifically verified, with CUR revealing an outstanding performanceon prevention, treatment and diagnosis of AD. However, in this success story of CUR, there is the fact that its bioavailability is too lower. To remove this problem, new formulations such as nanoCUR are developed. CUR nanoformulations are a therapeutic alternative in a new discovery phase, being nontoxic for other body cells.

Regarding nanocarriers formulation for CUR delivery, SLNs, NLCs, liposomes, LCNs and macrocyclic host macromolecules reported interesting characteristics that need to be more studied to a better to understand their mechanism of action and effectiveness. Future studies need to test this CUR nanoformulation, and different combinations and formulation, in brain diseases. New efforts are needed to test new CUR nanomedicine formulations, with better CUR bioavailability, in brain diseases.

Author Contributions: All authors contributed equally to the manuscript. Conceptualization, J.S.-R.; validation investigation, resources, data curation, writing—all authors; review and editing, N.M., M.M., D.C., and J.S.-R.; All authors have read and agreed to the published version of the manuscript.

Funding: This research received no external funding.

Acknowledgments: This work was supported by CONICYT PIA/APOYO CCTE AFB170007.N. Martins would like to thank the Portuguese Foundation for Science and Technology (FCT–Portugal) for the Strategic project ref. UID/BIM/04293/2013 and "NORTE2020—Programa Operacional Regional do Norte" (NORTE-01-0145-FEDER-000012).

Conflicts of Interest: The authors declare no conflict of interest.

References

1. Hatcher, H.; Planalp, R.; Cho, J.; Torti, F.M.; Torti, S.V. Curcumin: From ancient medicine to current clinical trials. *Cell. Mol. Life Sci.* **2008**, *65*, 1631–1652. [CrossRef] [PubMed]
2. Farooqui, T.; Farooqui, A.A. Chapter 2—Curcumin: Historical Background, Chemistry, Pharmacological Action, and Potential Therapeutic Value. In *Curcumin for Neurological and Psychiatric Disorders*; Farooqui, T., Farooqui, A.A., Eds.; Academic Press: New York, NY, USA, 2019; pp. 23–44. [CrossRef]
3. Anand, P.; Thomas, S.G.; Kunnumakkara, A.B.; Sundaram, C.; Harikumar, K.B.; Sung, B.; Tharakan, S.T.; Misra, K.; Priyadarsini, I.K.; Rajasekharan, K.N.; et al. Biological activities of curcumin and its analogues (Congeners) made by man and Mother Nature. *Biochem. Pharmacol.* **2008**, *76*, 1590–1611. [CrossRef] [PubMed]
4. Vogel, A.; Pelletier, J. Examen chimique de la racine de Curcuma. *J. Pharm.* **1815**, *1*, 289–300.
5. Gupta, S.C.; Patchva, S.; Koh, W.; Aggarwal, B.B. Discovery of curcumin, a component of golden spice, and its miraculous biological activities. *Clin. Exp. Pharmacol. Physiol.* **2012**, *39*, 283–299. [CrossRef] [PubMed]
6. Menon, V.P.; Sudheer, A.R. Antioxidant and anti-inflammatory properties of curcumin. *Adv. Exp. Med. Biol.* **2007**, *595*, 105–125. [CrossRef] [PubMed]
7. Yeung, A.W.K.; Horbanczuk, M.; Tzvetkov, N.T.; Mocan, A.; Carradori, S.; Maggi, F.; Marchewka, J.; Sut, S.; Dall'Acqua, S.; Gan, R.Y.; et al. Curcumin: Total-Scale Analysis of the Scientific Literature. *Molecules* **2019**, *24*, 1393. [CrossRef]
8. Khajehdehi, P.; Zanjaninejad, B.; Aflaki, E.; Nazarinia, M.; Azad, F.; Malekmakan, L.; Dehghanzadeh, G.R. Oral supplementation of turmeric decreases proteinuria, hematuria, and systolic blood pressure in patients suffering from relapsing or refractory lupus nephritis: A randomized and placebo-controlled study. *J. Ren. Nutr.* **2012**, *22*, 50–57. [CrossRef]
9. Akazawa, N.; Choi, Y.; Miyaki, A.; Tanabe, Y.; Sugawara, J.; Ajisaka, R.; Maeda, S. Curcumin ingestion and exercise training improve vascular endothelial function in postmenopausal women. *Nutr. Res.* **2012**, *32*, 795–799. [CrossRef]
10. Wojcik, M.; Krawczyk, M.; Wojcik, P.; Cypryk, K.; Wozniak, L.A. Molecular Mechanisms Underlying Curcumin-Mediated Therapeutic Effects in Type 2 Diabetes and Cancer. *Oxid. Med. Cell. Longev.* **2018**, *2018*. [CrossRef]
11. Chandran, B.; Goel, A. A randomized, pilot study to assess the efficacy and safety of curcumin in patients with active rheumatoid arthritis. *Phytother. Res.* **2012**, *26*, 1719–1725. [CrossRef]
12. Kumar, S.; Ahuja, V.; Sankar, M.J.; Kumar, A.; Moss, A.C. Curcumin for maintenance of remission in ulcerative colitis. *Cochrane Database Syst. Rev.* **2012**, *10*. [CrossRef]

13. Cole, G.M.; Teter, B.; Frautschy, S.A. Neuroprotective effects of curcumin. *Adv. Exp. Med. Biol.* **2007**, *595*, 197–212. [CrossRef] [PubMed]
14. Trebatická, J.; Ďuračková, Z. Psychiatric Disorders and Polyphenols: Can They Be Helpful in Therapy? *Oxid. Med. Cell. Longev.* **2015**, *2015*, 248529. [CrossRef] [PubMed]
15. Bhat, A.; Mahalakshmi, A.M.; Ray, B.; Tuladhar, S.; Hediyal, T.A.; Manthiannem, E.; Padamati, J.; Chandra, R.; Chidambaram, S.B.; Sakharkar, M.K. Benefits of curcumin in brain disorders. *BioFactors* **2019**, *45*, 666–689. [CrossRef]
16. Ng, T.P.; Chiam, P.C.; Lee, T.; Chua, H.C.; Lim, L.; Kua, E.H. Curry consumption and cognitive function in the elderly. *Am. J. Epidemiol.* **2006**, *164*, 898–906. [CrossRef]
17. Tai, Y.H.; Lin, Y.Y.; Wang, K.C.; Chang, C.L.; Chen, R.Y.; Wu, C.C.; Cheng, I.H. Curcuminoid submicron particle ameliorates cognitive deficits and decreases amyloid pathology in Alzheimer's disease mouse model. *Oncotarget* **2018**, *9*, 10681–10697. [CrossRef]
18. McClure, R.; Ong, H.; Janve, V.; Barton, S.; Zhu, M.; Li, B.; Dawes, M.; Jerome, W.G.; Anderson, A.; Massion, P.; et al. Aerosol Delivery of Curcumin Reduced Amyloid-beta Deposition and Improved Cognitive Performance in a Transgenic Model of Alzheimer's Disease. *J. Alzheimers Dis.* **2017**, *55*, 797–811. [CrossRef]
19. Ng, Q.X.; Koh, S.S.H.; Chan, H.W.; Ho, C.Y.X. Clinical Use of Curcumin in Depression: A Meta-Analysis. *J. Am. Med. Dir. Assoc.* **2017**, *18*, 503–508. [CrossRef]
20. WHO. *Neurological Disorders: Public Health Challenges*; World Health Organization (WHO) Press: Geneva, Switzerland, 2006.
21. Gomez-Pinilla, F.; Nguyen, T.T. Natural mood foods: The actions of polyphenols against psychiatric and cognitive disorders. *Nutr. Neurosci.* **2012**, *15*, 127–133. [CrossRef]
22. Williams, C.M.; El Mohsen, M.A.; Vauzour, D.; Rendeiro, C.; Butler, L.T.; Ellis, J.A.; Whiteman, M.; Spencer, J.P. Blueberry-induced changes in spatial working memory correlate with changes in hippocampal CREB phosphorylation and brain-derived neurotrophic factor (BDNF) levels. *Free Radic. Biol. Med.* **2008**, *45*, 295–305. [CrossRef]
23. Salehi, B.; Shivaprasad Shetty, M.; V Anil Kumar, N.; Živković, J.; Calina, D.; Oana Docea, A.; Emamzadeh-Yazdi, S.; Sibel Kılıç, C.; Goloshvili, T.; Nicola, S. Veronica Plants—Drifting from Farm to Traditional Healing, Food Application, and Phytopharmacology. *Molecules* **2019**, *24*, 2454. [CrossRef] [PubMed]
24. Salehi, B.; Sharifi-Rad, J.; Capanoglu, E.; Adrar, N.; Catalkaya, G.; Shaheen, S.; Jaffer, M.; Giri, L.; Suyal, R.; Jugran, A.K. Cucurbita Plants: From Farm to Industry. *Appl. Sci.* **2019**, *9*, 3387. [CrossRef]
25. Salehi, B.; Capanoglu, E.; Adrar, N.; Catalkaya, G.; Shaheen, S.; Jaffer, M.; Giri, L.; Suyal, R.; Jugran, A.K.; Calina, D. Cucurbits Plants: A Key Emphasis to Its Pharmacological Potential. *Molecules* **2019**, *24*, 1854. [CrossRef] [PubMed]
26. Carroll, R.E.; Benya, R.V.; Turgeon, D.K.; Vareed, S.; Neuman, M.; Rodriguez, L.; Kakarala, M.; Carpenter, P.M.; McLaren, C.; Meyskens, F.L., Jr.; et al. Phase IIa clinical trial of curcumin for the prevention of colorectal neoplasia. *Cancer Prev. Res. (Phila.)* **2011**, *4*, 354–364. [CrossRef] [PubMed]
27. Ullah, F.; Liang, A.; Rangel, A.; Gyengesi, E.; Niedermayer, G. High bioavailability curcumin: An anti-inflammatory and neurosupportive bioactive nutrient for neurodegenerative diseases characterized by chronic neuroinflammation. *Arch. Toxicol.* **2017**, *91*, 1623–1634. [CrossRef] [PubMed]
28. Jakubek, M.; Kejík, Z.; Kaplánek, R.; Hromádka, R.; Šandriková, V.; Sýkora, D.; Antonyová, V.; Urban, M.; Dytrych, P.; Mikula, I. Strategy for improved therapeutic efficiency of curcumin in the treatment of gastric cancer. *Biomed. Pharmacother.* **2019**, *118*, 109278. [CrossRef]
29. Ghalandarlaki, N.; Alizadeh, A.M. Nanotechnology-applied curcumin for different diseases therapy. *BioMed Res. Int.* **2014**, *2014*. [CrossRef]
30. Maiti, P.; Dunbar, G.L. Use of Curcumin, a Natural Polyphenol for Targeting Molecular Pathways in Treating Age-Related Neurodegenerative Diseases. *Int. J. Mol. Sci.* **2018**, *19*, 1637. [CrossRef]
31. Aqil, F.; Munagala, R.; Jeyabalan, J.; Vadhanam, M.V. Bioavailability of phytochemicals and its enhancement by drug delivery systems. *Cancer Lett.* **2013**, *334*, 133–141. [CrossRef]
32. Schiborr, C.; Kocher, A.; Behnam, D.; Jandasek, J.; Toelstede, S.; Frank, J. The oral bioavailability of curcumin from micronized powder and liquid micelles is significantly increased in healthy humans and differs between sexes. *Mol. Nutr. Food Res.* **2014**, *58*, 516–527. [CrossRef]

33. Zhu, L.N.; Mei, X.; Zhang, Z.G.; Xie, Y.P.; Lang, F. Curcumin intervention for cognitive function in different types of people: A systematic review and meta-analysis. *Phytother. Res.* **2019**, *33*, 524–533. [CrossRef] [PubMed]
34. Iqbal, M.; Sharma, S.D.; Okazaki, Y.; Fujisawa, M.; Okada, S. Dietary supplementation of curcumin enhances antioxidant and phase II metabolizing enzymes in ddY male mice: Possible role in protection against chemical carcinogenesis and toxicity. *Pharmacol. Toxicol.* **2003**, *92*, 33–38. [CrossRef] [PubMed]
35. Nie, D.; Bian, Z.; Yu, A.; Chen, Z.; Liu, Z.; Huang, C. Ground and excited state intramolecular proton transfer controlled intramolecular charge separation and recombination: A new type of charge and proton transfer reaction. *Chem. Phys.* **2008**, *348*, 181–186. [CrossRef]
36. Jovanovic, S.V.; Steenken, S.; Boone, C.W.; Simic, M.G. H-Atom Transfer Is A Preferred Antioxidant Mechanism of Curcumin. *J. Am. Chem. Soc.* **1999**, *121*, 9677–9681. [CrossRef]
37. Paramera, E.I.; Konteles, S.J.; Karathanos, V.T. Microencapsulation of curcumin in cells of Saccharomyces cerevisiae. *Food Chem.* **2011**, *125*, 892–902. [CrossRef]
38. Serafini, M.M.; Catanzaro, M.; Rosini, M.; Racchi, M.; Lanni, C. Curcumin in Alzheimer's disease: Can we think to new strategies and perspectives for this molecule? *Pharmacol. Res.* **2017**, *124*, 146–155. [CrossRef]
39. Pari, L.; Tewas, D.; Eckel, J. Role of curcumin in health and disease. *Arch. Physiol. Biochem.* **2008**, *114*, 127–149. [CrossRef]
40. Reddy, P.H.; Manczak, M.; Yin, X.; Grady, M.C.; Mitchell, A.; Tonk, S.; Kuruva, C.S.; Bhatti, J.S.; Kandimalla, R.; Vijayan, M. Protective effects of Indian spice curcumin against amyloid-β in Alzheimer's disease. *J. Alzheimers Dis.* **2018**, *61*, 843–866. [CrossRef]
41. Ringman, J.M.; Frautschy, S.A.; Cole, G.M.; Masterman, D.L.; Cummings, J.L. A potential role of the curry spice curcumin in Alzheimer's disease. *Curr. Alzheimer Res.* **2005**, *2*, 131–136. [CrossRef]
42. Zbarsky, V.; Datla, K.P.; Parkar, S.; Rai, D.K.; Aruoma, O.I.; Dexter, D.T. Neuroprotective properties of the natural phenolic antioxidants curcumin and naringenin but not quercetin and fisetin in a 6-OHDA model of Parkinson's disease. *Free Radic. Res.* **2005**, *39*, 1119–1125. [CrossRef]
43. Jagatha, B.; Mythri, R.B.; Vali, S.; Bharath, M.S. Curcumin treatment alleviates the effects of glutathione depletion in vitro and in vivo: Therapeutic implications for Parkinson's disease explained via in silico studies. *Free Radic. Biol. Med.* **2008**, *44*, 907–917. [CrossRef] [PubMed]
44. Xie, L.; Li, X.-K.; Takahara, S. Curcumin has bright prospects for the treatment of multiple sclerosis. *Int. Immunopharmacol.* **2011**, *11*, 323–330. [CrossRef] [PubMed]
45. Qureshi, M.; Al-Suhaimi, E.A.; Wahid, F.; Shehzad, O.; Shehzad, A. Therapeutic potential of curcumin for multiple sclerosis. *Neurol. Sci* **2018**, *39*, 207–214. [CrossRef] [PubMed]
46. Abdolahi, M.; Tafakhori, A.; Togha, M.; Okhovat, A.A.; Siassi, F.; Eshraghian, M.R.; Sedighiyan, M.; Djalali, M.; Honarvar, N.M.; Djalali, M. The synergistic effects of ω-3 fatty acids and nano-curcumin supplementation on tumor necrosis factor (TNF)-α gene expression and serum level in migraine patients. *Immunogenetics* **2017**, *69*, 371–378. [CrossRef] [PubMed]
47. Bulboacă, A.E.; Bolboacă, S.D.; Stănescu, I.C.; Sfrângeu, C.A.; Porfire, A.; Tefas, L.; Bulboacă, A.C. The effect of intravenous administration of liposomal curcumin in addition to sumatriptan treatment in an experimental migraine model in rats. *Int. J. Nanomed.* **2018**, *13*, 3093. [CrossRef]
48. He, Q.; Jiang, L.; Man, S.; Wu, L.; Hu, Y.; Chen, W. Curcumin reduces neuronal loss and inhibits the NLRP3 inflammasome activation in an epileptic rat model. *Curr. Neurovasc. Res.* **2018**, *15*, 186–192. [CrossRef]
49. Drion, C.; van Scheppingen, J.; Arena, A.; Geijtenbeek, K.; Kooijman, L.; van Vliet, E.; Aronica, E.; Gorter, J. Effects of rapamycin and curcumin on inflammation and oxidative stress in vitro and in vivo—In search of potential anti-epileptogenic strategies for temporal lobe epilepsy. *J. Neuroinflamm.* **2018**, *15*, 212. [CrossRef]
50. Kalani, A.; Kamat, P.K.; Kalani, K.; Tyagi, N. Epigenetic impact of curcumin on stroke prevention. *Metab. Brain Dis.* **2015**, *30*, 427–435. [CrossRef]
51. Lan, C.; Chen, X.; Zhang, Y.; Wang, W.; Wang, W.E.; Liu, Y.; Cai, Y.; Ren, H.; Zheng, S.; Zhou, L. Curcumin prevents strokes in stroke-prone spontaneously hypertensive rats by improving vascular endothelial function. *BMC Cardiovasc. Disord.* **2018**, *18*, 43. [CrossRef]
52. Dong, W.; Yang, B.; Wang, L.; Li, B.; Guo, X.; Zhang, M.; Jiang, Z.; Fu, J.; Pi, J.; Guan, D. Curcumin plays neuroprotective roles against traumatic brain injury partly via Nrf2 signaling. *Toxicol. Appl. Pharmacol.* **2018**, *346*, 28–36. [CrossRef]

53. Laird, M.D.; Sukumari-Ramesh, S.; Swift, A.E.B.; Meiler, S.E.; Vender, J.R.; Dhandapani, K.M. Curcumin attenuates cerebral edema following traumatic brain injury in mice: A possible role for aquaporin-4? *J. Neurochem.* **2010**, *113*, 637–648. [CrossRef] [PubMed]
54. Requejo-Aguilar, R.; Alastrue-Agudo, A.; Cases-Villar, M.; Lopez-Mocholi, E.; England, R.; Vicent, M.J.; Moreno-Manzano, V. Combined polymer-curcumin conjugate and ependymal progenitor/stem cell treatment enhances spinal cord injury functional recovery. *Biomaterials* **2017**, *113*, 18–30. [CrossRef] [PubMed]
55. Aggarwal, B.B. Targeting inflammation-induced obesity and metabolic diseases by curcumin and other nutraceuticals. *Annu. Rev. Nutr.* **2010**, *30*, 173–199. [CrossRef] [PubMed]
56. Acar, A.; Akil, E.; Alp, H.; Evliyaoglu, O.; Kibrisli, E.; Inal, A.; Unan, F.; Tasdemir, N. Oxidative damage is ameliorated by curcumin treatment in brain and sciatic nerve of diabetic rats. *Int. J. Neurosci.* **2012**, *122*, 367–372. [CrossRef] [PubMed]
57. Babu, A.; Mohammed, S.; Harikumar, K. Antioxidant Properties of Curcumin: Impact on Neurological Disorders. In *Curcumin for Neurological and Psychiatric Disorders*; Elsevier: London, UK, 2019; pp. 155–167.
58. Tang, Y.; Chen, A. Curcumin eliminates the effect of advanced glycation end-products (AGEs) on the divergent regulation of gene expression of receptors of AGEs by interrupting leptin signaling. *Lab. Investig.* **2014**, *94*, 503. [CrossRef] [PubMed]
59. Paul, S.; Mahanta, S. Association of heat-shock proteins in various neurodegenerative disorders: Is it a master key to open the therapeutic door? *Mol. Cell. Biochem.* **2014**, *386*, 45–61. [CrossRef] [PubMed]
60. Surh, Y.-J.; Chun, K.-S.; Cha, H.-H.; Han, S.S.; Keum, Y.-S.; Park, K.-K.; Lee, S.S. Molecular mechanisms underlying chemopreventive activities of anti-inflammatory phytochemicals: Down-regulation of COX-2 and iNOS through suppression of NF-κB activation. *Mutat. Res. Fundament. Mol. Mech. Mutagen.* **2001**, *480*, 243–268. [CrossRef]
61. Armstrong, R.A. Plaques and tangles and the pathogenesis of Alzheimer's disease. *Folia Neuropathol.* **2006**, *44*.
62. Tang, M.; Taghibiglou, C. The mechanisms of action of curcumin in Alzheimer's disease. *J. Alzheimers Dis.* **2017**, *58*, 1003–1016. [CrossRef]
63. Schneider, L.S.; Mangialasche, F.; Andreasen, N.; Feldman, H.; Giacobini, E.; Jones, R.; Mantua, V.; Mecocci, P.; Pani, L.; Winblad, B. Clinical trials and late-stage drug development for Alzheimer's disease: An appraisal from 1984 to 2014. *J. Intern. Med.* **2014**, *275*, 251–283. [CrossRef]
64. Nakia, B.; Tony, B. Alzheimer's disease and the neuroprotective effects of dietary curcumin. *J. Psychol. Clin. Psychiatry* **2016**, *6*, 00354.
65. Chandra, V.; Pandav, R.; Dodge, H.; Johnston, J.; Belle, S.; DeKosky, S.; Ganguli, M. Incidence of Alzheimer's disease in a rural community in India: The Indo–US study. *Neurology* **2001**, *57*, 985–989. [CrossRef] [PubMed]
66. Vas, C.J.; Pinto, C.; Panikker, D.; Noronha, S.; Deshpande, N.; Kulkarni, L.; Sachdeva, S. Prevalence of dementia in an urban Indian population. *Int. Psychogeriatr.* **2001**, *13*, 439–450. [CrossRef] [PubMed]
67. Yanagisawa, D.; Shirai, N.; Amatsubo, T.; Taguchi, H.; Hirao, K.; Urushitani, M.; Morikawa, S.; Inubushi, T.; Kato, M.; Kato, F. Relationship between the tautomeric structures of curcumin derivatives and their Aβ-binding activities in the context of therapies for Alzheimer's disease. *Biomaterials* **2010**, *31*, 4179–4185. [CrossRef]
68. Zhang, X.; Tian, Y.; Li, Z.; Tian, X.; Sun, H.; Liu, H.; Moore, A.; Ran, C. Design and synthesis of curcumin analogues for in vivo fluorescence imaging and inhibiting copper-induced cross-linking of amyloid beta species in Alzheimer's disease. *J. Am. Chem. Soc.* **2013**, *135*, 16397–16409. [CrossRef]
69. Zheng, K.; Dai, X.; Wu, X.; Wei, Z.; Fang, W.; Zhu, Y.; Zhang, J.; Chen, X. Curcumin ameliorates memory decline via inhibiting BACE1 expression and β-Amyloid pathology in 5× FAD transgenic mice. *Mol. Neurobiol.* **2017**, *54*, 1967–1977. [CrossRef]
70. Xiong, Z.; Hongmei, Z.; Lu, S.; Yu, L. Curcumin mediates presenilin-1 activity to reduce β-amyloid production in a model of Alzheimer's disease. *Pharmacol. Rep.* **2011**, *63*, 1101–1108. [CrossRef]
71. Reinke, A.A.; Gestwicki, J.E. Structure–activity Relationships of amyloid beta-aggregation inhibitors based on curcumin: Influence of linker length and flexibility. *Chem. Biol. Drug Des.* **2007**, *70*, 206–215. [CrossRef]
72. Thapa, A.; Vernon, B.C.; De la Peña, K.; Soliz, G.; Moreno, H.A.; López, G.P.; Chi, E.Y. Membrane-mediated neuroprotection by curcumin from amyloid-β-peptide-induced toxicity. *Langmuir* **2013**, *29*, 11713–11723. [CrossRef]
73. Cai, H.-Y.; Yang, J.-T.; Wang, Z.-J.; Zhang, J.; Yang, W.; Wu, M.-N.; Qi, J.-S. Lixisenatide reduces amyloid plaques, neurofibrillary tangles and neuroinflammation in an APP/PS1/tau mouse model of Alzheimer's disease. *Biochem. Biophys. Res. Commun.* **2018**, *495*, 1034–1040. [CrossRef]

74. Guillozet-Bongaarts, A.L.; Garcia-Sierra, F.; Reynolds, M.R.; Horowitz, P.M.; Fu, Y.; Wang, T.; Cahill, M.E.; Bigio, E.H.; Berry, R.W.; Binder, L.I. Tau truncation during neurofibrillary tangle evolution in Alzheimer's disease. *Neurobiol. Aging* **2005**, *26*, 1015–1022. [CrossRef]
75. Wegmann, S.; Bennett, R.E.; Delorme, L.; Robbins, A.B.; Hu, M.; McKenzie, D.; Kirk, M.J.; Schiantarelli, J.; Tunio, N.; Amaral, A.C. Experimental evidence for the age dependence of tau protein spread in the brain. *Sci. Adv.* **2019**, *5*, eaaw6404. [CrossRef] [PubMed]
76. Patil, S.P.; Tran, N.; Geekiyanage, H.; Liu, L.; Chan, C. Curcumin-induced upregulation of the anti-tau cochaperone BAG2 in primary rat cortical neurons. *Neurosci. Lett.* **2013**, *554*, 121–125. [CrossRef] [PubMed]
77. Huang, H.-C.; Tang, D.; Xu, K.; Jiang, Z.-F. Curcumin attenuates amyloid-β-induced tau hyperphosphorylation in human neuroblastoma SH-SY5Y cells involving PTEN/Akt/GSK-3β signaling pathway. *J. Recept. Signal Transduct.* **2014**, *34*, 26–37. [CrossRef] [PubMed]
78. Liu, B.; Hong, J.-S. Role of microglia in inflammation-mediated neurodegenerative diseases: Mechanisms and strategies for therapeutic intervention. *J. Pharmacol. Exp. Ther.* **2003**, *304*, 1–7. [CrossRef]
79. Walker, D.G.; Lue, L.-F. Immune phenotypes of microglia in human neurodegenerative disease: Challenges to detecting microglial polarization in human brains. *Alzheimers Res. Ther.* **2015**, *7*, 56. [CrossRef]
80. Haque, M.E.; Kim, I.-S.; Jakaria, M.; Akther, M.; Choi, D.-K. Importance of GPCR-Mediated Microglial Activation in Alzheimer's Disease. *Front. Cell. Neurosci.* **2018**, *12*. [CrossRef]
81. Shi, X.; Zheng, Z.; Li, J.; Xiao, Z.; Qi, W.; Zhang, A.; Wu, Q.; Fang, Y. Curcumin inhibits Aβ-induced microglial inflammatory responses in vitro: Involvement of ERK1/2 and p38 signaling pathways. *Neurosci. Lett.* **2015**, *594*, 105–110. [CrossRef]
82. Porro, C.; Cianciulli, A.; Trotta, T.; Lofrumento, D.D.; Panaro, M.A. Curcumin Regulates Anti-Inflammatory Responses by JAK/STAT/SOCS Signaling Pathway in BV-2 Microglial Cells. *Biology* **2019**, *8*, 51. [CrossRef]
83. Liu, Z.-J.; Li, Z.-H.; Liu, L.; Tang, W.-X.; Wang, Y.; Dong, M.-R.; Xiao, C. Curcumin attenuates beta-amyloid-induced neuroinflammation via activation of peroxisome proliferator-activated receptor-gamma function in a rat model of Alzheimer's disease. *Front. Pharmacol.* **2016**, *7*, 261. [CrossRef]
84. Zhang, L.; Fiala, M.; Cashman, J.; Sayre, J.; Espinosa, A.; Mahanian, M.; Zaghi, J.; Badmaev, V.; Graves, M.C.; Bernard, G.; et al. Curcuminoids enhance amyloid-β uptake by macrophages of Alzheimer's disease patients. *J. Alzheimers Dis.* **2006**, *10*, 1–7. [CrossRef] [PubMed]
85. Tsatsakis, A.; Docea, A.O.; Calina, D.; Tsarouhas, K.; Zamfira, L.-M.; Mitrut, R.; Sharifi-Rad, J.; Kovatsi, L.; Siokas, V.; Dardiotis, E. A mechanistic and pathophysiological approach for stroke associated with drugs of abuse. *J. Clin. Med.* **2019**, *8*, 1295. [CrossRef] [PubMed]
86. Collins, L.M.; Toulouse, A.; Connor, T.J.; Nolan, Y.M. Contributions of central and systemic inflammation to the pathophysiology of Parkinson's disease. *Neuropharmacology* **2012**, *62*, 2154–2168. [CrossRef] [PubMed]
87. Stephenson, J.; Nutma, E.; van der Valk, P.; Amor, S. Inflammation in CNS neurodegenerative diseases. *Immunology* **2018**, *154*, 204–219. [CrossRef]
88. Padureanu, R.; Albu, C.V.; Mititelu, R.R.; Bacanoiu, M.V.; Docea, A.O.; Calina, D.; Padureanu, V.; Olaru, G.; Sandu, R.E.; Malin, R.D. Oxidative Stress and Inflammation Interdependence in Multiple Sclerosis. *J. Clin. Med.* **2019**, *8*, 1815. [CrossRef]
89. Tarafdar, A.; Pula, G. The role of NADPH oxidases and oxidative stress in neurodegenerative disorders. *Int. J. Mol. Sci.* **2018**, *19*, 3824. [CrossRef]
90. Hsieh, H.-L.; Yang, C.-M. Role of redox signaling in neuroinflammation and neurodegenerative diseases. *BioMed Res. Int.* **2013**, *2013*. [CrossRef]
91. Mosley, R.L.; Benner, E.J.; Kadiu, I.; Thomas, M.; Boska, M.D.; Hasan, K.; Laurie, C.; Gendelman, H.E. Neuroinflammation, oxidative stress, and the pathogenesis of Parkinson's disease. *Clin. Neurosci. Res.* **2006**, *6*, 261–281. [CrossRef]
92. Von Bernhardi, R.; Eugenin, J. Alzheimer's disease: Redox dysregulation as a common denominator for diverse pathogenic mechanisms. *Antioxid. Redox Signal.* **2012**, *16*, 974–1031. [CrossRef]
93. Ak, T.; Gülçin, İ. Antioxidant and radical scavenging properties of curcumin. *Chem. Biol. Interact.* **2008**, *174*, 27–37. [CrossRef]
94. Abrahams, S.; Haylett, W.L.; Johnson, G.; Carr, J.A.; Bardien, S. Antioxidant Effects of Curcumin in Models of Neurodegeneration, Ageing, Oxidative and NITROSATIVE Stress: A Review. *Neuroscience* **2019**. [CrossRef] [PubMed]

95. Gibellini, L.; Bianchini, E.; De Biasi, S.; Nasi, M.; Cossarizza, A.; Pinti, M. Natural compounds modulating mitochondrial functions. *Evid. Based Complementary Altern. Med.* **2015**, *2015*. [CrossRef] [PubMed]
96. Trujillo, J.; Granados-Castro, L.F.; Zazueta, C.; Andérica-Romero, A.C.; Chirino, Y.I.; Pedraza-Chaverrí, J. Mitochondria as a target in the therapeutic properties of curcumin. *Arch. Pharm.* **2014**, *347*, 873–884. [CrossRef] [PubMed]
97. Nawab, A.; Li, G.; Liu, W.; Lan, R.; Wu, J.; Zhao, Y.; Kang, K.; Kieser, B.; Sun, C.; Tang, S. Effect of Dietary Curcumin on the Antioxidant Status of Laying Hens under High-Temperature Conditions. *Braz. J. Poult. Sci.* **2019**, *21*. [CrossRef]
98. Nussbaum, L.; Hogea, L.M.; Călina, D.; Andreescu, N.; Grădinaru, R.; Ștefănescu, R.; Puiu, M. Modern treatment approaches in psychoses. Pharmacogenetic, neuroimagistic and clinical implications. *Farmacia* **2017**, *65*, 75–81.
99. Buga, A.-M.; Docea, A.O.; Albu, C.; Malin, R.D.; Branisteanu, D.E.; Ianosi, G.; Ianosi, S.L.; Iordache, A.; Calina, D. Molecular and cellular stratagem of brain metastases associated with melanoma. *Oncol. Lett.* **2019**, *17*, 4170–4175. [CrossRef]
100. Xu, Y.; Quinn, C.C. Transition between synaptic branch formation and synaptogenesis is regulated by the lin-4 microRNA. *Dev. Biol.* **2016**, *420*, 60–66. [CrossRef]
101. Sarnat, H.B.; Flores-Sarnat, L. Precocious and delayed neocortical synaptogenesis in fetal holoprosencephaly. *Clin. Neuropathol.* **2013**, *32*, 255–268. [CrossRef]
102. Dubourg, C.; Carré, W.; Hamdi-Rozé, H.; Mouden, C.; Roume, J.; Abdelmajid, B.; Amram, D.; Baumann, C.; Chassaing, N.; Coubes, C. Mutational spectrum in holoprosencephaly shows that FGF is a new major signaling pathway. *Hum. Mutat.* **2016**, *37*, 1329–1339. [CrossRef]
103. Dabrowski, A.; Terauchi, A.; Strong, C.; Umemori, H. Distinct sets of FGF receptors sculpt excitatory and inhibitory synaptogenesis. *Development* **2015**, *142*, 1818–1830. [CrossRef]
104. Gupta, S.C.; Prasad, S.; Kim, J.H.; Patchva, S.; Webb, L.J.; Priyadarsini, I.K.; Aggarwal, B.B. Multitargeting by curcumin as revealed by molecular interaction studies. *Nat. Prod. Rep.* **2011**, *28*, 1937–1955. [CrossRef] [PubMed]
105. Dong, S.; Zeng, Q.; Mitchell, E.S.; Xiu, J.; Duan, Y.; Li, C.; Tiwari, J.K.; Hu, Y.; Cao, X.; Zhao, Z. Curcumin enhances neurogenesis and cognition in aged rats: Implications for transcriptional interactions related to growth and synaptic plasticity. *PLoS ONE* **2012**, *7*, e31211. [CrossRef] [PubMed]
106. Cole, G.M.; Teter, B.; Frautschy, S.A. Neuroprotective effects of curcumin. In *The Molecular Targets and Therapeutic Uses of Curcumin in Health and Disease*; Springer: Boston, MA, USA, 2007; pp. 197–212.
107. Zatta, P.; Drago, D.; Bolognin, S.; Sensi, S.L. Alzheimer's disease, metal ions and metal homeostatic therapy. *Trends Pharmacol. Sci.* **2009**, *30*, 346–355. [CrossRef] [PubMed]
108. Wanninger, S.; Lorenz, V.; Subhan, A.; Edelmann, F.T. Metal complexes of curcumin–synthetic strategies, structures and medicinal applications. *Chem. Soc. Rev.* **2015**, *44*, 4986–5002. [CrossRef]
109. Shehzad, A.; Islam, S.U.; Lee, Y.S. Curcumin and Inflammatory Brain Diseases. In *Curcumin for Neurological and Psychiatric Disorders*; Elsevier: London, UK, 2019; pp. 437–458.
110. Berk, Z. Chapter 11—Extraction. In *Food Process Engineering and Technology*, 3rd ed.; Berk, Z., Ed.; Elsevier: London, UK, 2018; pp. 289–310.
111. Mandal, V.; Dewanjee, S.; Sahu, R.; Mandal, S.C. Design and optimization of ultrasound assisted extraction of curcumin as an effective alternative for conventional solid liquid extraction of natural products. *Nat. Prod. Commun.* **2009**, *4*, 95–100. [CrossRef]
112. Moghtaderi, H.; Sepehri, H.; Attari, F. Combination of arabinogalactan and curcumin induces apoptosis in breast cancer cells in vitro and inhibits tumor growth via overexpression of p53 level in vivo. *Biomed. Pharmacother.* **2017**, *88*, 582–594. [CrossRef]
113. Padhye, S.; Chavan, D.; Pandey, S.; Deshpande, J.; Swamy, K.V.; Sarkar, F.H. Perspectives on chemopreventive and therapeutic potential of curcumin analogs in medicinal chemistry. *Mini Rev. Med. Chem.* **2010**, *10*, 372–387. [CrossRef]
114. Stagos, D.; Amoutzias, G.D.; Matakos, A.; Spyrou, A.; Tsatsakis, A.M.; Kouretas, D. Chemoprevention of liver cancer by plant polyphenols. *Food Chem. Toxicol.* **2012**, *50*, 2155–2170. [CrossRef]
115. Kakarala, M.; Brenner, D.E.; Korkaya, H.; Cheng, C.; Tazi, K.; Ginestier, C.; Liu, S.; Dontu, G.; Wicha, M.S. Targeting breast stem cells with the cancer preventive compounds curcumin and piperine. *Breast Cancer Res. Treat.* **2010**, *122*, 777–785. [CrossRef]

116. Cioboată, R.; Găman, A.; Traşcă, D.; Ungureanu, A.; Docea, A.O.; Tomescu, P.; Gherghina, F.; Arsene, A.L.; Badiu, C.; Tsatsakis, A.M.; et al. Pharmacological management of non-alcoholic fatty liver disease: Atorvastatin versus pentoxifylline. *Exp. Ther. Med.* **2017**, *13*, 2375–2381. [CrossRef]
117. Wojciechowski, V.V.; Calina, D.; Tsarouhas, K.; Pivnik, A.V.; Sergievich, A.A.; Kodintsev, V.V.; Filatova, E.A.; Ozcagli, E.; Docea, A.O.; Arsene, A.L.; et al. A guide to acquired vitamin K coagulophathy diagnosis and treatment: The Russian perspective. *DARU J. Pharm. Sci.* **2017**, *25*, 10. [CrossRef] [PubMed]
118. Oyemitan, I.A.; Elusiyan, C.A.; Onifade, A.O.; Akanmu, M.A.; Oyedeji, A.O.; McDonald, A.G. Neuropharmacological profile and chemical analysis of fresh rhizome essential oil of Curcuma longa (turmeric) cultivated in Southwest Nigeria. *Toxicol. Rep.* **2017**, *4*, 391–398. [CrossRef] [PubMed]
119. Zhou, H.; Beevers, C.S.; Huang, S. The targets of curcumin. *Curr. Drug Targets* **2011**, *12*, 332–347. [CrossRef] [PubMed]
120. Wahlang, B.; Pawar, Y.B.; Bansal, A.K. Identification of permeability-related hurdles in oral delivery of curcumin using the Caco-2 cell model. *Eur. J. Pharm. Biopharm.* **2011**, *77*, 275–282. [CrossRef] [PubMed]
121. Anand, P.; Kunnumakkara, A.B.; Newman, R.A.; Aggarwal, B.B. Bioavailability of curcumin: Problems and promises. *Mol. Pharm.* **2007**, *4*, 807–818. [CrossRef] [PubMed]
122. Kidd, P.M. Bioavailability and activity of phytosome complexes from botanical polyphenols: The silymarin, curcumin, green tea, and grape seed extracts. *Altern. Med. Rev.* **2009**, *14*, 226–246.
123. Maiti, K.; Mukherjee, K.; Gantait, A.; Saha, B.P.; Mukherjee, P.K. Curcumin-phospholipid complex: Preparation, therapeutic evaluation and pharmacokinetic study in rats. *Int. J. Pharm.* **2007**, *330*, 155–163. [CrossRef]
124. Marczylo, T.H.; Verschoyle, R.D.; Cooke, D.N.; Morazzoni, P.; Steward, W.P.; Gescher, A.J. Comparison of systemic availability of curcumin with that of curcumin formulated with phosphatidylcholine. *Cancer Chemother. Pharmacol.* **2007**, *60*, 171–177. [CrossRef]
125. Tsatsakis, A.; Stratidakis, A.K.; Goryachaya, A.V.; Tzatzarakis, M.N.; Stivaktakis, P.D.; Docea, A.O.; Berdiaki, A.; Nikitovic, D.; Velonia, K.; Shtilman, M.I.; et al. In vitro blood compatibility and in vitro cytotoxicity of amphiphilic poly-N-vinylpyrrolidone nanoparticles. *Food Chem. Toxicol.* **2019**, *127*, 42–52. [CrossRef]
126. Bhawana; Basniwal, R.K.; Buttar, H.S.; Jain, V.K.; Jain, N. Curcumin nanoparticles: Preparation, characterization, and antimicrobial study. *J. Agric. Food Chem.* **2011**, *59*, 2056–2061. [CrossRef]
127. Bisht, S.; Feldmann, G.; Soni, S.; Ravi, R.; Karikar, C.; Maitra, A.; Maitra, A. Polymeric nanoparticle-encapsulated curcumin ("nanocurcumin"): A novel strategy for human cancer therapy. *J. Nanobiotechnology.* **2007**, *5*, 3. [CrossRef] [PubMed]
128. Tonnesen, H.H.; Masson, M.; Loftsson, T. Studies of curcumin and curcuminoids. XXVII. Cyclodextrin complexation: Solubility, chemical and photochemical stability. *Int. J. Pharm.* **2002**, *244*, 127–135. [CrossRef]
129. Paolino, D.; Vero, A.; Cosco, D.; Pecora, T.M.; Cianciolo, S.; Fresta, M.; Pignatello, R. Improvement of Oral Bioavailability of Curcumin upon Microencapsulation with Methacrylic Copolymers. *Front. Pharmacol.* **2016**, *7*, 485. [CrossRef] [PubMed]
130. Mourtas, S.; Lazar, A.N.; Markoutsa, E.; Duyckaerts, C.; Antimisiaris, S.G. Multifunctional nanoliposomes with curcumin-lipid derivative and brain targeting functionality with potential applications for Alzheimer disease. *Eur. J. Med. Chem.* **2014**, *80*, 175–183. [CrossRef]
131. Li, L.; Braiteh, F.S.; Kurzrock, R. Liposome-encapsulated curcumin: In vitro and in vivo effects on proliferation, apoptosis, signaling, and angiogenesis. *Cancer* **2005**, *104*, 1322–1331. [CrossRef] [PubMed]
132. Ross, C.; Taylor, M.; Fullwood, N.; Allsop, D. Liposome delivery systems for the treatment of Alzheimer's disease. *Int. J. Nanomed.* **2018**, *13*, 8507–8522. [CrossRef] [PubMed]
133. Zhao, L.; Du, J.; Duan, Y.; Zang, Y.; Zhang, H.; Yang, C.; Cao, F.; Zhai, G. Curcumin loaded mixed micelles composed of Pluronic P123 and F68: Preparation, optimization and in vitro characterization. *Colloids Surf. B Biointerfaces* **2012**, *97*, 101–108. [CrossRef] [PubMed]
134. Lin, C.C.; Lin, H.Y.; Chi, M.H.; Shen, C.M.; Chen, H.W.; Yang, W.J.; Lee, M.H. Preparation of curcumin microemulsions with food-grade soybean oil/lecithin and their cytotoxicity on the HepG2 cell line. *Food Chem.* **2014**, *154*, 282–290. [CrossRef] [PubMed]
135. Teixeira, C.C.; Mendonca, L.M.; Bergamaschi, M.M.; Queiroz, R.H.; Souza, G.E.; Antunes, L.M.; Freitas, L.A. Microparticles Containing Curcumin Solid Dispersion: Stability, Bioavailability and Anti-Inflammatory Activity. *AAPS PharmSciTech* **2016**, *17*, 252–261. [CrossRef]

136. Parikh, A.; Kathawala, K.; Li, J.; Chen, C.; Shan, Z.; Cao, X.; Zhou, X.F.; Garg, S. Curcumin-loaded self-nanomicellizing solid dispersion system: Part II: In vivo safety and efficacy assessment against behavior deficit in Alzheimer disease. *Drug Deliv. Transl. Res.* **2018**, *8*, 1406–1420. [CrossRef]
137. Vaz, G.R.; Hadrich, G.; Bidone, J.; Rodrigues, J.L.; Falkembach, M.C.; Putaux, J.L.; Hort, M.A.; Monserrat, J.M.; Varela Junior, A.S.; Teixeira, H.F.; et al. Development of Nasal Lipid Nanocarriers Containing Curcumin for Brain Targeting. *J. Alzheimers Dis.* **2017**, *59*, 961–974. [CrossRef] [PubMed]
138. Del Prado-Audelo, M.L.; Magaña, J.J.; Mejía-Contreras, B.A.; Borbolla-Jiménez, F.V.; Giraldo-Gomez, D.M.; Piña-Barba, M.C.; Quintanar-Guerrero, D.; Leyva-Gómez, G. In vitro cell uptake evaluation of curcumin-loaded PCL/F68 nanoparticles for potential application in neuronal diseases. *J. Drug Deliv. Sci. Technol.* **2019**, *52*, 905–914. [CrossRef]
139. Wang, Z.H.; Wang, Z.Y.; Sun, C.S.; Wang, C.Y.; Jiang, T.Y.; Wang, S.L. Trimethylated chitosan-conjugated PLGA nanoparticles for the delivery of drugs to the brain. *Biomaterials* **2010**, *31*, 908–915. [CrossRef] [PubMed]
140. Pinzaru, I.; Coricovac, D.; Dehelean, C.; Moacă, E.-A.; Mioc, M.; Baderca, F.; Sizemore, I.; Brittle, S.; Marti, D.; Calina, C.D.; et al. Stable PEG-coated silver nanoparticles—A comprehensive toxicological profile. *Food Chem. Toxicol.* **2018**, *111*, 546–556. [CrossRef] [PubMed]
141. Marin, E.; Briceno, M.I.; Torres, A.; Caballero-George, C. New Curcumin-Loaded Chitosan Nanocapsules: In Vivo Evaluation. *Planta Med.* **2017**, *83*, 877–883. [CrossRef] [PubMed]
142. Kalani, A.; Chaturvedi, P. Curcumin-primed and curcumin-loaded exosomes: Potential neural therapy. *Neural Regen. Res.* **2017**, *12*, 205. [CrossRef] [PubMed]
143. Wang, H.; Sui, H.; Zheng, Y.; Jiang, Y.; Shi, Y.; Liang, J.; Zhao, L. Curcumin-primed exosomes potently ameliorate cognitive function in AD mice by inhibiting hyperphosphorylation of the Tau protein through the AKT/GSK-3β pathway. *Nanoscale* **2019**, *11*, 7481–7496. [CrossRef]
144. Cheng, K.K.; Chan, P.S.; Fan, S.; Kwan, S.M.; Yeung, K.L.; Wang, Y.X.; Chow, A.H.; Wu, E.X.; Baum, L. Curcumin-conjugated magnetic nanoparticles for detecting amyloid plaques in Alzheimer's disease mice using magnetic resonance imaging (MRI). *Biomaterials* **2015**, *44*, 155–172. [CrossRef]
145. Huo, X.; Zhang, Y.; Jin, X.; Li, Y.; Zhang, L. A novel synthesis of selenium nanoparticles encapsulated PLGA nanospheres with curcumin molecules for the inhibition of amyloid beta aggregation in Alzheimer's disease. *J. Photochem. Photobiol. B* **2019**, *190*, 98–102. [CrossRef]
146. Blanco, E.; Shen, H.; Ferrari, M. Principles of nanoparticle design for overcoming biological barriers to drug delivery. *Nat. Biotechnol.* **2015**, *33*, 941–951. [CrossRef]
147. Henrich-Noack, P.; Nikitovic, D.; Neagu, M.; Docea, A.O.; Engin, A.B.; Gelperina, S.; Shtilman, M.; Mitsias, P.; Tzanakakis, G.; Gozes, I.; et al. The blood-brain barrier and beyond: Nano-based neuropharmacology and the role of extracellular matrix. *Nanomedicine* **2019**, *17*, 359–379. [CrossRef] [PubMed]
148. Garcia-Alloza, M.; Borrelli, L.A.; Rozkalne, A.; Hyman, B.T.; Bacskai, B.J. Curcumin labels amyloid pathology in vivo, disrupts existing plaques, and partially restores distorted neurites in an Alzheimer mouse model. *J. Neurochem.* **2007**, *102*, 1095–1104. [CrossRef]
149. Tosi, G.; Pederzoli, F.; Belletti, D.; Vandelli, M.A.; Forni, F.; Duskey, J.T.; Ruozi, B. Chapter 2—Nanomedicine in Alzheimer's disease: Amyloid beta targeting strategy. In *Nanoneuroprotection and Nanoneurotoxicology*; Sharma, H.S., Aruna, S., Eds.; Elsevier: London, UK, 2019; Volume 245.
150. Bukhari, S.N.; Jantan, I.; Masand, V.H.; Mahajan, D.T.; Sher, M.; Naeem-ul-Hassan, M.; Amjad, M.W. Synthesis of alpha, beta-unsaturated carbonyl based compounds as acetylcholinesterase and butyrylcholinesterase inhibitors: Characterization, molecular modeling, QSAR studies and effect against amyloid beta-induced cytotoxicity. *Eur. J. Med. Chem.* **2014**, *83*, 355–365. [CrossRef] [PubMed]
151. Si, G.; Zhou, S.; Xu, G.; Wang, J.; Wu, B.; Zhou, S. A curcumin-based NIR fluorescence probe for detection of amyloid-beta (Aβ) plaques in Alzheimer's disease. *Dyes Pigm.* **2019**, *163*, 509–515. [CrossRef]
152. Mishra, S.; Palanivelu, K. The effect of curcumin (turmeric) on Alzheimer's disease: An overview. *Ann. Indian Acad. Neurol.* **2008**, *11*, 13–19. [CrossRef] [PubMed]
153. Fan, Y.; Yi, J.; Zhang, Y.; Yokoyama, W. Fabrication of curcumin-loaded bovine serum albumin (BSA)-dextran nanoparticles and the cellular antioxidant activity. *Food Chem.* **2018**, *239*, 1210–1218. [CrossRef]
154. Nakagawa, Y.; Chiba, K. Diversity and plasticity of microglial cells in psychiatric and neurological disorders. *Pharmacol. Ther.* **2015**, *154*, 21–35. [CrossRef]

155. Fan, C.; Song, Q.; Wang, P.; Li, Y.; Yang, M.; Liu, B.; Yu, S.Y. Curcumin Protects Against Chronic Stress-induced Dysregulation of Neuroplasticity and Depression-like Behaviors via Suppressing IL-1beta Pathway in Rats. *Neuroscience* **2018**, *392*, 92–106. [CrossRef]
156. Hucklenbroich, J.; Klein, R.; Neumaier, B.; Graf, R.; Fink, G.R.; Schroeter, M.; Rueger, M.A. Aromatic-turmerone induces neural stem cell proliferation in vitro and in vivo. *Stem Cell Res. Ther.* **2014**, *5*, 100. [CrossRef]
157. Calsolaro, V.; Edison, P. Neuroinflammation in Alzheimer's disease: Current evidence and future directions. *Alzheimers Dement.* **2016**, *12*, 719–732. [CrossRef]
158. Yang, F.; Lim, G.P.; Begum, A.N.; Ubeda, O.J.; Simmons, M.R.; Ambegaokar, S.S.; Chen, P.P.; Kayed, R.; Glabe, C.G.; Frautschy, S.A.; et al. Curcumin inhibits formation of amyloid beta oligomers and fibrils, binds plaques, and reduces amyloid in vivo. *J. Biol. Chem.* **2005**, *280*, 5892–5901. [CrossRef] [PubMed]
159. Salehi, B.; Stojanovic-Radic, Z.; Matejic, J.; Sharifi-Rad, M.; Anil Kumar, N.V.; Martins, N.; Sharifi-Rad, J. The therapeutic potential of curcumin: A review of clinical trials. *Eur. J. Med. Chem.* **2019**, *163*, 527–545. [CrossRef] [PubMed]
160. Karunaweera, N.; Raju, R.; Gyengesi, E.; Munch, G. Plant polyphenols as inhibitors of NF-kappaB induced cytokine production-a potential anti-inflammatory treatment for Alzheimer's disease? *Front. Mol. Neurosci.* **2015**, *8*, 24. [CrossRef] [PubMed]
161. Jones, S.V.; Kounatidis, I. Nuclear Factor-Kappa B and Alzheimer Disease, Unifying Genetic and Environmental Risk Factors from Cell to Humans. *Front. Immunol.* **2017**, *8*, 1805. [CrossRef]
162. Xu, Y.; Ku, B.; Cui, L.; Li, X.; Barish, P.A.; Foster, T.C.; Ogle, W.O. Curcumin reverses impaired hippocampal neurogenesis and increases serotonin receptor 1A mRNA and brain-derived neurotrophic factor expression in chronically stressed rats. *Brain Res.* **2007**, *1162*, 9–18. [CrossRef]
163. Rainey-Smith, S.R.; Brown, B.M.; Sohrabi, H.R.; Shah, T.; Goozee, K.G.; Gupta, V.B.; Martins, R.N. Curcumin and cognition: A randomised, placebo-controlled, double-blind study of community-dwelling older adults. *Br. J. Nutr.* **2016**, *115*, 2106–2113. [CrossRef]
164. Small, G.W.; Siddarth, P.; Li, Z.; Miller, K.J.; Ercoli, L.; Emerson, N.D.; Martinez, J.; Wong, K.P.; Liu, J.; Merrill, D.A.; et al. Memory and Brain Amyloid and Tau Effects of a Bioavailable Form of Curcumin in Non-Demented Adults: A Double-Blind, Placebo-Controlled 18-Month Trial. *Am. J. Geriatr. Psychiatry.* **2018**, *26*, 266–277. [CrossRef]
165. Zhang, R.; Miller, R.G.; Madison, C.; Jin, X.; Honrada, R.; Harris, W.; Katz, J.; Forshew, D.A.; McGrath, M.S. Systemic immune system alterations in early stages of Alzheimer's disease. *J. Neuroimmunol.* **2013**, *256*, 38–42. [CrossRef]
166. Solito, E.; Sastre, M. Microglia function in Alzheimer's disease. *Front. Pharmacol.* **2012**, *3*, 14. [CrossRef]
167. Teter, B.; Morihara, T.; Lim, G.P.; Chu, T.; Jones, M.R.; Zuo, X.; Paul, R.M.; Frautschy, S.A.; Cole, G.M. Curcumin restores innate immune Alzheimer's disease risk gene expression to ameliorate Alzheimer pathogenesis. *Neurobiol. Dis.* **2019**, *127*, 432–448. [CrossRef]
168. Fiala, M.; Liu, P.T.; Espinosa-Jeffrey, A.; Rosenthal, M.J.; Bernard, G.; Ringman, J.M.; Sayre, J.; Zhang, L.; Zaghi, J.; Dejbakhsh, S.; et al. Innate immunity and transcription of MGAT-III and Toll-like receptors in Alzheimer's disease patients are improved by bisdemethoxycurcumin. *Proc. Natl. Acad. Sci. USA* **2007**, *104*, 12849–12854. [CrossRef] [PubMed]
169. Reglodi, D.; Renaud, J.; Tamas, A.; Tizabi, Y.; Socias, S.B.; Del-Bel, E.; Raisman-Vozari, R. Novel tactics for neuroprotection in Parkinson's disease: Role of antibiotics, polyphenols and neuropeptides. *Prog. Neurobiol.* **2017**, *155*, 120–148. [CrossRef] [PubMed]
170. Kundu, P.; Das, M.; Tripathy, K.; Sahoo, S.K. Delivery of Dual Drug Loaded Lipid Based Nanoparticles across the Blood-Brain Barrier Impart Enhanced Neuroprotection in a Rotenone Induced Mouse Model of Parkinson's Disease. *ACS Chem. Neurosci.* **2016**, *7*, 1658–1670. [CrossRef] [PubMed]
171. Dolati, S.; Babaloo, Z.; Jadidi-Niaragh, F.; Ayromlou, H.; Sadreddini, S.; Yousefi, M. Multiple sclerosis: Therapeutic applications of advancing drug delivery systems. *Biomed. Pharmacother.* **2017**, *86*, 343–353. [CrossRef] [PubMed]
172. Natarajan, C.; Bright, J.J. Curcumin inhibits experimental allergic encephalomyelitis by blocking IL-12 signaling through Janus kinase-STAT pathway in T lymphocytes. *J. Immunol.* **2002**, *168*, 6506–6513. [CrossRef] [PubMed]

173. Mohajeri, M.; Sadeghizadeh, M.; Najafi, F.; Javan, M. Polymerized nano-curcumin attenuates neurological symptoms in EAE model of multiple sclerosis through down regulation of inflammatory and oxidative processes and enhancing neuroprotection and myelin repair. *Neuropharmacology* **2015**, *99*, 156–167. [CrossRef]
174. Wang, Y.J.; Pan, M.H.; Cheng, A.L.; Lin, L.I.; Ho, Y.S.; Hsieh, C.Y.; Lin, J.K. Stability of curcumin in buffer solutions and characterization of its degradation products. *J. Pharm. Biomed. Anal.* **1997**, *15*, 1867–1876. [CrossRef]
175. Sharma, R.A.; Steward, W.P.; Gescher, A.J. Pharmacokinetics and pharmacodynamics of curcumin. In *The Molecular Targets and Therapeutic Uses of Curcumin in Health and Disease*; Aggarwal, B.B., Surh, Y.-J., Shishodia, S., Eds.; Springer: Boston, MA, USA, 2007; pp. 453–470. [CrossRef]
176. Sadegh Malvajerd, S.; Azadi, A.; Izadi, Z.; Kurd, M.; Dara, T.; Dibaei, M.; Sharif Zadeh, M.; Akbari Javar, H.; Hamidi, M. Brain Delivery of Curcumin Using Solid Lipid Nanoparticles and Nanostructured Lipid Carriers: Preparation, Optimization, and Pharmacokinetic Evaluation. *ACS Chem. Neurosci.* **2019**, *10*, 728–739. [CrossRef]
177. Lombardo, D.; Kiselev, M.A.; Caccamo, M.T. Smart Nanoparticles for Drug Delivery Application: Development of Versatile Nanocarrier Platforms in Biotechnology and Nanomedicine. *J. Nanomater.* **2019**, *2019*, 26. [CrossRef]
178. Tosi, G.; Costantino, L.; Ruozi, B.; Forni, F.; Vandelli, M.A. Polymeric nanoparticles for the drug delivery to the central nervous system. *Expert Opin. Drug Deliv.* **2008**, *5*, 155–174. [CrossRef]
179. Cai, Q.; Wang, L.; Deng, G.; Liu, J.; Chen, Q.; Chen, Z. Systemic delivery to central nervous system by engineered PLGA nanoparticles. *Am. J. Transl. Res.* **2016**, *8*, 749–764. [PubMed]
180. Tsai, Y.M.; Jan, W.C.; Chien, C.F.; Lee, W.C.; Lin, L.C.; Tsai, T.H. Optimised nano-formulation on the bioavailability of hydrophobic polyphenol, curcumin, in freely-moving rats. *Food Chem.* **2011**, *127*, 918–925. [CrossRef] [PubMed]
181. Tsai, Y.M.; Chien, C.F.; Lin, L.C.; Tsai, T.H. Curcumin and its nano-formulation: The kinetics of tissue distribution and blood-brain barrier penetration. *Int. J. Pharm.* **2011**, *416*, 331–338. [CrossRef] [PubMed]
182. Doggui, S.; Sahni, J.K.; Arseneault, M.; Dao, L.; Ramassamy, C. Neuronal uptake and neuroprotective effect of curcumin-loaded PLGA nanoparticles on the human SK-N-SH cell line. *J. Alzheimers Dis.* **2012**, *30*, 377–392. [CrossRef]
183. Djiokeng Paka, G.; Doggui, S.; Zaghmi, A.; Safar, R.; Dao, L.; Reisch, A.; Klymchenko, A.; Roullin, V.G.; Joubert, O.; Ramassamy, C. Neuronal Uptake and Neuroprotective Properties of Curcumin-Loaded Nanoparticles on SK-N-SH Cell Line: Role of Poly(lactide-co-glycolide) Polymeric Matrix Composition. *Mol. Pharm.* **2016**, *13*, 391–403. [CrossRef]
184. Mulik, R.S.; Monkkonen, J.; Juvonen, R.O.; Mahadik, K.R.; Paradkar, A.R. ApoE3 mediated polymeric nanoparticles containing curcumin: Apoptosis induced in vitro anticancer activity against neuroblastoma cells. *Int. J. Pharm.* **2012**, *437*, 29–41. [CrossRef]
185. Mulik, R.S.; Monkkonen, J.; Juvonen, R.O.; Mahadik, K.R.; Paradkar, A.R. ApoE3 mediated poly(butyl) cyanoacrylate nanoparticles containing curcumin: Study of enhanced activity of curcumin against beta amyloid induced cytotoxicity using in vitro cell culture model. *Mol. Pharm.* **2010**, *7*, 815–825. [CrossRef]
186. Karewicz, A.; Bielska, D.; Loboda, A.; Gzyl-Malcher, B.; Bednar, J.; Jozkowicz, A.; Dulak, J.; Nowakowska, M. Curcumin-containing liposomes stabilized by thin layers of chitosan derivatives. *Colloids Surf. B Biointerfaces* **2013**, *109*, 307–316. [CrossRef]
187. Yadav, A.; Lomash, V.; Samim, M.; Flora, S.J. Curcumin encapsulated in chitosan nanoparticles: A novel strategy for the treatment of arsenic toxicity. *Chem. Biol. Interact.* **2012**, *199*, 49–61. [CrossRef]
188. Yang, R.; Zheng, Y.; Wang, Q.; Zhao, L. Curcumin-loaded chitosan-bovine serum albumin nanoparticles potentially enhanced Abeta 42 phagocytosis and modulated macrophage polarization in Alzheimer's disease. *Nanoscale Res. Lett.* **2018**, *13*, 330. [CrossRef]
189. Chiappetta, D.A.; Sosnik, A. Poly(ethylene oxide)-poly(propylene oxide) block copolymer micelles as drug delivery agents: Improved hydrosolubility, stability and bioavailability of drugs. *Eur. J. Pharm. Biopharm.* **2007**, *66*, 303–317. [CrossRef] [PubMed]
190. Lombardo, D.; Munao, G.; Calandra, P.; Pasqua, L.; Caccamo, M.T. Evidence of pre-micellar aggregates in aqueous solution of amphiphilic PDMS-PEO block copolymer. *Phys. Chem. Chem. Phys.* **2019**, *21*, 11983–11991. [CrossRef] [PubMed]

191. Nance, E.A.; Woodworth, G.F.; Sailor, K.A.; Shih, T.Y.; Xu, Q.; Swaminathan, G.; Xiang, D.; Eberhart, C.; Hanes, J. A dense poly(ethylene glycol) coating improves penetration of large polymeric nanoparticles within brain tissue. *Sci. Transl. Med.* **2012**, *4*, 149ra119. [CrossRef]
192. Suk, J.S.; Xu, Q.; Kim, N.; Hanes, J.; Ensign, L.M. PEGylation as a strategy for improving nanoparticle-based drug and gene delivery. *Adv. Drug Deliv. Rev.* **2016**, *99*, 28–51. [CrossRef] [PubMed]
193. Joseph, A.; Wood, T.; Chen, C.-C.; Corry, K.; Snyder, J.M.; Juul, S.E.; Parikh, P.; Nance, E. Curcumin-loaded polymeric nanoparticles for neuroprotection in neonatal rats with hypoxic-ischemic encephalopathy. *Nano Res.* **2018**, *11*, 5670–5688. [CrossRef]
194. Song, Z.; Feng, R.; Sun, M.; Guo, C.; Gao, Y.; Li, L.; Zhai, G. Curcumin-loaded PLGA-PEG-PLGA triblock copolymeric micelles: Preparation, pharmacokinetics and distribution in vivo. *J. Colloid Interface Sci.* **2011**, *354*, 116–123. [CrossRef]
195. Mathew, A.; Fukuda, T.; Nagaoka, Y.; Hasumura, T.; Morimoto, H.; Yoshida, Y.; Maekawa, T.; Venugopal, K.; Kumar, D.S. Curcumin loaded-PLGA nanoparticles conjugated with Tet-1 peptide for potential use in Alzheimer's disease. *PLoS ONE* **2012**, *7*, e32616. [CrossRef]
196. Paka, G.D.; Ramassamy, C. Optimization of Curcumin-Loaded PEG-PLGA Nanoparticles by GSH Functionalization: Investigation of the Internalization Pathway in Neuronal Cells. *Mol. Pharm.* **2017**, *14*, 93–106. [CrossRef]
197. Huang, N.; Lu, S.; Liu, X.G.; Zhu, J.; Wang, Y.J.; Liu, R.T. PLGA nanoparticles modified with a BBB-penetrating peptide co-delivering Abeta generation inhibitor and curcumin attenuate memory deficits and neuropathology in Alzheimer's disease mice. *Oncotarget* **2017**, *8*, 81001–81013. [CrossRef]
198. Ebrahim Attia, A.B.; Ong, Z.Y.; Hedrick, J.L.; Lee, P.P.; Ee, P.L.R.; Hammond, P.T.; Yang, Y.-Y. Mixed micelles self-assembled from block copolymers for drug delivery. *Curr. Opin. Colloid Interface Sci.* **2011**, *16*, 182–194. [CrossRef]
199. Ji, S.; Lin, X.; Yu, E.; Dian, C.; Yan, X.; Li, L.; Zhang, M.; Zhao, W.; Dian, L. Curcumin-Loaded Mixed Micelles: Preparation, Characterization, and In Vitro Antitumor Activity. *J. Nanotechnol.* **2018**, *2018*, 9. [CrossRef]
200. Puri, A.; Loomis, K.; Smith, B.; Lee, J.H.; Yavlovich, A.; Heldman, E.; Blumenthal, R. Lipid-based nanoparticles as pharmaceutical drug carriers: From concepts to clinic. *Crit. Rev. Ther. Drug Carrier Syst.* **2009**, *26*, 523–580. [CrossRef] [PubMed]
201. Katsaras, J.; Gutberlet, T. *Lipid Bilayers. Structure and Interactions*; Springer: Berlin/Heidelberg, Germany, 2001. [CrossRef]
202. Kiselev, M.A.; Lombardo, D. Structural characterization in mixed lipid membrane systems by neutron and X-ray scattering. *Biochim. Biophys. Acta Gen. Subj.* **2017**, *1861*, 3700–3717. [CrossRef] [PubMed]
203. Lombardo, D.; Calandra, P.; Barreca, D.; Magazu, S.; Kiselev, M.A. Soft Interaction in Liposome Nanocarriers for Therapeutic Drug Delivery. *Nanomaterials* **2016**, *6*, 125. [CrossRef]
204. Mishra, V.; Bansal, K.K.; Verma, A.; Yadav, N.; Thakur, S.; Sudhakar, K.; Rosenholm, J.M. Solid Lipid Nanoparticles: Emerging Colloidal Nano Drug Delivery Systems. *Pharmaceutics* **2018**, *10*, 191. [CrossRef]
205. Khosa, A.; Reddi, S.; Saha, R.N. Nanostructured lipid carriers for site-specific drug delivery. *Biomed. Pharmacother.* **2018**, *103*, 598–613. [CrossRef]
206. Naseri, N.; Valizadeh, H.; Zakeri-Milani, P. Solid Lipid Nanoparticles and Nanostructured Lipid Carriers: Structure, Preparation and Application. *Adv. Pharm. Bull.* **2015**, *5*, 305–313. [CrossRef]
207. Gastaldi, L.; Battaglia, L.; Peira, E.; Chirio, D.; Muntoni, E.; Solazzi, I.; Gallarate, M.; Dosio, F. Solid lipid nanoparticles as vehicles of drugs to the brain: Current state of the art. *Eur. J. Pharm. Biopharm.* **2014**, *87*, 433–444. [CrossRef]
208. Ganesan, P.; Kim, B.; Ramalaingam, P.; Karthivashan, G.; Revuri, V.; Park, S.; Kim, J.S.; Ko, Y.T.; Choi, D.K. Antineuroinflammatory Activities and Neurotoxicological Assessment of Curcumin Loaded Solid Lipid Nanoparticles on LPS-Stimulated BV-2 Microglia Cell Models. *Molecules* **2019**, *24*, 1170. [CrossRef]
209. Maiti, P.; Dunbar, G.L. Comparative Neuroprotective Effects of Dietary Curcumin and Solid Lipid Curcumin Particles in Cultured Mouse Neuroblastoma Cells after Exposure to Abeta42. *Int. J. Alzheimers Dis.* **2017**, *2017*. [CrossRef]
210. Sadegh Malvajerd, S.; Izadi, Z.; Azadi, A.; Kurd, M.; Derakhshankhah, H.; Sharifzadeh, M.; Akbari Javar, H.; Hamidi, M. Neuroprotective Potential of Curcumin-Loaded Nanostructured Lipid Carrier in an Animal Model of Alzheimer's Disease: Behavioral and Biochemical Evidence. *J. Alzheimers Dis.* **2019**, *69*, 671–686. [CrossRef] [PubMed]

211. Chen, Y.; Pan, L.; Jiang, M.; Li, D.; Jin, L. Nanostructured lipid carriers enhance the bioavailability and brain cancer inhibitory efficacy of curcumin both in vitro and in vivo. *Drug Deliv.* **2016**, *23*, 1383–1392. [CrossRef] [PubMed]
212. Kaur, I.P.; Bhandari, R.; Bhandari, S.; Kakkar, V. Potential of solid lipid nanoparticles in brain targeting. *J. Control. Release* **2008**, *127*, 97–109. [CrossRef] [PubMed]
213. Bozzuto, G.; Molinari, A. Liposomes as nanomedical devices. *Int. J. Nanomed.* **2015**, *10*, 975–999. [CrossRef] [PubMed]
214. Vieira, D.B.; Gamarra, L.F. Getting into the brain: Liposome-based strategies for effective drug delivery across the blood-brain barrier. *Int. J. Nanomed.* **2016**, *11*, 5381–5414. [CrossRef]
215. Daraee, H.; Etemadi, A.; Kouhi, M.; Alimirzalu, S.; Akbarzadeh, A. Application of liposomes in medicine and drug delivery. *Artif. Cells Nanomed. Biotechnol.* **2016**, *44*, 381–391. [CrossRef]
216. Lombardo, D.; Calandra, P.; Bellocco, E.; Lagana, G.; Barreca, D.; Magazu, S.; Wanderlingh, U.; Kiselev, M.A. Effect of anionic and cationic polyamidoamine (PAMAM) dendrimers on a model lipid membrane. *Biochim. Biophys. Acta* **2016**, *1858*, 2769–2777. [CrossRef]
217. Lombardo, D.; Calandra, P.; Magazu, S.; Wanderlingh, U.; Barreca, D.; Pasqua, L.; Kiselev, M.A. Soft nanoparticles charge expression within lipid membranes: The case of amino terminated dendrimers in bilayers vesicles. *Colloids Surf. B Biointerfaces* **2018**, *170*, 609–616. [CrossRef]
218. Balducci, C.; Mancini, S.; Minniti, S.; La Vitola, P.; Zotti, M.; Sancini, G.; Mauri, M.; Cagnotto, A.; Colombo, L.; Fiordaliso, F.; et al. Multifunctional liposomes reduce brain beta-amyloid burden and ameliorate memory impairment in Alzheimer's disease mouse models. *J. Neurosci.* **2014**, *34*, 14022–14031. [CrossRef]
219. Lazar, A.N.; Mourtas, S.; Youssef, I.; Parizot, C.; Dauphin, A.; Delatour, B.; Antimisiaris, S.G.; Duyckaerts, C. Curcumin-conjugated nanoliposomes with high affinity for Abeta deposits: Possible applications to Alzheimer disease. *Nanomedicine* **2013**, *9*, 712–721. [CrossRef]
220. Gao, J.Q.; Lv, Q.; Li, L.M.; Tang, X.J.; Li, F.Z.; Hu, Y.L.; Han, M. Glioma targeting and blood-brain barrier penetration by dual-targeting doxorubincin liposomes. *Biomaterials* **2013**, *34*, 5628–5639. [CrossRef] [PubMed]
221. Chen, Z.L.; Huang, M.; Wang, X.R.; Fu, J.; Han, M.; Shen, Y.Q.; Xia, Z.; Gao, J.Q. Transferrin-modified liposome promotes alpha-mangostin to penetrate the blood-brain barrier. *Nanomedicine* **2016**, *12*, 421–430. [CrossRef] [PubMed]
222. Chen, H.; Tang, L.; Qin, Y.; Yin, Y.; Tang, J.; Tang, W.; Sun, X.; Zhang, Z.; Liu, J.; He, Q. Lactoferrin-modified procationic liposomes as a novel drug carrier for brain delivery. *Eur. J. Pharm. Sci.* **2010**, *40*, 94–102. [CrossRef] [PubMed]
223. Lindgren, M.; Hallbrink, M.; Prochiantz, A.; Langel, U. Cell-penetrating peptides. *Trends Pharmacol. Sci.* **2000**, *21*, 99–103. [CrossRef]
224. Vives, E.; Richard, J.P.; Rispal, C.; Lebleu, B. TAT peptide internalization: Seeking the mechanism of entry. *Curr. Protein Pept. Sci.* **2003**, *4*, 125–132. [CrossRef]
225. Sancini, G.; Gregori, M.; Salvati, E.; Cambianica, L.; Re, F.; Ornaghi, F.; Canovi, M.; Fracasso, C.; Cagnotto, A.; Colombo, M.; et al. Functionalization with TAT-Peptide Enhances Blood-Brain Barrier Crossing In vitro of Nanoliposomes Carrying a Curcumin-Derivative to Bind Amyloid-B Peptide. *J. Nanomed. Nanotechnol.* **2013**, *4*, 1–8. [CrossRef]
226. Taylor, M.; Moore, S.; Mourtas, S.; Niarakis, A.; Re, F.; Zona, C.; La Ferla, B.; Nicotra, F.; Masserini, M.; Antimisiaris, S.G.; et al. Effect of curcumin-associated and lipid ligand-functionalized nanoliposomes on aggregation of the Alzheimer's Abeta peptide. *Nanomedicine* **2011**, *7*, 541–550. [CrossRef]
227. Madheswaran, T.; Kandasamy, M.; Bose, R.J.; Karuppagounder, V. Current potential and challenges in the advances of liquid crystalline nanoparticles as drug delivery systems. *Drug Discov. Today* **2019**, *24*, 1405–1412. [CrossRef]
228. Wei, L.; Li, X.; Guo, F.; Liu, X.; Wang, Z. Structural properties, in vitro release and radical scavenging activity of lecithin based curcumin-encapsulated inverse hexagonal (HII) liquid crystals. *Colloids Surf.* **2018**, *539*, 124–131. [CrossRef]
229. Angelova, A.; Drechsler, M.; Garamus, V.M.; Angelov, B. Liquid Crystalline Nanostructures as PEGylated Reservoirs of Omega-3 Polyunsaturated Fatty Acids: Structural Insights toward Delivery Formulations against Neurodegenerative Disorders. *ACS Omega* **2018**, *3*, 3235–3247. [CrossRef]
230. Baskaran, R.; Madheswaran, T.; Sundaramoorthy, P.; Kim, H.M.; Yoo, B.K. Entrapment of curcumin into monoolein-based liquid crystalline nanoparticle dispersion for enhancement of stability and anticancer activity. *Int. J. Nanomed.* **2014**, *9*, 3119–3130. [CrossRef] [PubMed]

231. Coisne, C.; Tilloy, S.; Monflier, E.; Wils, D.; Fenart, L.; Gosselet, F. Cyclodextrins as Emerging Therapeutic Tools in the Treatment of Cholesterol-Associated Vascular and Neurodegenerative Diseases. *Molecules* **2016**, *21*, 1748. [CrossRef] [PubMed]
232. Ramdani, L.; Bourboulou, R.; Belkouch, M.; Jebors, S.; Tauran, Y.; Parizot, C.; Suwinska, K.; Coleman, A.W.; Duyckaerts, C.; Lazar, A.N. Multifunctional Curcumin-Nanocarriers Based on Host-Guest Interactions for Alzheimer Disease Diagnostic. *J. Nanomed. Nanotechnol.* **2015**, *6*. [CrossRef]
233. Quitschke, W.W.; Steinhauff, N.; Rooney, J. The effect of cyclodextrin-solubilized curcuminoids on amyloid plaques in Alzheimer transgenic mice: Brain uptake and metabolism after intravenous and subcutaneous injection. *Alzheimers Res. Ther.* **2013**, *5*, 16. [CrossRef] [PubMed]
234. Cheng, K.K.; Yeung, C.F.; Ho, S.W.; Chow, S.F.; Chow, A.H.; Baum, L. Highly stabilized curcumin nanoparticles tested in an in vitro blood-brain barrier model and in Alzheimer's disease Tg2576 mice. *AAPS J.* **2013**, *15*, 324–336. [CrossRef] [PubMed]
235. Mendes, M.; Sousa, J.J.; Pais, A.; Vitorino, C. Targeted Theranostic Nanoparticles for Brain Tumor Treatment. *Pharmaceutics* **2018**, *10*, 181. [CrossRef] [PubMed]
236. Ramanathan, S.; Archunan, G.; Sivakumar, M.; Tamil Selvan, S.; Fred, A.L.; Kumar, S.; Gulyas, B.; Padmanabhan, P. Theranostic applications of nanoparticles in neurodegenerative disorders. *Int. J. Nanomed.* **2018**, *13*, 5561–5576. [CrossRef]
237. Ghorbani, M.; Bigdeli, B.; Jalili-Baleh, L.; Baharifar, H.; Akrami, M.; Dehghani, S.; Goliaei, B.; Amani, A.; Lotfabadi, A.; Rashedi, H.; et al. Curcumin-lipoic acid conjugate as a promising anticancer agent on the surface of goldiron oxide nanocomposites: A pH-sensitive targeted drug delivery system for brain cancer theranostics. *Eur. J. Pharm. Sci.* **2018**, *114*, 175–188. [CrossRef]
238. Gamage, N.H.; Jing, L.; Worsham, M.J.; Ali, M.M. Targeted Theranostic Approach for Glioma Using Dendrimer-Based Curcumin Nanoparticle. *J. Nanomed. Nanotechnol.* **2016**, *7*. [CrossRef]
239. Jaruszewski, K.M.; Curran, G.L.; Swaminathan, S.K.; Rosenberg, J.T.; Grant, S.C.; Ramakrishnan, S.; Lowe, V.J.; Poduslo, J.F.; Kandimalla, K.K. Multimodal nanoprobes to target cerebrovascular amyloid in Alzheimer's disease brain. *Biomaterials* **2014**, *35*, 1967–1976. [CrossRef]
240. Pasqua, L.; Leggio, A.; Sisci, D.; Ando, S.; Morelli, C. Mesoporous Silica Nanoparticles in Cancer Therapy: Relevance of the Targeting Function. *Mini Rev. Med. Chem.* **2016**, *16*, 743–753. [CrossRef] [PubMed]
241. Bagheri, E.; Ansari, L.; Abnous, K.; Taghdisi, S.M.; Charbgoo, F.; Ramezani, M.; Alibolandi, M. Silica based hybrid materials for drug delivery and bioimaging. *J. Control. Release* **2018**, *277*, 57–76. [CrossRef] [PubMed]
242. Vallet-Regi, M.; Colilla, M.; Izquierdo-Barba, I.; Manzano, M. Mesoporous Silica Nanoparticles for Drug Delivery: Current Insights. *Molecules* **2017**, *23*, 47. [CrossRef] [PubMed]
243. Pasqua, L.; De Napoli, I.E.; De Santo, M.; Greco, M.; Catizzone, E.; Lombardo, D.; Montera, G.; Comandè, A.; Nigro, A.; Morelli, C.; et al. Mesoporous silica-based hybrid materials for bone-specific drug delivery. *Nanoscale Adv.* **2019**, *1*, 3269–3278. [CrossRef]
244. Jambhrunkar, S.; Karmakar, S.; Popat, A.; Yu, M.; Yu, C. Mesoporous silica nanoparticles enhance the cytotoxicity of curcumin. *RSC Adv.* **2014**, *4*, 709–712. [CrossRef]
245. Ceresa, C.; Nicolini, G.; Rigolio, R.; Bossi, M.; Pasqua, L.; Cavaletti, G. Functionalized mesoporous silica nanoparticles: A possible strategy to target cancer cells reducing peripheral nervous system uptake. *Curr. Med. Chem.* **2013**, *20*, 2589–2600. [CrossRef] [PubMed]
246. Nigro, A.; Pellegrino, M.; Greco, M.; Comande, A.; Sisci, D.; Pasqua, L.; Leggio, A.; Morelli, C. Dealing with Skin and Blood-Brain Barriers: The Unconventional Challenges of Mesoporous Silica Nanoparticles. *Pharmaceutics* **2018**, *10*, 250. [CrossRef]
247. Lungare, S.; Hallam, K.; Badhan, R.K. Phytochemical-loaded mesoporous silica nanoparticles for nose-to-brain olfactory drug delivery. *Int. J. Pharm.* **2016**, *513*, 280–293. [CrossRef]
248. Ahmadi Nasab, N.; Hassani Kumleh, H.; Beygzadeh, M.; Teimourian, S.; Kazemzad, M. Delivery of curcumin by a pH-responsive chitosan mesoporous silica nanoparticles for cancer treatment. *Artif. Cells Nanomed. Biotechnol.* **2018**, *46*, 75–81. [CrossRef]

Journal of
Clinical Medicine

MDPI

Review

Potential Therapeutic Targets of Quercetin and Its Derivatives: Its Role in the Therapy of Cognitive Impairment

Md. Jakaria [1,2], Shofiul Azam [1] Song-Hee Jo [1], In-Su Kim [1,3], Raju Dash [4] and Dong-Kug Choi [1,3,*]

1 Department of Applied Life Sciences and Integrated Bioscience, Graduate School, Konkuk University, Chungju 27478, Korea; pharmajakaria@rocketmail.com (M.J.); shofiul_azam@hotmail.com (S.A.); wowsong333@naver.com (S.-H.J.); kis5497@hanmail.net (I.-S.K.)
2 The Florey Institute of Neuroscience and Mental Health, The University of Melbourne, Parkville, Victoria 3010, Australia
3 Department of Integrated Bioscience and Biotechnology, College of Biomedical and Health Sciences, and Research Institute of Inflammatory Diseases (RID), Konkuk University, Chungju 27478, Korea
4 Department of Anatomy, Dongguk University Graduate School of Medicine, Gyeongju 38066, Korea; rajudash.bgctub@gmail.com
* Correspondence: choidk@kku.ac.kr; Tel.: +82-43-840-3610

Received: 16 September 2019; Accepted: 21 October 2019; Published: 25 October 2019

Abstract: Quercetin (QC) is a flavonoid and crucial bioactive compound found in a variety of vegetables and fruits. In preclinical studies, QC has demonstrated broad activity against several diseases and disorders. According to recent investigations, QC is a potential therapeutic candidate for the treatment of nervous system illnesses because of its protective role against oxidative damage and neuroinflammation. QC acts on several molecular signals, including ion channels, neuroreceptors, and inflammatory receptor signaling, and it also regulates neurotrophic and anti-oxidative signaling molecules. While the study of QC in neurological disorders has focused on numerous target molecules, the role of QC on certain molecular targets such as G-protein coupled and nuclear receptors remains to be investigated. Our analysis presents several molecular targets of QC and its derivatives that demonstrate the pharmacological potential against cognitive impairment. Consequently, this article may guide future studies using QC and its analogs on specific signaling molecules. Finding new molecular targets of QC and its analogs may ultimately assist in the treatment of cognitive impairment.

Keywords: quercetin; nervous system; molecular signals; pharmacological potential; cognitive impairment

1. Introduction

Cognitive impairment is very common in various neurological disorders, which affect the thinking, communication, understanding, and memory of a person. A patient's cognitive function might be affected in several neurodegenerative diseases (NDDs) such as Alzheimer's disease (AD), Parkinson's disease (PD), multiple sclerosis, or stroke [1]. The common pathological characterization of these disorders is one of the progressive dysfunctions and neuronal injury, leading to a slow and irreversible deterioration in brain function. These multifactorial and debilitating disorders affect approximately 30 million individuals worldwide [2].

Due to the complexity in the mechanistic progression of cognitive impaired disorders, illuminating the proper disease pathophysiology and therapeutics of cognitive impairment remains a foremost challenge [3]. No curative treatment for cognitive impairment currently exists, an alternative would be to find ways to attenuate cognitive impairment in older people, which, in turn, could delay the onset of cognitive impairment [4]. Numerous phytochemicals have received significant attention as potential agents in treating neurodegenerative conditions, as adjuncts to modern medicines [1,5–7]. Quercetin (QC), a readily available natural polyphenol, is one such phyotochemical, which is abundant in vegetables and fruits, and considered to be the main flavonoid in our daily diet [8]. QC displays broad spectrum properties against inflammation and cancer [9]. It is also a crucial bioactive compound, protective against injuries to the nervous, hepatic, cardiovascular, and urinary systems [10–12]. In a recent study on a mild traumatic brain injury (TBI)-induced mouse model, the treatment with QC significantly reduced anxiety-like behaviors of mice. QC treatment also ameliorated the dysregulation of the hypothalamic–pituitary–adrenal axis in TBI-induced mice and decreased levels of adrenocorticotropic hormones and corticosterones [13]. The protective role of QC against cognitive impairment has been demonstrated in several studies [9,10,14], just as recent advances have led to an increased understanding of the processes underlying cognitive impairment [15]. The identification of molecules that contribute to the pathological progression of disease is crucial in the therapy and drug discovery process, therefore, in this article, we discuss several potential targets where QC displays pharmacological activity against cognitive impairment along with an overview of QC chemistry and biopharmaceutics.

2. Overview of Quercetin

Among the over 4000 naturally occurring phenolic compounds in plants, QC was isolated and defined as biologically active by Szent-Gyorgyi in 1936 [16]. QC (5,7,3′,4′-hydroxyflavonol) is found in onions, curly kale, leeks, broccoli, apples, tea, capers, and blueberries, with onion (as 300 mg/kg of fresh onion) often contributing the most to total QC intake [17]. QC is a promising dietary component in the prevention of lifestyle diseases due to its wide-ranging effects [18]. In addition, we have published that methanol extract of red onion protects against lipopolysaccharide (LPS) and 1-methyl-4-phenylpyridinium, and upregulates the antioxidant enzymes that could potentially be used in the therapy of NDDs [19].

QC is naturally available as derivatives either in glycosidic form (primarily bound to glucose and rutinose), bound to ethers, and, very rarely, as a sulfate and prenyl substituent [20,21]. QC O-glycosides are QC derivatives with at least one O-glycosidic bond primarily glycosylated at the hydroxyl group of C-3 carbon with galactose, glucose, xylose or rhamnose [10]. The backbone of the QC chemical structure (Figure 1) and QC derivatives, with their potential targets for neuroprotection are listed in Table 1 [22]. Another glycosylation site is the hydroxyl group of C-7 carbon, for example, QC 7-O-glucoside, which is accessible in beans [23]. Ether derivatives of QC are formed between the OH group of QC and an alcohol molecule, typically methanol. QC ether derivatives are connected to sugar moiety groups, including 7-methoxy-3-glucoside and QC 30-methoxy-3-galactoside, which occurs widely in nature [24]. The presence of the five-hydroxyl group makes QC a highly lipophilic compound, although solubility of QC-derivatives is dependent on the type of substituent molecules existing in the OH group. C-methyl, O-methyl and prenyl derivatives of QC are lipophilic in nature [21]. Glycosylation of QC raises hydrophilicity, and these glycosylated derivatives are cytosol soluble, simply transported to all fragments of the plants and frequently deposited in vacuoles [21,25].

The unique structure of QC allows it to demonstrate a potent antioxidant action. The functional groups of QC are accountable for the stability and antioxidant activity; these are 3- and 5-OH groups, in conjugation with the 4-oxo group and the orthodihydroxy or catechol group [26]. QC gives a proton to free radicals, for example, 2,2-diphenyl-1-picrylhydrazyl and converts itself into a quinone intermediate, which is steadied by the electrons donated by these functional groups [27]. QC derivatives such as C3 and C4__OH glycoside derivatives display reduced H- donating capability. The decreasing potential of C3__OH derivatives of QC is greater when compared to its aglycone form [28].

Aglycone QC bioavailability is poor, and in human plasma, free QC has been not found after oral ingestion of QC [29]. As stated earlier, QC occurs in the form of glycosides in fruits and vegetables. Upon dietetic intake, QC glycosides are quickly hydrolyzed in the epithelial cells, with the help of β-glucosidase enzyme or by bacterial action in the colon, to make QC aglycone, which is readily absorbed in the large intestine. QC aglycone is then transported to the liver via portal circulation, where it starts glucuronidation, O-methylation, and/or sulphation to form its conjugates QC-3-glucuronide, QC-30-sulphate, and iso-rhamnetin-3-glucuronide [26,30,31]. The nature and binding site of glycosides at the position of 3, 5, 7, or 40 determine the extent of absorption. Wittig et al. [32] displayed that fried onion consumption exhibited only the presence of QC glucuronides and not QC aglycone or glucoside, which designates that the conjugated form of QC is more extensively found in plasma than its aglycone form. QC intake with fat-enriched diets and emulsifiers elevated the QC metabolite accumulation in blood plasma by suggestively delaying its excretion [33].

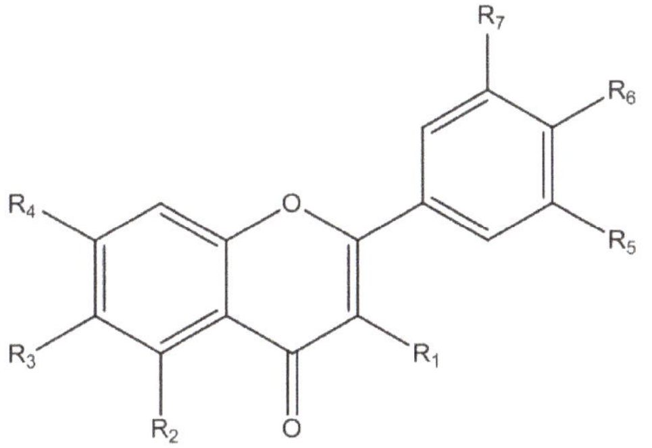

Figure 1. The chemical structure of quercetin (QC). The changing of functional groups makes derivatives of QC.

Metabolites of QC follow two dissimilar approaches of excretion such as part of biliary secretions into the small intestine or the urine [34]. Any QC absorption in the small intestine appears futile, as it is degraded by microflora, along with that secreted in the bile; the subsequent aglycone endures ring fission, leading to hydroxycinnamates and phenolic acid production [35]. QC metabolites follow a slow elimination rate (the range of half-lives are 11 to 28 h) [33]. A lower dose of QC can be more methylated than higher doses in humans [36]. Additionally, sulphation is usually a greater affinity, lower capacity pathway than glucuronidation; an elevate in the amount of QC swallowed may lead to a shift from sulphation toward glucuronidation. An extensive amount of research utilizing QC aglycone in vitro has been done due to the very low concentrations of aglycone found in plasma.

Harwood et al. have extensively reviewed the safety of QC [37]. Briefly, QC is not categorized as mutagenic or carcinogenic in vivo [38], albeit it has been found to hinder CYP3A4, an enzyme that breaks down numerous frequently prescribed drugs [39]. Thus, QC should not be ingested in combination with drugs including colchicine and alprazolam (Xanax), which depend on this pathway for appropriate metabolism [40].

The dietary intake of all flavonoids has been estimated to be approximately 200–350 mg/d, and that of flavonols, approximately 20 mg/d, with QC accounting for nearly 50% of this total (given a daily intake of approximately 10 mg/d) [41]. The results of a Japanese study reinforced these approximations, as daily intake of QC was determined to be 16 mg [19]. QC aglycone is sold as a nutritional supplement, with a suggested dosage of 1 g/d [37]. Over-the-counter supplemental QC is available in 250 and 1500 mg capsules and is marketed as being helpful for a variety of ailments such as eye disorders, asthma, gout, arthritis, allergies, bacterial infections, hypertension, and neurodegenerative disorders [42].

Table 1. Several derivatives of QC with their potential targets for neuroprotective therapy.

Sl	Common Name	Substituents							Sources	Targets in Neuroprotection	Ability to crossBBB	References
		R1	R2	R3	R4	R5	R6	R7				
1	Quercetin 3′-O-(3-chloropivaloyl) (quercetin pivaloyl ester)	OH	OH	H	OH	H	OH	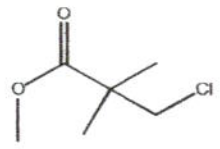	Synthetically modified quercetin	Toll-like receptor (TLR)-4	+	[43]
2	3, 5, 7, 3′, 4′-pentahydroxyflavon (quercetin)	OH	OH	H	OH	OH	OH	H	Elderberries, cranberries, coriander leaves, canned capers	Nuclear factor erythroid 2-related factor 2-antioxidant responsive element (Nrf2-ARE) and antioxidant/ anti-inflammatory enzyme paraoxonase 2 (PON2) enzyme	+	[13,44]
3	Quercetin 3-O-glucoside (isoquercetin)	O-Glc	OH	H	OH	OH	OH	H	Mango fruits, beans, plums, onions	TLR-2 and 4	+	[44–47]
4	Quercetin 3-O-rhamnoside (quercitrin)	O-Rha	OH	H	OH	OH	OH	H	Mango–fruits, pepper–fruits, cranberry, lingonberry	TLR-2 and 4	–	[28,45,47]
5	Quercetin 3-O-rhamnosyl-(1–6)-glucoside (rutin)	O-X	OH	H	OH	OH	OH	H	Plums, cherries, tomatoes, buckwheat leaves, buckwheat seeds, chokeberry	–	+	[48–50]
6	Quercetin 7-O-glucoside	OH	OH	H	O-Glc	OH	OH	H	Beans	–	–	[23]
7	Quercetin 3-O-rhamnoside-7-O-glucoside	O-Y	OH	H	Glc	OH	OH	H	Pepper fruits	–	–	[28]
8	Quercetin 3-sulfate-7-O-arabinoside	O-Sul	OH	H	O-Ara	OH	OH	H	Salt bush	–	–	[21]
9	Quercetin 3-O-glucoside-3′-sulfate	O-Glc	OH	H	OH	O-Sul	OH	H	Corn flower	TLR-2 and 4	–	[47,51]
10	Quercetin 5-methyl ether (azaleatin)	OH	O-M	H	OH	OH	OH	H	Flowers of *Rhododendron mucronatum*, *Plumbago capensis*, *Ceratostigmawillmottiana*, *Carya pecan*, leaves of *Eucryphia*	Extracellular signal-regulated kinase 1/2 (ERK)-pathway	–	[13,52]

Table 1. *Cont.*

Sl	Common Name	Substituents							Sources	Targets in Neuroprotection	Ability to crossBBB	References
		R1	R2	R3	R4	R5	R6	R7				
11	Quercetin 7-methyl ether (rhamnetin)	OH	OH	H	O-M	OH	OH	H	Cloves, berries from buckthorn family, such as *Rhamnusinfectorius, R. cathartica*	–	+	[13,53]
12	Quercetin 3′-methyl ether (isohramnetin)	OH	OH	H	OH	O-M	OH	H	Honey	TLR-2 and 4	+	[47,54,55]
13	Quercetin 4′-methyl ether (tamarixetin)	OH	OH	H	OH	OH	O-M	H	*Artemisia annua*	TLR-4 and myeloid differentiation primary response 88	+	[13,55,56]
14	Quercetin 7-methoxy-3-O-glucoside	O-Glc	OH	H	O-M	OH	OH	H	Honey	–	–	[54]
15	Quercetin 3′-methoxy-3-O-galactoside	O-Gal	OH	H	OH	O-M	OH	H	Sage	–	–	[24]
16	6, 5′-Di-C-prenylquercetin	OH	OH	Z	OH	OH	OH	Z	Paper mullberry	–	–	[57]
17	Quercetin-3-O-glucuronide	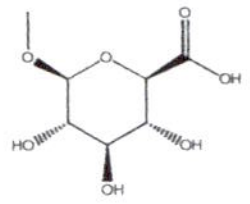	OH	H	OH	H	OH	OH	Red wine	Cyclic AMP response element binding protein (CREB) phosphorylation and ↓amyloid beta $(A\beta)_{1\text{-}40}$	+	[58,59]
18	7-O-galloylquercetin	OH	OH	H	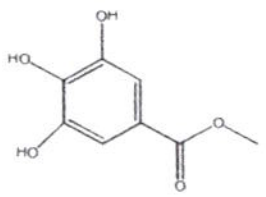	H	OH	OH	Semisynthetic flavonoid	Activate Nrf2/ARE and ↑antioxidant enzyme NAD(P)H quinone oxidoreducase-1 (NQO1)	–	[60]

3. Potential Therapeutic Targets of Quercetin

3.1. Voltage-Gated Ion Channels

Several studies have demonstrated the potential role of QC action on voltage-gated ion channels. In one such study, the polyphenols QC, catechin, and resveratrol from red grapes were found to prevent peak INa, with half maximal inhibitory concentration (IC50s) of 19.4, 76.8, and 77.3 μM, correspondingly. Resveratrol and QC reduced the voltage-gated sodium channel (VGSC) long QT mutant R1623Q-induced late INa. Resveratrol and QC also blocked anemonia viridis toxin 2 (ATX II)-induced late INa, with IC50s of 26.1 μM and 24.9 μM, correspondingly. The inhibitory action of QC on cardiac VGSCs may thus potentially contribute to the cardioprotective effectiveness of products containing red grape extract [61].

QC may hold potential as an agent to treat cerebral ischemia and vascular dementia due to its inhibitory effect on the sodium channel [62]. In a study conducted on chronic cerebral ischemia in rats, QC (5 mg/kg i.p. for 14 d) improved the cognitive performance of ischemic rats on the Morris water maze test. In electrophysiological experiments, QC attenuated the prevention of long-term potentiation in ischemic rats. Also, in acutely isolated rat hippocampal CA1 pyramidal neurons, QC (0.3, 3.0, and 30.0 μM) reduced the amplitude of voltage-dependent sodium currents in a voltage- and dose-dependent way [62].

QC affects the release of glutamate in rat cerebral cortex nerve terminals (synaptosomes). Treatment with QC prevented glutamate release evoked by 4-aminopyridine (4-AP), which is a K+ channel blocker but chelating extracellular Ca^{2+} ions inhibited this effect. QC reduced the depolarization-induced elevate in the cytosolic free Ca^{2+}, while it did not alter 4-AP-mediated depolarization and Na+ influx. The QC-mediated prevention of glutamate release was reversed by antagonizing the Cav2.2 (N-type) and Cav2.1 (P/Q-type) channels. The combined prevention of protein kinase C (PKC) and protein kinase A (PKA) also blocked the antagonistic action of QC on evoked release of glutamate. In addition, QC declined the 4-AP-induced phosphorylation of PKC and PKA. As per these findings that QC-mediated inhibitory action on glutamate release from rat cortical synaptosomes is connected both to a decrease in presynaptic voltage-dependent entry of Ca^{2+} and to the prevention of the activity of PKC and PKA [63].

QC protects against bupivacaine-induced neurotoxicity in SH-SY5Y cells. Treatment with QC (50 μM) significantly prevented bupivacaine-intoxicated cell apoptosis and declined intracellular Ca^{2+} concentration in SH-SY5Y cells. QC treatment also normalized Cav3.1 protein expression. Thus, QC-treatment decreased bupivacaine-intoxicated toxicity, probably via inhibition of the T-type calcium channel. QC-mediated this action may indicate its potential in the treatment of local anesthetic agent-mediated toxicity [64].

3.2. Neuroreceptors

3.2.1. Dopamine Receptors

QC displayed protective activity in several models of toxic agent-induced PD. In a 6-hydroxydopamine (6-OHDA)-intoxicated PD model, QC showed neuroprotective activity by displaying effects against oxidative stress [65,66]. The treatment with QC (30 mg/kg body weight, over 14 days) markedly elevated the glutathione and striatal dopamine levels compared with 6-OHDA-induced group [65]. QC also showed protective activity against 1-methyl-4-phenyl-1,2,3,6-tetrahydropyridine (MPTP)-induced PD-like syndromes, where it prevents MPTP-induced loss of dopamine in the mice brain [67]. In addition to 6-OHDA and MPTP, QC treatment also ameliorated acrylamide-induced memory impairment by increasing dopamine content [49]. While QC showed protective activity in PD models, only a few studies have investigated its effect on dopamine receptors. In one study, the D2 agonist quinpirole (0.2 mg/kg) potentiated QC (200 mg/kg) antinociceptive activity, but dopamine D1 receptor agonist, SKF38393 (10 and 15 mg/kg), was unsuccessful in modifying the QC-mediated antinociceptive effect. QC (200 mg/kg) prevented reserpine-intoxicated (2 mg/kg, 4 h) hyperalgesia, which was inverted by sulpiride. Thus, a role of alpha2-adrenoreceptors and dopamine D2 receptors is hypothesized in the antinociceptive effect of QC [68].

In a polychlorinated biphenyl (PCB/Aroclor-1254)-induced rat model, QC ameliorated against PCB-treated impairment of dopaminergic receptor expressions in the hippocampus [69]. Upon PCB induction, hydrogen peroxide was generated, and lipid peroxidation was induced in the hippocampus, which led to a disturbance of ATPases and dopamine receptor expressions [69]. PCB also caused an alteration in the expression of tyrosine hydroxylase (TH). Changes in the dopaminergic receptor expressions at mRNA and protein levels evidently represent the adverse role of PCBs on the dopaminergic system, which may, in turn, influence cognitive impairment. The reduction in calcium voltage-gated channel subunit alpha1 D gene expression indicates there may also be an alteration in neurotransmitter release and signal transduction [69]. Administering QC reinstated the biochemical and morphological changes in the PCB-intoxicated hippocampus [69].

The exposure of cadmium in rat corpus striatum and PC12 cells leads to a selective reduction in dopamine (DA)-D2 receptors, which affected the post-synaptic PKA/ protein phosphatase 1 regulatory subunit 1B/type 1 protein phosphatase alpha and β arrestin/protein kinase B (Akt)/glycogen synthase kinase 3β signaling concomitantly. The antagonism of PKA and c in vitro reveals that both pathways are independently moderated by DA-D2 receptors and are connected to the cadmium-induced motor abnormalities. Ultrastructural deviations in the corpus striatum confirmed neuronal collapse and loss of synapses on cadmium induction. According to the molecular docking hypothesis, the direct interaction of cadmium with the dopamine on DA-D2 receptor competitive sites may be connected to the decrease in DA-D2 receptors. As treatment with QC ameliorated cadmium-induced behavioral and neurochemical variations, QC may be a potential agent to ameliorate cadmium-induced dopaminergic dysfunctions [70].

3.2.2. Glutaminergic Receptors

QC acts on ionotropic glutamate receptors, and it is reported to exhibit neuroprotective activity in a dexamethasone-induced cognitive deficit mouse model. The administration of dexamethasone changed the expression of N-methyl-D-aspartate (NMDA) receptors in the hippocampus, while pretreatment with QC protected against a reduction in NMDA receptor expression [71]. In addition, QC pretreatment demonstrated antidepressant activity in an olfactory bulbectomy mouse model that involved the NMDA receptor; the administration of NMDA reversed QC-mediated antidepressant activity [72]. According to the computational study, QC may be a potential ligand of the α-amino-3-hydroxy-5-methyl-4-isoxazolepropionic acid (AMPA) receptor as it shows a superior docking score [73]. QC action on the glutamate-treated inward current (IGlu) in Xenopus oocytes that heterologously express human AMPA receptor and stargazin, was examined. The two-electrode voltage clamp technique was employed to measure IGlu. In oocytes inserted with cRNAs coding for AMPA receptor (GluA1) and stargazin, QC-mediated prevention of IGlu was in a concentration- and reversible-dependent manner. The activity of QC on IGlu was ameliorated by elevating glutamate concentration, and the activity was membrane holding potential dependent. These findings indicate that QC interacts with the AMPA receptor, which was heterologously expressed in Xenopus oocytes. The action of QC on the IGlu of the AMPA receptor may show potential for neuroprotective therapy [73]. In a recent study, QC ameliorated kainic acid (KA)-induced seizures in mice. Pretreatment with QC (100 mg/kg) significantly elevated gene expression of the GluA1 subunit of AMPA and the GluN2A and GluN2B subunits of NMDA only 7 d after KA intoxication, in comparison with the control and KA groups. Enhancement in the QC-mediated gene expressions of AMPA and NMDA receptor subunits may be indicating its protective effect on the synaptic plasticity and memory [74].

3.2.3. Acetylcholine Receptors

Several studies have revealed QC's actions on nicotinic acetylcholine receptors. In a study on α9α10 nicotinic acetylcholine receptor-dependent ion currents, the action of QC was examined utilizing the two-electrode voltage clamp technique. The treatment with acetylcholine evoked inward currents (IACh) in oocytes heterologously expressing the α9α10 nicotinic acetylcholine receptor. IACh was prevented by QC treatment in a concentration-dependent and reversible manner. The pre-application of QC on IACh was stronger than its co-application, and the IC50 of QC was 45.4 ± 10.1 μM. QC-mediated prevention of IACh was not affected by the concentration of acetylcholine and was independent of membrane-holding potential. While the preventive action of QC was significantly weakened in the absence of extracellular Ca^{2+}, the QC effect was independent of extracellular Ca^{2+} concentration, suggesting that extracellular Ca^{2+} availability might be required for QC-mediated action and might play a critical role in QC-treated α9α10 nicotinic acetylcholine receptor regulation [75].

In another study, the treatment with acetylcholine elicited an IACh in oocytes expressing both muscle types of nicotinic acetylcholine receptors. QC cotreatment with acetylcholine protected IACh. QC pretreatment further protected IACh in oocytes expressing adult and fetal muscle-type nicotinic acetylcholine receptors. IACh prevention by QC was reversible and concentration-dependent, and the IC50 of QC was 18.9 ± 1.2 μM in oocytes expressing adult muscle-type nicotinic acetylcholine receptors. The prevention of IACh by QC was voltage independent and noncompetitive. According to these results, QC may have the potential to regulate the action of human muscle-type nicotinic acetylcholine receptors. QC-treated muscle-type nicotinic acetylcholine receptor regulation might be coupled with the regulation of neuromuscular junction action [76].

The actions of QC on heteromeric neuronal α3β4 nicotinic acetylcholine receptor channel action expressed in Xenopus oocytes after injection of cRNA encoding bovine neuronal α3 and β4 subunits have also been studied. Acetylcholine treatment provoked an IACh in oocytes expressing α3β4 nicotinic acetylcholine receptors, while cotreatment with QC and acetylcholine prevented IACh in oocytes expressing α3β4 nicotinic acetylcholine receptors. The prevention of IACh by QC was in a concentration-dependent and reversible manner. In oocytes expressing the α3β4 nicotinic acetylcholine receptor, the IC50 of QC was 14.9 ± 0.8 μM, and the antagonism of IACh by QC was voltage independent and noncompetitive. Therefore, QC might control the α3β4 nicotinic acetylcholine receptor, which may have pharmacological importance in the treatment of nervous system disorders [77].

It has been found that QC can elevate α7 nicotinic acetylcholine receptor (α7 nAChR)-dependent ion currents [78]. The action of QC glycosides on the acetylcholine-mediated peak IACh in Xenopus oocytes expressing the α7 nAChR has been studied. In oocytes injected with α7 nAChR copy RNA, QC increased IACh, while QC glycosides prevented IACh. As QC glycosides mediated inhibition of IACh, the mediation effect increased when the QC glycosides were pre-applied, and the preventive actions were concentration dependent. The order of IACh prevention by QC glycosides was Rutin≥Rham1>Rham2. QC glycoside-mediated IACh improvement was not affected by ACh concentration and appeared to be voltage independent. Additionally, QC-mediated IACh prevention can be ameliorated when QC is co-treated with Rham1 and rutin, demonstrating that QC glycosides could interfere with QC-mediated α7 nAChR regulation and that the carbohydrate numbers in the QC glycoside plays a crucial role in the disruption of QC-mediated effect. Thus, QC and QC glycosides control the α7 nAChR in a differential manner [79].

In a 2014 study, muscarinic acetylcholine receptor-active compounds were shown to have potential use in the treatment of AD [80]. As this computational study demonstrated the interaction of QC with the M1 muscarinic acetylcholine receptor [80], QC may represent a possible agent in the treatment of the disease.

3.2.4. Serotonergic Receptors

A few studies have addressed the action of QC on serotonin receptors. In one such study in 2014, QC administered with ascorbic acid was found to prevent monoamine oxidase-A activity in SH-SY5Y cells by targeting mitochondria [81]. This combination also employed operative vasodilator actions in isolated pulmonary artery and prevented proliferation of cells and induced apoptosis in human pulmonary artery smooth muscle cells. QC-treated, these actions were connected to the decrease in expression of serotonin 2A receptor (5-HT_{2A}) receptor and Akt and S6 phosphorylation and partly restored Kv currents. Thus, QC could be valuable in the management of pulmonary hypertension [82]. In oocytes injected with 5-HT_{3A} receptor cRNA, QC inhibited the 5-HT-treated inward peak current (IC50: 64.7 ± 2.2 μM) in a competitive and voltage-dependent manner. QC cooperates with the pre-transmembrane domain 1 (pre-TM1) of the 5-HT3A receptor because point mutations of pre-transmembrane domain 1 (pre-TM1) including R222T and R222A—but not R222D, R222E, and R222K—abolished prevention [83].

3.2.5. Gamma-aminobutyric acid-ergic Receptors

Several investigations have focused on the anxiolytic activity of QC. For example, in a behavioral study using a mouse model, QC displayed significant anxiolytic activity. A gamma-aminobutyric acid (GABA)A-ρ agonist (trans-4-aminocrotonic acid, 20 mg/kg) antagonized the anxiolytic-like activities of QC. On the other hand, WAY-100635 (a 5-HT1A antagonist, 0.3 mg/kg) and flumazenil (a GABAA antagonist, 10 mg/kg) did not antagonize a QC-mediated anxiolytic effect. Therefore, the promoting anxiolytic-like activity of QC may be mediated by the GABAergic nervous system [84]. In another study, GABAAρ1 receptor responses were prevented by QC in a dose-dependent, fast, and reversible way. This antagonistic effect was inhibited in the existence of ascorbic acid, but not by thiol reagents changing the extracellular Cys-loop of these receptors. An amino-acid residue positioned near the ρ1 subunit GABA binding site (H141) is involved in the allosteric modulation of GABAAρ1 receptors by numerous agents such as ascorbic acid. QC likewise prevented GABA-evoked actions mediated by mutant H141DGABAAρ1 and wild-type receptors, nonetheless inhibition employed by ascorbic acid on QC actions was diminished in mutant receptors. Therefore, antagonistic actions of QC on GABAAρ1 receptors are arbitrated via a redox-independent allosteric mechanism [85].

The action of QC on the GABAA α5 receptor gene has been studied in a mouse model of KA-induced seizures. QC (50 or 100 mg/kg) treatment reduced, in a dose-dependent manner, the behavioral seizure score in mice with KA-induced seizures. Two hours after the end of the 7-d treatment regimen, GABAA α5 receptor gene expression was increased in the hippocampus by KA induction. Treatment with QC (50 mg and 100 mg/kg) reduced the KA-induced increase of GABAA α5 expression. According to these results, the expression of the GABAAα5 receptor could be a potential target of QC to reduce or to serve as a marker of seizure severity [86].

Recently, QC has been shown to reduce prefrontal cortical GABAergic transmission and to alleviate the hyperactivity induced by the glutamatergic NMDA receptor antagonist MK-801. In cultured cortical neurons, QC noticeably decreased the GABA-activated currents in a noncompetitive manner. In mouse prefrontal cortical slices, the treatment with QC moderately prevented spontaneous and electrically evoked GABAergic inhibitory postsynaptic currents. The prefrontal-specific and systemic delivery of QC resulted in a decline in basal locomotor movement, apart from alleviating MK-801-induced hyperactivity. QC action was not fully dependent on GABAA α5, as knockdown of the α5-subunit in the prefrontal cortex elevated the MK-801-evoked psychotic symptom but reserved the QC-mediated action. Thus, QC may be a negative allosteric GABAA receptor modulator employing antipsychotic action and could be potential in the therapeutic development for psychiatric disorders [87]. QC-mediated action on GABA receptor is portrayed in Figure 2.

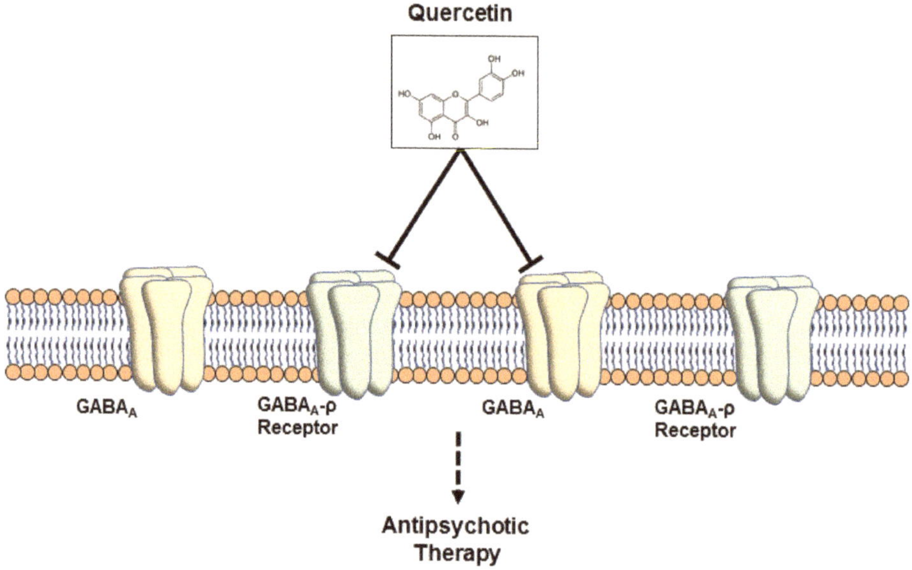

Figure 2. Antipsychotic activity of QC through GABA receptors. QC acts on the GABAA receptor and is possibly suitable for antipsychotic therapy.

3.2.6. Glycinergic Receptors

QC acts on the human glycine receptor alpha 1 channel expressed in Xenopus oocytes utilizing a two-electrode voltage clamp technique. In one study, it was found to reversibly inhibit glycine-induced current (I(Gly)) [88]. QC-treated inhibition depended on its dose, with an IC50 of 21.5 ± 0.2 μM, and was sensitive to membrane voltages. This QC-induced inhibition of I(Gly) was nearly eliminated upon the site-directed mutations of S267 to S267Y but not S267A, S267F, S267G, S267K, S267L, and S267T at transmembrane domain 2 (TM2). In contrast, QC increased I(Gly) in comparison with the wild-type receptor in site-directed mutant receptors including S267 to S267I, S267R, and S267V. The value of half maximal effective concentration (EC50) was 22.6 ± 1.4, 25.5 ± 4.2, and 14.5 ± 3.1 μM for S267I, S267R, and S267V, correspondingly. Therefore, QC may have the potential to regulate human glycine receptor alpha 1 via communication with amino acid residue alpha267 [88].

In cultured rat hippocampal neurons, the actions of QC on native glycine receptors (GlyRs) were examined. QC depressed glycine-induced current I(Gly) in a revocable and concentration-dependent manner, with an IC50 value is 10.7 ± 0.24 μM with a Hill coefficient of 1.08 ± 0.12. QC depressed maximum I(Gly) and suggestively altered the EC50 for glycine and the Hill coefficient. As per kinetic analysis, QC enhanced the desensitization rates. Remarkably, after the end of the glycine-with-QC co-application, a transient rebound occurred. The actions of QC also displayed voltage dependence, being greater at positive membrane potentials. Thus, QC could be a potential open channel blocker. In addition, in the sequential application protocol, QC prevented the peak amplitude of I(Gly) to a macroscopic degree while reducing GlyR desensitization. These effects implied that QC has a depressant action on the GlyR channel's opening, which may be triggered by an allosteric mechanism. QC outstandingly prevented the recombinant-induced current mediated amplitude by alpha2, alpha2beta, alpha3, and alpha3beta GlyRs, nonetheless had no action on the alpha1 and alpha1beta GlyRs that were expressed in HEK293T cells. In addition, QC action on I(Gly) in spinal neurons during development in vitro were also studied. In spinal neurons, the degree of blockade by QC on I(Gly) was less manifested than in hippocampal neurons in a development-dependent way. Thus, QC has conceivable actions in the processing of information within a neuronal network by preventing I(Gly) and may be valuable as a pharmacological probe for recognizing the subunit types of GlyRs [89].

3.3. Miscellaneous Targets

3.3.1. Toll-Like Receptors and Cytokine Receptors

In several studies, QC produces its anti-inflammatory activity by acting on TLR4 and cytokines. In LPS-triggered signaling via TLR4, QC suppresses the nuclear factor of kappa light polypeptide gene enhancer in B degradation, with subsequent activation of nuclear factor-kappa B (NF-κB) as well as activation of phosphorylation of p38 and Akt in bone marrow-derived macrophages. In tumor necrosis factor-α (TNF-α)-induced signaling, QC significantly repressed the interleukin (IL)-6 production and NF-κB activation [90].

QC protected against LPS-induced expressions of cell surface molecules such as cluster of differentiation (CD)80, CD86, and major histocompatibility complex class I/II and pro-inflammatory cytokines such as IL-1β, TNF-α, IL-6 and IL-12p70 but protecting action was inhibited toll-interacting protein silencing in RAW264.7 cells. In addition, QC treatment inhibited LPS-induced activation of mitogen-activated protein kinase (MAPK), including p38, c-Jun N-terminal kinase (JNK), and ERK1/2 and the NF-κB (p65) translocations via toll-interacting proteins. QC treatment also displayed a significant reduction in prostaglandin E2 and cyclooxygenase-2 levels as well as inducible nitric oxide synthase (iNOS)-mediated production of nitric oxide (NO) production by LPS induction [91].

The treatment of QC prevented the NF-κB nuclear translocation and cytokine release. In addition, QC prevents the release of TNF-α by acting on the NF-κB signaling pathway. Additionally, oxidized low-density lipoprotein-induced inflammation was also connected to the p38MAPK, ERK1/2, and JNK, and Akt pathway activations, and the QC-mediated action may also be related to protecting from the activation of these pathways. In addition, QC suggestively downregulated the increase TLRs and TNF-α expression at mRNA level in high carbohydrate diet-fed atherosclerotic rats. As QC displays a preventive action on the TLR-mediated MAPK and NF-κB signaling pathways, it could be a potential agent in the protection and management of atherosclerosis by decreasing detrimental vascular inflammation [92].

QC displayed anti-inflammatory activity in BV-2 microglial cells. It pointedly prevented LPS-induced NO release and expression of iNOS. QC notably prevented NF-κB activation by protecting from the degradation of nuclear factor of kappa light polypeptide gene enhancer in B-cells inhibitor, alpha [93]. QC also showed anti-inflammatory effects in another study conducted on BV-2 microglial cells, where QC was 10-fold more potent than cyanidin in the inhibition of LPS-induced NO release [94].

3.3.2. Neurotrophic Factors

Several studies have reported the activity of QC on neurotrophic factors. Brain-derived neurotrophic factor (BDNF) is a vital neurotrophin that plays an important role in the survival of neuronal cells. In a recent study, QC (20 and 50 mg/kg) significantly enhanced the mRNA BDNF expression compared with that of a control group and produced neuroprotective effects [95]. In addition, QC derived from *Ginkgo biloba* extract (EGb 761) stimulates depression-related signaling pathways involving BDNF/phosphorylation of CREB/postsynaptic density proteins-95 [96]. QC declines Aβ in neurons collected from the double transgenic AD mice (TgAPPswe/PS1e9). The administration of QC increases BDNF expression and reduces Aβ oligomers in the hippocampus of the TgAPPswe/PS1e9, which correlated with mouse cognitive improvement [96]. In another study, QC treatment reduced cell apoptosis in the focal cerebral ischemia rat brain in a way of a mechanism that may be related to the activation of the BDNF–tropomyosin receptor kinase B–phosphoinositide 3-kinases/Akt signaling pathway [97]. QC meaningfully activated the Akt and 3-phosphoinositide-dependent protein kinase 1 (PDK1) in MN9D dopaminergic neuronal cell lines. Regarding the blocking or siRNA, knockdown of PDK1 prevented the Akt activation. Therefore, Akt is a downstream signaling protein of PDK1 in the QC-mediated neuroprotection. QC also enhanced CREB phosphorylation and elevated the mitochondrial bioenergetics ability and prevented 6-hydroxydopamine-intoxicated toxicity in MN9D cells. In a MitoPark transgenic mouse model of PD, the attenuation of cognitive deficits, depletion of striatal dopamine and TH neuronal cell loss were accompanied by QC administration [8].

In PC12 cells, QC dose-dependently stimulated nerve growth factor (NGF)-induced neurite outgrowth. QC-mediated stimulatory action was abolished by the knockdown of Na-K-Cl cotransporter (NKCC1) via RNAi methods; QC stimulated NKCC1 activity without any elevation in the NKCC1 protein expression. The action of QC on neurite outgrowth was dependent on extracellular Cl-. Thus, QC stimulates NGF-induced neurite outgrowth via increasing Cl- incorporation into the intracellular space by stimulating NKCC1 [98]. Furthermore, QC, like the extract of *Ginkgo folium*, could enhance the effect of NGF in cultured PC12 cells. QC potentiates neurite outgrowth and phosphorylation of ERK1/2 [99].

QC protects against neurodegeneration in a model of diabetic retinopathy [100]. Treatment with QC suggestively elevated the neurotrophic factors (BDNF, NGF) and prevented a rise in caspase-3 activity and cytochrome c level in the diabetic retina. In addition, the expression of B-cell lymphoma 2 (Bcl-2) was increased in the QC-treated diabetic retina. Therefore, QC may have the pharmacological potential to protect against neuronal damage in the diabetic retina by attenuating the expression of neurotrophic factors and correspondingly by preventing the neuronal apoptosis [100]. QC-mediated action on neurotrophic signaling leading to neuronal survival and protection are portrayed in Figure 3.

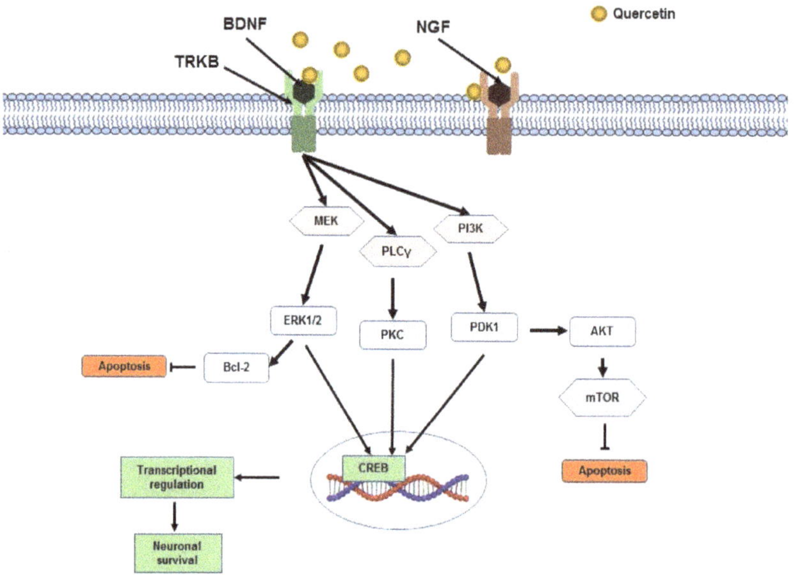

Figure 3. Molecular pathways regarding neuronal survival on which QC seems to assess their effects within the brain. QC-mediated action on neurotrophic factors BDNF and NGF. QC activates BDNF-TrkB and its associated signaling pathway, which ultimately, results in phosphorylation of CREB, and the CREB-mediated neuronal survival effect [101]. BDNF: Brain-derived neurotrophic factor; TRKB: Tropomyosin receptor kinase B; NGF: Nerve growth factor; PLCγ: Phospholipase C gamma; PI3K: Phosphatidylinositol 3-kinase; PKC: Protein kinase C; ERK: Extracellular signal-regulated kinase 1/2; PDK1: 3-phosphoinositide-dependent protein kinase 1; mTOR: Mammalian target of rapamycin; Akt: Protein Kinase B; Bcl-2: B-cell lymphoma 2; CREB: Cyclic AMP response element binding protein.

3.3.3. Apolipoprotein E

Apolipoprotein E (APOE) is encoded by the APOE gene which consists of 299 amino acid proteins. Change of a single amino acid of the APOE protein is due to the three common polymorphisms in the APOE gene—$\epsilon 2$, $\epsilon 3$, and $\epsilon 4$. With the change to the APOE $\epsilon 2$, $\epsilon 3$, and $\epsilon 4$ alleles, the likelihood of evolving cerebral amyloid angiopathy and AD is greater. This relationship is observed in a dose-dependent manner. APOE $\epsilon 4$ is mainly connected to an elevated risk for AD, whereas APOE $\epsilon 2$ is associated with a decreased risk. The actions of the APOE genotype on the risk of these disorders are likely to be arbitrated by differential properties of APOE on the accumulation of Aβ in the brain and its vasculature. Interestingly, the response pattern to AD treatment might differ with APOE genotype [102]. QC-enriched diets induced hepatic paraoxonase/arylesterase 1 gene expression, with a propensity for superior induction in APOE $\epsilon 3$ in comparison with APOE $\epsilon 4$ mice. In addition, hepatic mRNA and protein levels of β-glucuronidase and sulfatase, both enzymes centrally connected to the deconjugation of QC conjugates, were lesser in APOE $\epsilon 4$ in comparison with APOE $\epsilon 3$ mice. Peroxisome proliferator-activated receptor gamma (which partially controls the expression of the paraoxonase/arylesterase 1 gene) mRNA levels were lesser in APOE $\epsilon 4$ in comparison with APOE $\epsilon 3$ mice [103].

QC displayed blood pressure-lowering actions in overweight/obese carriers of the APOE $\epsilon 3$/APOE $\epsilon 4$ genotype but not in carriers of the $\epsilon 4$ allele [104]. Elevated APOE in the brain may be an operative therapeutic approach for AD. QC can also meaningfully increase APOE levels by hindering APOE degradation in immortalized astrocytes. In the 5xFAD mouse model, QC significantly elevated brain APOE, and declined insoluble Aβ levels in the cortex. Therefore, QC increases APOE levels via a novel mechanism and may be developed as a novel class of drug for AD therapy [105]. More research should be designed to reveal the in-depth mechanism of QC on APOE.

3.3.4. Nuclear Factor Erythroid 2-Related Factor 2-Antioxidant Responsive Element

In recent times, the antioxidant activity of QC focusing on the Nrf2-ARE pathway have been addressed by several investigations in the models of neurological disorders. QC protected PC12 cells from 1-methyl-4-phenylpyridinium-induced oxidative stress and degeneration by Nrf2-mediated upregulation of the heme oxygenase-1 (HO-1), NQO1 and glutathione [106]. QC also protected against high-glucose-induced oxidative stress in SH-SY5Y cells. Under the chronic high-glucose conditions, it enhanced Glo-1 functions in central neurons which may be mediated by activation of the Nrf2/ARE pathway. In addition, QC-treated PKC activation increased phosphorylation of Nrf2. Moreover, glycogen synthase kinase-3β inhibition may be connected to the QC-mediated Nrf2/ARE pathway activation [107].

In LPS-induced murine BV-2 microglial cells, QC produced a greater stimulating effect on Nrf2-induced increase expression of heme-oxygenase-1 (HO-1) protein than cyanidin. QC upregulated Nrf2/HO-1 activity in terms of endotoxic stress. QC upregulated HO-1 against endotoxic stress via the participation of MAPKs [94].

QC displayed neuroprotective activity in manganese-, domoic acid- and d-galactose-induced neurotoxicity models [108–110]. In a model of Mn-intoxicated inflammatory and apoptosis response in SK-N-MC cells and Sprague Dawley rats, QC-mediated protective actions that may be connected to the stimulation of HO-1/Nrf2 and prevention of the NF-κB pathway [108]. In domoic acid-intoxicated memory impairment, QC treatment activated Nrf2-ARE and decreased protein carbonylation and reactive oxygen species in mice. Moreover, the activity of AMP-activated protein kinase (AMPK) was suggestively elevated in the QC-treated group [109]. QC also inhibited changes in the cell morphology and apoptosis in the hippocampus along with elevated the expression of Nrf2, HO-1, and superoxidase dismutase in D-galactose-induced mice. Brusatol (a Nrf2 inhibitor) treatment reversed the QC-mediated HO-1 and superoxidase dismutase expression and protection of cells [110]. The action of QC on Nf2-ARE signaling pathway leading to neuroprotection is displayed in Figure 4.

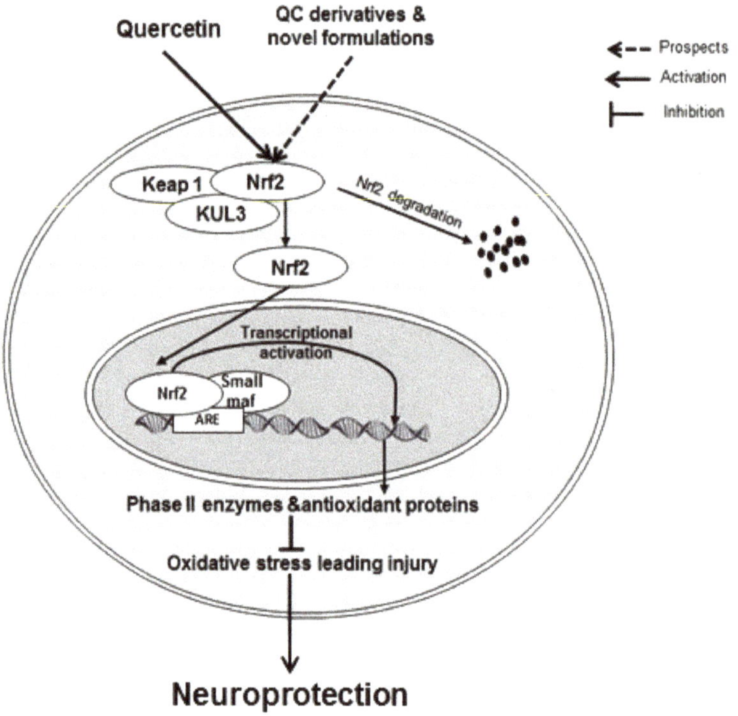

Figure 4. QC prevents oxidative stress leading to damage by activating the Nrf2 pathway. QC-mediated Nrf2 activation leads to transcriptional activation of antioxidant response elements. This activation results in prevention against oxidative damage and ultimately leads to amelioration of cognitive impairment. Keap1: Kelch-like ECH-associated protein 1; Nrf2-ARE: Nuclear factor erythroid 2.

3.3.5. Sirtuins

In the numerous molecular pathways, seven types of sirtuins (SIRT1 to SIRT7) are involved in diversity, with different cellular localization and molecular targets in mammals [111]. Of these, sirtuin 1 (SIRT1) mostly localizes in the nucleus and acts as a deacetylase for histones and other targets. SIRT1 protects cells from apoptosis and promotes the differentiation of stem cells. SIRT2 is prevalent in the cytoplasm and has been found to accumulate in neurons, while other SIRTs localize primarily in the mitochondria [111]. Sirtuin 6 (SIRT6) is crucial in regulating various cellular processes such as glucose metabolism and genomic stability [112]. Sirtuins has physiological role on the progression of NDDs by modulating transcriptional activity along with directly deacetylating proteotoxic species. Targeting sirtuin proteins are crucial in finding nonprotective agents for several NDDs such as PD, Huntington's disease, AD, spinal and bulbar muscular atrophy, and amyotrophic lateral sclerosis [113–115].

As per several studies, QC has actions on SIRT1, and in an investigation, the beneficial action of QC on lipid and glucose metabolism disorder were connected to the upregulation of SIRT1 expression and its impact on the Akt signaling pathway [116]. In another study, QC suppresses oxidized low-density lipoprotein-induced endothelial oxidative damages by regulating the NADPH oxidase/AMPK/Akt/endothelial nitric oxide synthase signaling pathway and stimulating SIRT1 action [117]. In addition, QC might suppress adipose tissue macrophage inflammation and infiltration through the AMPKα1/SIRT1 pathway in high-fat diet-fed mice [118]. A recent study addressed the neuroprotective action of QC via the SIRT1-mediated pathway, where QC plays a crucial role against excitotoxic neurodegeneration which is potential for the therapy of motor neuron disorders [119]. QC displayed the highest antioxidant activity compared to other tested polyphenols in an in vitro comparative study. Polyphenols can improve the expression of SIRT1 as well as the activation of AMPK [120]. In an investigation on QC derivatives, diquercetin and 2-chloro-1,4-naphtoquinone-quercetin were recognized as auspicious SIRT6 inhibitors with IC50 130 μM and 55 μM, respectively. 2-Chloro-1,4-naphtoquinone-quercetin inhibited SIRT2 (IC50: 14 μM). The Michaelis constant (Km) value of nicotinamide adenine dinucleotide (NAD+) are elevated by diquercetin, while 2-chloro-1,4-naphthoquinone-quercetin elevated the Km value of the acetylated substrate. The binding site of the nicotinamide moiety are preferred by diquercetin, but 2-chloro-1,4-naphtoquinone-quercetin docked with the substrate binding site as per molecular docking studies. Overall, diquercetin competes with NAD+, while 2-chloro-1,4-naphthoquinone-quercetin competes with the SIRT6 (acetylated substrate in the catalytic site) [112]. QC actions on sirtuin proteins are presented in Figure 5.

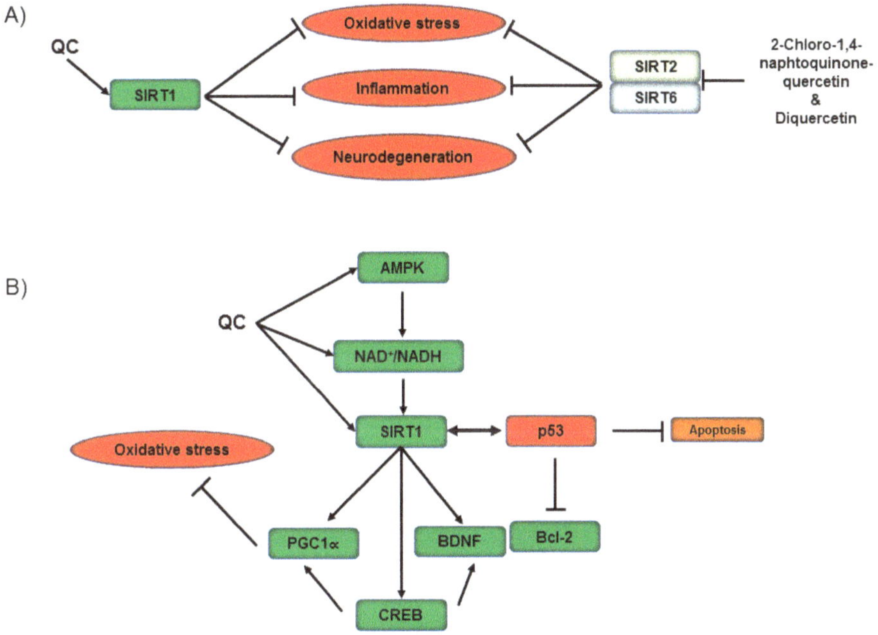

Figure 5. QC-mediated regulation of sirtuins for the therapy of cognitive impairment. The action of QC on several sirtuin proteins, leads to protective action. (**A**) QC-mediated activation of SIRT1 and 2-chloro-1,4-naphtoquinone-quercetin- and diquercetin-mediated prevention may have potential in the prevention of oxidative stress, inflammation and neurodegeneration. (**B**) QC-mediated stimulation of SIRT1 and regulation of AMPK and NAD+/NADH may have potential against oxidative stress and apoptosis. QC: Quercetin; SIRT: Sirtuin; AMPK: AMP-activated protein kinase; NAD: nicotinamide adenine dinucleotide; BDNF: Brain-derived neurotrophic factor; Bcl-2: B-cell lymphoma 2; CREB: Cyclic AMP response element binding protein.

4. Closing Remarks

We have recently published that the methanol extract of red onion displays anti-inflammatory activity against LPS-induced BV-2 microglial cells via preventing several inflammatory markers. In addition, the extract also upregulated anti-apoptotic markers and several antioxidant enzymes in N27-A cells [19]. Considering the data, we are interested in QC, which is one of the major components of red onion extract. As a phytochemical constituent, QC has demonstrated its pharmacological role in the models of several chronic diseases and disorders. Several recent studies have proved its potential therapeutic activity in neurological disorders. In our discussion, we present its role in modulating several signals focusing on neurodegenerative diseases. The role of QC on sodium and calcium channel signaling may have the potential to protect against neuronal damage in neurodegenerative diseases. QC also acts on several molecules in the dopaminergic signal pathway that may be helpful in basic research on disorders such as PD, schizophrenia, and attention deficit hyperactivity disorder. QC is a potentially bioactive compound against cognitive deficits, as it shows a role in acetylcholinergic, serotonergic, and glycinergic systems. Further study on these systems may help find the molecular role of QC in preventing cognitive impairment.

The action of QC on TLR-4 and cytokine signals may indicate its potential role against several neuroinflammatory conditions, as toll-like and cytokine receptors are considered crucial targets to the discovery of anti-inflammatory agents to treat neuroinflammatory conditions. To date, the role of QC has only been studied on TLR-4; investigations into its role in other TLRs should be conducted.

An essential action of QC is on Nrf2-ARE signals. Further studies should be designed to correlate these signals with other receptors. QC also produces suggestive effects on several neurotrophic factors, effects that range from neuronal survival to neuronal protection. Additionally, QC and its derivatives have actions on sirtuins. The QC-mediated activation of SIRT1 and it-mediated inhibition of SIRT6 may be potential in neuroprotective therapy. It would be fascinating to study the expression patterns of these neurotrophic factors after knockdown and knockout of potential receptors.

Finally, the ability of QC to modulate several drug targets may be an attractive research focus in the quest to discover treatments for neurodegenerative diseases. Some of this research has already been conducted, and, according to recent studies, the role of QC in nuclear receptors, (e.g., estrogen receptors and peroxisome proliferator-activated receptors) should be investigated. While GPCRs are considered crucial targets in the treatment of neurological disorders, QC's role in numerous GPCRs such as metabotropic glutamate, cannabinoid, and opioid receptors remains to be studied. Thus, a target-based study of QC and its analogs may help establish potential therapies for the treatment of several neurodegenerative conditions.

QC has actions on multiple targets; however, it cannot cross the BBB due to its water insolubility and low oral bioavailability, a major stumbling block in central nervous system therapeutics. Several novel deliveries of QC have been conducted to enhance its bioavailability. QC nanoparticle and nano emulsion protected ischemia [121,122] and QC nanoparticles prevented neuroinflammation in rodent models [123]. The study of novel deliveries of QC and its derivatives on several receptors for neuroprotective therapy would be interesting areas of research. In addition, the designing of QC derivatives considering the pharmacokinetic limitations would also be fascinating for the therapy of cognitive impairment. Another important area of research would be conducting studies of QC, its derivatives and novel formulations on patients with cognitive impairment at the clinical level. Preclinical studies are needed to find its potential derivatives and novel formulations.

Author Contributions: M.J. and D.-K.C.: Conceived and designed the study; M.J.: Performed the literature review, produced figures and wrote the manuscript; S.A.: Compiled the table and S.-H.J.: Performed the literature review; M.J., R.D. and I.-S.K.: Edited the manuscript; D.-K.C.: Supervised and handled the correspondence. All authors read and approved the final manuscript.

Funding: This work was supported by the Basic Science Research Program through the National Research Foundation of Korea funded by the Ministry of Education, Science and Technology (NRF-2017R1A2A2A07001035).

Conflicts of Interest: The authors declare no conflict of interest.

Abbreviations

6-OHDA	6-hydroxydopamine
AD	Alzheimer's disease
Akt	Protein Kinase B
AMPA	α-amino-3-hydroxy-5-methyl-4-isoxazolepropionic acid
APOE	Apolipoprotein E
Aβ	Amyloid beta
BBB	Blood-brain barrier
Bcl-2	B-cell lymphoma 2
BDNF	Brain-derived neurotrophic factor
CD	Cluster of differentiation
CREB	Cyclic AMP response element binding protein
ERK	Extracellular signal-regulated kinase 1/2
GABA	Gamma-aminobutyric acid
IACh	Inward currents
IL	Interleukin
iNOS	Inducible nitric oxide synthase
Keap1	Kelch-like ECH-associated protein 1
MAPK	Mitogen-activated protein kinase
MPTP	1-methyl-4-phenyl-1,2,3,6-tetrahydropyridine
mTOR	Mammalian target of rapamycin
NDDs	Neurodegenerative diseases
NF-κB	Nuclear factor-kappa B
NGF	Nerve growth factor
NKCC1	Na-K-Cl cotransporter
NMDA	N-methyl-D-aspartate
NO	Nitric oxide
NQO1	NAD(P)H quinone oxidoreducase-1
Nrf2-ARE	Nuclear factor erythroid 2-related factor 2-antioxidant responsive element
PD	Parkinson's disease
PDK1	3-phosphoinositide-dependent protein kinase 1
PI3K	Phosphatidylinositol 3-kinase
PKC	Protein kinase C
PLCγ	Phospholipase C gamma
QC	Quercetin
SIRT	Sirtuin
TLR	Toll-like receptor
TrkB	Tropomyosin receptor kinase B
α7 nAChR	α7 nicotinic acetylcholine receptor
HO-1	Heme-oxygenase-1

References

1. Jakaria, M.; Haque, M.E.; Kim, J.; Cho, D.-Y.; Kim, I.-S.; Choi, D.-K. Active ginseng components in cognitive impairment: Therapeutic potential and prospects for delivery and clinical study. *Oncotarget* **2018**, *9*, 33601–33620. [CrossRef] [PubMed]
2. Jakaria, M.; Kim, J.; Karthivashan, G.; Park, S.-Y.; Ganesan, P.; Choi, D.-K. Emerging signals modulating potential of ginseng and its active compounds focusing on neurodegenerative diseases. *J. Ginseng Res.* **2019**, *43*, 163–171. [CrossRef] [PubMed]
3. Jakaria, M.; Park, S.-Y.; Haque, M.E.; Karthivashan, G.; Kim, I.-S.; Ganesan, P.; Choi, D.-K. Neurotoxic Agent-Induced Injury in Neurodegenerative Disease Model: Focus on Involvement of Glutamate Receptors. *Front. Mol. Neurosci.* **2018**, *11*, 307. [CrossRef] [PubMed]
4. Amieva, H.; Meillon, C.; Helmer, C.; Barberger-Gateau, P.; Dartigues, J.F. Ginkgo biloba extract and long-term cognitive decline: A 20-year follow-up population-based study. *PLoS ONE* **2013**, *8*, e52755. [CrossRef]

5. Jakaria, M.; Cho, D.Y.; EzazulHaque, M.; Karthivashan, G.; Kim, I.S.; Ganesan, P.; Choi, D.K. Neuropharmacological Potential and Delivery Prospects of Thymoquinone for Neurological Disorders. *Oxid. Med. Cell. Longev.* **2018**, *2018*, 1209801. [CrossRef]
6. Uddin, M.S.; Al Mamun, A.; Kabir, M.T.; Jakaria, M.; Mathew, B.; Barreto, G.E.; Ashraf, G.M. Nootropic and Anti-Alzheimer's Actions of Medicinal Plants: Molecular Insight into Therapeutic Potential to Alleviate Alzheimer's Neuropathology. *Mol. Neurobiol.* **2018**, *56*, 4925–4944. [CrossRef]
7. Jakaria, M.; Haque, M.E.; Cho, D.Y.; Azam, S.; Kim, I.S.; Choi, D.K. Molecular Insights into NR4A2(Nurr1): An Emerging Target for Neuroprotective Therapy Against Neuroinflammation and Neuronal Cell Death. *Mol. Neurobiol.* **2019**, *56*, 5799–5814. [CrossRef]
8. Ay, M.; Luo, J.; Langley, M.; Jin, H.; Anantharam, V.; Kanthasamy, A.; Kanthasamy, A.G. Molecular mechanisms underlying protective effects of quercetin against mitochondrial dysfunction and progressive dopaminergic neurodegeneration in cell culture and MitoPark transgenic mouse models of Parkinson's Disease. *J. Neurochem.* **2017**, *141*, 766–782. [CrossRef]
9. Dajas, F. Life or death: Neuroprotective and anticancer effects of quercetin. *J. Ethnopharmacol.* **2012**, *143*, 383–396. [CrossRef]
10. Suganthy, N.; Devi, K.P.; Nabavi, S.F.; Braidy, N.; Nabavi, S.M. Bioactive effects of quercetin in the central nervous system: Focusing on the mechanisms of actions. *Biomed. Pharmacother. = Biomed. Pharmacother.* **2016**, *84*, 892–908. [CrossRef]
11. Tinay, I.; Sener, T.E.; Cevik, O.; Cadirci, S.; Toklu, H.; Cetinel, S.; Sener, G.; Tarcan, T. Antioxidant Agent Quercetin Prevents Impairment of Bladder Tissue Contractility and Apoptosis in a Rat Model of Ischemia/Reperfusion Injury. *Lower Urin. Tract Symptoms* **2017**, *9*, 117–123. [CrossRef] [PubMed]
12. Bondonno, N.; Bondonno, C.; Hodgson, J.; Ward, N.C.; Croft, K.D. The Efficacy of Quercetin in Cardiovascular Health. *Curr. Nutr. Rep.* **2015**, *4*, 290–303. [CrossRef]
13. Kosari-Nasab, M.; Shokouhi, G.; Ghorbanihaghjo, A.; Mesgari-Abbasi, M.; Salari, A.A. Quercetin mitigates anxiety-like behavior and normalizes hypothalamus–pituitary–adrenal axis function in a mouse model of mild traumatic brain injury. *Behav. Pharmacol.* **2019**, *30*, 282–289. [CrossRef] [PubMed]
14. Costa, L.G.; Garrick, J.M.; Roquè, P.J.; Pellacani, C. Mechanisms of Neuroprotection by Quercetin: Counteracting Oxidative Stress and More. *Oxid. Med. Cell. Longev.* **2016**, *2016*, 2986796. [CrossRef]
15. Trippier, P.C.; Jansen Labby, K.; Hawker, D.D.; Mataka, J.J.; Silverman, R.B. Target- and Mechanism-Based Therapeutics for Neurodegenerative Diseases: Strength in Numbers. *J. Med. Chem.* **2013**, *56*, 3121–3147. [CrossRef]
16. RusznyÁK, S.T.; Szent-GyÖRgyi, A. Vitamin P: Flavonols as Vitamins. *Nature* **1936**, *138*, 27. [CrossRef]
17. Sampson, L.; Rimm, E.; Hollman, P.C.; de Vries, J.H.; Katan, M.B. Flavonol and flavone intakes in US health professionals. *J. Am. Diet. Assoc.* **2002**, *102*, 1414–1420. [CrossRef]
18. Nishimuro, H.; Ohnishi, H.; Sato, M.; Ohnishi-Kameyama, M.; Matsunaga, I.; Naito, S.; Ippoushi, K.; Oike, H.; Nagata, T.; Akasaka, H.; et al. Estimated daily intake and seasonal food sources of quercetin in Japan. *Nutrients* **2015**, *7*, 2345–2358. [CrossRef]
19. Jakaria, M.; Azam, S.; Cho, D.Y.; Haque, M.E.; Kim, I.S.; Choi, D.K. The Methanol Extract of Allium cepa L. Protects Inflammatory Markers in LPS-Induced BV-2 Microglial Cells and Upregulates the Antiapoptotic Gene and Antioxidant Enzymes in N27-A Cells. *Antioxidants* **2019**, *8*, 348. https://www.ncbi.nlm.nih.gov/pubmed/31480531. [CrossRef]
20. Harborne, J.B. Flavonoids in the environment: Structure-activity relationships. *Prog. Clin. Biol. Res.* **1988**, *280*, 17–27.
21. Williams, C.A.; Grayer, R.J. Anthocyanins and other flavonoids. *Nat. Prod. Rep.* **2004**, *21*, 539–573. [CrossRef] [PubMed]
22. Wiczkowski, W.A.; Piskuła, M. Food flavonoids. *Pol. J. Food Nutr. Sci.* **2004**, *13*, 101–114.
23. Chang, Q.; Wong, Y.-S. Identification of Flavonoids in Hakmeitau Beans (Vigna sinensis) by High-Performance Liquid Chromatography– Electrospray Mass Spectrometry (LC-ESI/MS). *J. Agric. Food Chem.* **2004**, *52*, 6694–6699. [CrossRef] [PubMed]
24. Lu, Y.; Foo, L.Y. Polyphenolics of Salvia—A review. *Phytochemistry* **2002**, *59*, 117–140. [CrossRef]
25. Rice-Evans, C.; Miller, N.; Paganga, G. Antioxidant properties of phenolic compounds. *Trends Plant Sci.* **1997**, *2*, 152–159. [CrossRef]
26. Hollman, P.; Katan, M. Absorption, metabolism and health effects of dietary flavonoids in man. *Biomed. Pharmacother.* **1997**, *51*, 305–310. [CrossRef]

27. Mariani, C.; Braca, A.; Vitalini, S.; De Tommasi, N.; Visioli, F.; Fico, G. Flavonoid characterization and in vitro antioxidant activity of Aconitum anthoraL. (Ranunculaceae). *Phytochemistry* **2008**, *69*, 1220–1226. [CrossRef]
28. Materska, M.; Perucka, I. Antioxidant activity of the main phenolic compounds isolated from hot pepper fruit (Capsicum annuum L.). *J. Agric. Food Chem.* **2005**, *53*, 1750–1756. [CrossRef]
29. Janisch, K.M.; Williamson, G.; Needs, P.; Plumb, G.W. Properties of quercetin conjugates: Modulation of LDL oxidation and binding to human serum albumin. *Free Radic. Res.* **2004**, *38*, 877–884. [CrossRef]
30. Murota, K.; Terao, J. Antioxidative flavonoid quercetin: Implication of its intestinal absorption and metabolism. *Arch. Biochem. Biophys.* **2003**, *417*, 12–17. [CrossRef]
31. Manach, C.; Scalbert, A.; Morand, C.; Remesy, C.; Jimenez, L. Polyphenols: Food sources and bioavailability. *Am. J. Clin. Nutr.* **2004**, *79*, 727–747. [CrossRef] [PubMed]
32. Wittig, J.; Herderich, M.; Graefe, E.U.; Veit, M. Identification of quercetin glucuronides in human plasma by high-performance liquid chromatography-tandem mass spectrometry. *J. Chromatography. B Biomed. Sci. Appl.* **2001**, *753*, 237–243. [CrossRef]
33. Azuma, K.; Ippoushi, K.; Ito, H.; Higashio, H.; Terao, J. Combination of lipids and emulsifiers enhances the absorption of orally administered quercetin in rats. *J. Agric. Food Chem.* **2002**, *50*, 1706–1712. [CrossRef] [PubMed]
34. Mullen, W.; Edwards, C.A.; Crozier, A. Absorption, excretion and metabolite profiling of methyl-, glucuronyl-, glucosyl- and sulpho-conjugates of quercetin in human plasma and urine after ingestion of onions. *Br. J. Nutr.* **2006**, *96*, 107–116. [CrossRef]
35. Del Rio, D.; Rodriguez-Mateos, A.; Spencer, J.P.E.; Tognolini, M.; Borges, G.; Crozier, A. Dietary (poly)phenolics in human health: Structures, bioavailability, and evidence of protective effects against chronic diseases. *Antioxid. Redox Signal.* **2013**, *18*, 1818–1892. [CrossRef]
36. DuPont, M.S.; Mondin, Z.; Williamson, G.; Price, K.R. Effect of variety, processing, and storage on the flavonoid glycoside content and composition of lettuce and endive. *J. Agric. Food Chem.* **2000**, *48*, 3957–3964. [CrossRef]
37. Harwood, M.; Danielewska-Nikiel, B.; Borzelleca, J.F.; Flamm, G.W.; Williams, G.M.; Lines, T.C. A critical review of the data related to the safety of quercetin and lack of evidence of in vivo toxicity, including lack of genotoxic/carcinogenic properties. *Food Chem. Toxicol.* **2007**, *45*, 2179–2205. https://www.ncbi.nlm.nih.gov/pubmed/17698276. [CrossRef]
38. Knab, A.M.; Shanely, R.A.; Henson, D.A.; Jin, F.; Heinz, S.A.; Austin, M.D.; Nieman, D.C. Influence of quercetin supplementation on disease risk factors in community-dwelling adults. *J. Am. Diet. Assoc.* **2011**, *111*, 542–549. [CrossRef]
39. Choi, J.S.; Piao, Y.J.; Kang, K.W. Effects of quercetin on the bioavailability of doxorubicin in rats: Role of CYP3A4 and P-gp inhibition by quercetin. *Arch. Pharm. Res.* **2011**, *34*, 607–613. [CrossRef]
40. Turnbull, F. Effects of different blood-pressure-lowering regimens on major cardiovascular events: Results of prospectively-designed overviews of randomised trials. *Lancet (London, England)* **2003**, *362*, 1527–1535.
41. Kawabata, K.; Mukai, R.; Ishisaka, A. Quercetin and related polyphenols: New insights and implications for their bioactivity and bioavailability. *Food Funct.* **2015**, *6*, 1399–1417. [CrossRef] [PubMed]
42. Larson, A.J.; Symons, J.D.; Jalili, T. Quercetin: A Treatment for Hypertension?-A Review of Efficacy and Mechanisms. *Pharmaceuticals* **2010**, *3*, 237–250. [CrossRef] [PubMed]
43. Mrvová, N.; Škandík, M.; Kuniaková, M.; Račková, L. Modulation of BV-2 microglia functions by novel quercetin pivaloyl ester. *Neurochem. Int.* **2015**, *90*, 246–254. [CrossRef] [PubMed]
44. Ishisaka, A.; Ichikawa, S.; Sakakibara, H.; Piskula, M.K.; Nakamura, T.; Kato, Y.; Ito, M.; Miyamoto, K.-I.; Tsuji, A.; Kawai, Y.; et al. Accumulation of orally administered quercetin in brain tissue and its antioxidative effects in rats. *Free Radic. Biol. Med.* **2011**, *51*, 1329–1336. [CrossRef]
45. Berardini, N.; Fezer, R.; Conrad, J.; Beifuss, U.; Carle, R.; Schieber, A.J.J.O.A.; Chemistry, F. Screening of mango (Mangiferaindica L.) cultivars for their contents of flavonol O-and xanthone C-glycosides, anthocyanins, and pectin. *Agric. Food Chem.* **2005**, *53*, 1563–1570. [CrossRef]
46. Nemeth, K.; Piskula, M.J.C.R.I.F.S. Food content, processing, absorption and metabolism of onion flavonoids. *Nutrition* **2007**, *47*, 397–409. [CrossRef]
47. Keddy, P.G.W.; Dunlop, K.; Warford, J.; Samson, M.L.; Jones, Q.R.D.; Rupasinghe, H.P.V.; Robertson, G.S. Neuroprotective and anti-inflammatory effects of the flavonoid-enriched fraction AF4 in a mouse model of hypoxic-ischemic brain injury. *PLoS ONE* **2012**, *7*, 51324. [CrossRef]

48. Slimestad, R.; Verheul, M.J.J.O.A.; Chemistry, F. Seasonal variations in the level of plant constituents in greenhouse production of cherry tomatoes.). *Agric. Food Chem.* **2005**, *53*, 3114–3119. [CrossRef]
49. Uthra, C.; Shrivastava, S.; Jaswal, A.; Sinha, N.; Reshi, M.S.; Shukla, S. Therapeutic potential of quercetin against acrylamide induced toxicity in rats. *Biomed. Pharmacother.* **2017**, *86*, 705–714. [CrossRef]
50. Ferri, P.; Angelino, D.; Gennari, L.; Benedetti, S.; Ambrogini, P.; Del Grande, P.; Ninfali, P. Enhancement of flavonoid ability to cross the blood-brain barrier of rats by co-administration with alpha-tocopherol. *Food Funct.* **2015**, *6*, 394–400. [CrossRef]
51. Flamini, G.; Antognoli, E.; Morelli, I.J.P. Two flavonoids and other compounds from the aerial parts of Centaurea bracteata from Italy. *Phytochemistry* **2001**, *57*, 559–564. [CrossRef]
52. Li, J.; Mottamal, M.; Li, H.; Liu, K.; Zhu, F.; Cho, Y.-Y.; Sosa, C.P.; Zhou, K.; Bowden, G.T.; Bode, A.M.; et al. Quercetin-3-methyl ether suppresses proliferation of mouse epidermal JB6 P+ cells by targeting ERKs. *Carcinogenesis* **2011**, *33*, 459–465. [CrossRef] [PubMed]
53. Pandey, A.; Bhattacharya, P.; Paul, S.; Patnaik, R. Rhamnetin Attenuates Oxidative Stress and Matrix Metalloproteinase in Animal Model of Ischemia/Reperfusion: A Possible Antioxidant Therapy in Stroke. *Am. J. Neuroprot. Neuroregener.* **2013**, *5*, 1–7. [CrossRef]
54. Yao, L.; Datta, N.; Tomás-Barberán, F.A.; Ferreres, F.; Martos, I.; Singanusong, R.J.F.C. Flavonoids, phenolic acids and abscisic acid in Australian and New Zealand Leptospermum honeys. *Food Chem.* **2003**, *81*, 159–168. [CrossRef]
55. Rangel-Ordonez, L.; Noldner, M.; Schubert-Zsilavecz, M.; Wurglics, M. Plasma levels and distribution of flavonoids in rat brain after single and repeated doses of standardized Ginkgo biloba extract EGb 761(R). *Planta Med.* **2010**, *76*, 1683–1690. [CrossRef]
56. Park, H.J.; Lee, S.J.; Cho, J.; Gharbi, A.; Han, H.D.; Kang, T.H.; Kim, Y.; Lee, Y.; Park, W.S.; Jung, I.D.; et al. Tamarixetin Exhibits Anti-inflammatory Activity and Prevents Bacterial Sepsis by Increasing IL-10 Production. *J. Nat. Prod.* **2018**, *81*, 1435–1443. [CrossRef]
57. Son, K.H.; Kwon, S.J.; Chang, H.W.; Kim, H.P.; Kang, S.S. Papyriflavonol A, a new prenylated flavonol from Broussonetiapapyrifera. *Fitoterapia* **2001**, *72*, 456–458. [CrossRef]
58. Ho, L.; Ferruzzi, M.G.; Janle, E.M.; Wang, J.; Gong, B.; Chen, T.-Y.; Lobo, J.; Cooper, B.; Wu, Q.L.; Talcott, S.T.; et al. Identification of brain-targeted bioactive dietary quercetin-3-O-glucuronide as a novel intervention for Alzheimer's disease. *FASEB J.* **2013**, *27*, 769–781. [CrossRef]
59. Ishisaka, A.; Mukai, R.; Terao, J.; Shibata, N.; Kawai, Y. Specific localization of quercetin-3-O-glucuronide in human brain. *Arch. Biochem. Biophys.* **2014**, *557*, 11–17. [CrossRef]
60. Roubalová, L.; Biedermann, D.; Papoušková, B.; Vacek, J.; Kuzma, M.; Křen, V.; Ulrichová, J.; Dinkova-Kostova, A.T.; Vrba, J. Semisynthetic flavonoid 7-O-galloylquercetin activates Nrf2 and induces Nrf2-dependent gene expression in RAW264.7 and Hepa1c1c7 cells. *Chem. Biol. Interact.* **2016**, *260*, 58–66. [CrossRef]
61. Wallace, C.H.R.; Baczkó, I.; Jones, L.; Fercho, M.; Light, P.E. Inhibition of cardiac voltage-gated sodium channels by grape polyphenols. *Br. J. Pharmacol.* **2006**, *149*, 657–665. [CrossRef] [PubMed]
62. Yao, Y.; Han, D.D.; Zhang, T.; Yang, Z. Quercetin improves cognitive deficits in rats with chronic cerebral ischemia and inhibits voltage-dependent sodium channels in hippocampal CA1 pyramidal neurons. *Phytother. Res.* **2010**, *24*, 136–140. [CrossRef] [PubMed]
63. Lu, C.W.; Lin, T.Y.; Wang, S.J. Quercetin inhibits depolarization-evoked glutamate release in nerve terminals from rat cerebral cortex. *Neurotoxicology* **2013**, *39*, 1–9. [CrossRef] [PubMed]
64. Jin, C.; Wu, H.; Tang, C.; Ke, J.; Wang, Y. Protective effect of quercetin on bupivacaine-induced neurotoxicity via T-type calcium channel inhibition. *Trop. J. Pharm. Res.* **2017**, *16*, 1827–1833. [CrossRef]
65. Haleagrahara, N.; Siew, C.J.; Mitra, N.K.; Kumari, M. Neuroprotective effect of bioflavonoid quercetin in 6-hydroxydopamine-induced oxidative stress biomarkers in the rat striatum. *Neurosci. Lett.* **2011**, *500*, 139–143. [CrossRef]
66. Sriraksa, N.; Wattanathorn, J.; Muchimapura, S.; Tiamkao, S.; Brown, K.; Chaisiwamongkol, K. Cognitive-enhancing effect of quercetin in a rat model of Parkinson's disease induced by 6-hydroxydopamine. *Evid. Based Complement. Altern. Med.* **2012**, *2012*, 823206. [CrossRef]
67. Lv, C.; Hong, T.; Yang, Z.; Zhang, Y.; Wang, L.; Dong, M.; Zhao, J.; Mu, J.; Meng, Y. Effect of Quercetin in the 1-Methyl-4-phenyl-1, 2, 3, 6-tetrahydropyridine-Induced Mouse Model of Parkinson's Disease. *Evid. Based Complement Altern. Med.* **2012**, *2012*, 928643. [CrossRef]

68. Naidu, P.S.; Singh, A.; Kulkarni, S.K. D2-dopamine receptor and alpha2-adrenoreceptor-mediated analgesic response of quercetin. *Indian J. Exp. Biol.* **2003**, *41*, 1400–1404.
69. Selvakumar, K.; Bavithra, S.; Krishnamoorthy, G.; Ganesh, A.; Venkataraman, P.; Arunakaran, J. Impact of quercetin on PCBs (Aroclor-1254)-induced impairment of dopaminergic receptors expression in hippocampus of adult male Wistar rats. *Biomed. Prev. Nutr.* **2013**, *3*, 42–52. [CrossRef]
70. Gupta, R.; Shukla, R.K.; Pandey, A.; Sharma, T.; Dhuriya, Y.K.; Srivastava, P.; Singh, M.P.; Siddiqi, M.I.; Pant, A.B.; Khanna, V.K. Involvement of PKA/DARPP-32/PP1α and β- arrestin/Akt/GSK-3β Signaling in Cadmium-Induced DA-D2 Receptor-Mediated Motor Dysfunctions: Protective Role of Quercetin. *Sci. Rep.* **2018**, *8*, 2528. [CrossRef]
71. Tongjaroenbuangam, W.; Ruksee, N.; Chantiratikul, P.; Pakdeenarong, N.; Kongbuntad, W.; Govitrapong, P. Neuroprotective effects of quercetin, rutin and okra (Abelmoschusesculentus Linn.) in dexamethasone-treated mice. *Neurochem. Int.* **2011**, *59*, 677–685. [CrossRef] [PubMed]
72. Holzmann, I.; da Silva, L.M.; Correa da Silva, J.A.; Steimbach, V.M.; de Souza, M.M. Antidepressant-like effect of quercetin in bulbectomized mice and involvement of the antioxidant defenses, and the glutamatergic and oxidonitrergic pathways. *Pharmacol. Biochem. Behav.* **2015**, *136*, 55–63. [CrossRef] [PubMed]
73. Bagchi, P.; Anuradha, M.; Kar, A. Pharmacophore Screening and Docking studies of AMPA Receptor Implicated in AlzheimerÃ¢ Â Â s disease with Some CNS Acting Phytocompounds from Selected Ayurvedic Medicinal Plants. *Neuropsychiatry* **2018**, *8*, 1101–1114. [CrossRef]
74. Moghbelinejad, S.; Mohammadi, G.; Khodabandehloo, F.; Najafipour, R.; NaserpourFarivar, T.; Rashvand, Z.; Nassiri-Asl, M. The Role of Quercetin in Gene Expression of GluR1 Subunit of AMPA Receptors, and NR2A and NR2B Subunits of NMDA Receptors in Kainic Acid Model of Seizure in Mice. *Iran. Red Crescent Med. J.* **2016**, *19*, e42415. [CrossRef]
75. Lee, B.-H.; Choi, S.-H.; Shin, T.-J.; Pyo, M.K.; Hwang, S.-H.; Lee, S.-M.; Paik, H.-D.; Kim, H.-C.; Nah, S.-Y. Effects of quercetin on α9α10 nicotinic acetylcholine receptor-mediated ion currents. *Eur. J. Pharmacol.* **2011**, *650*, 79–85. [CrossRef]
76. Lee, B.-H.; Shin, T.-J.; Hwang, S.-H.; Choi, S.-H.; Kang, J.; Kim, H.-J.; Park, C.-W.; Lee, S.-H.; Nah, S.-Y. Inhibitory Effects of Quercetin on Muscle-type of Nicotinic Acetylcholine Receptor-Mediated Ion Currents Expressed in Xenopus Oocytes. *Korean J. Physiol. Pharmacol. Off. J. Korean Physiol. Soc. Korean Soc. Pharmacol.* **2011**, *15*, 195–201. [CrossRef]
77. Lee, B.-H.; Hwang, S.-H.; Choi, S.-H.; Shin, T.-J.; Kang, J.; Lee, S.-M.; Nah, S.-Y. Quercetin Inhibits α3β4 Nicotinic Acetylcholine Receptor-Mediated Ion Currents Expressed in Xenopus Oocytes. *Korean J. Physiol. Pharmacol. Off. J. Korean Physiol. Soc. Korean Soc. Pharmacol.* **2011**, *15*, 17–22. [CrossRef]
78. Lee, B.H.; Choi, S.H.; Shin, T.J.; Pyo, M.K.; Hwang, S.H.; Kim, B.R.; Lee, S.M.; Lee, J.H.; Kim, H.C.; Park, H.Y.; et al. Quercetin enhances human alpha7 nicotinic acetylcholine receptor-mediated ion current through interactions with Ca(2+) binding sites. *Mol. Cell.* **2010**, *30*, 245–253. [CrossRef]
79. Lee, B.-H.; Choi, S.-H.; Kim, H.-J.; Jung, S.-W.; Hwang, S.-H.; Pyo, M.-K.; Rhim, H.; Kim, H.-C.; Kim, H.-K.; Lee, S.-M.; et al. Differential Effects of Quercetin and Quercetin Glycosides on Human α7 Nicotinic Acetylcholine Receptor-Mediated Ion Currents. *Biomol. Ther.* **2016**, *24*, 410–417. [CrossRef]
80. Swaminathan, M.; Chee, F.C.; Chin, P.S.; Buckle, J.M.; Rahman, A.N.; Doughty, W.S.; Chung, Y.L. Flavonoids with M1 Muscarinic Acetylcholine Receptor Binding Activity. *Molecules* **2014**, *19*, 8933–8948. [CrossRef]
81. Bandaruk, Y.; Mukai, R.; Terao, J. Cellular uptake of quercetin and luteolin and their effects on monoamine oxidase-A in human neuroblastoma SH-SY5Y cells. *Toxicol. Rep.* **2014**, *1*, 639–649. [CrossRef] [PubMed]
82. Morales-Cano, D.; Menendez, C.; Moreno, E.; Moral-Sanz, J.; Barreira, B.; Galindo, P.; Pandolfi, R.; Jimenez, R.; Moreno, L.; Cogolludo, A.; et al. The Flavonoid Quercetin Reverses Pulmonary Hypertension in Rats. *PLoS ONE* **2014**, *9*, e114492. [CrossRef] [PubMed]
83. Lee, B.H.; Jeong, S.M.; Lee, J.H.; Kim, J.H.; Yoon, I.S.; Lee, J.H.; Choi, S.H.; Lee, S.M.; Chang, C.G.; Kim, H.C.; et al. Quercetin inhibits the 5-hydroxytryptamine type 3 receptor-mediated ion current by interacting with pre-transmembrane domain I. *Mol. Cell.* **2005**, *20*, 69–73.
84. Jung, J.W.; Lee, S. Anxiolytic effects of quercetin: Involvement of GABAergic system. *J. Life Sci.* **2014**, *24*, 290–296. [CrossRef]
85. Calero, C.I.; González, A.N.B.; Gasulla, J.; Alvarez, S.; Evelson, P.; Calvo, D.J. Quercetin antagonism of GABAAρ1 receptors is prevented by ascorbic acid through a redox-independent mechanism. *Eur. J. Pharmacol.* **2013**, *714*, 274–280. [CrossRef]

86. Moghbelinejad, S.; Alizadeh, S.; Mohammadi, G.; Khodabandehloo, F.; Rashvand, Z.; Najafipour, R.; Nassiri-Asl, M. The effects of quercetin on the gene expression of the GABA A receptor α5 subunit gene in a mouse model of kainic acid-induced seizure. *J. Physiol. Sci.* **2017**, *67*, 339–343. [CrossRef]
87. Fan, H.-R.; Du, W.-F.; Zhu, T.; Wu, Y.-J.; Liu, Y.-M.; Wang, Q.; Wang, Q.; Gu, X.; Shan, X.; Deng, S. Quercetin reduces cortical GABAergic transmission and alleviates MK-801-induced hyperactivity. *E Bio. Med.* **2018**, *34*, 201–213. [CrossRef]
88. Lee, B.-H.; Lee, J.-H.; Yoon, I.-S.; Lee, J.-H.; Choi, S.-H.; Pyo, M.K.; Jeong, S.M.; Choi, W.-S.; Shin, T.-J.; Lee, S.-M. Human glycine α1 receptor inhibition by quercetin is abolished or inversed by α267 mutations in transmembrane domain 2. *Brain Res.* **2007**, *1161*, 1–10. [CrossRef]
89. Sun, H.; Cheng, X.P.; You-Ye, Z.; Jiang, P.; Zhou, J.N. Quercetin subunit specifically reduces GlyR-mediated current in rat hippocampal neurons. *Neuroscience* **2007**, *148*, 548–559. [CrossRef]
90. Kaneko, M.; Takimoto, H.; Sugiyama, T.; Seki, Y.; Kawaguchi, K.; Kumazawa, Y. Suppressive effects of the flavonoids quercetin and luteolin on the accumulation of lipid rafts after signal transduction via receptors. *Immunopharmacol. Immunotoxicol.* **2008**, *30*, 867–882. [CrossRef]
91. Byun, E.B.; Yang, M.S.; Choi, H.G.; Sung, N.Y.; Song, D.S.; Sin, S.J.; Byun, E.H. Quercetin negatively regulates TLR4 signaling induced by lipopolysaccharide through Tollip expression. *Biochem. Biophys. Res. Commun.* **2013**, *431*, 698–705. [CrossRef] [PubMed]
92. Bhaskar, S.; Helen, A. Quercetin modulates toll-like receptor-mediated protein kinase signaling pathways in oxLDL-challenged human PBMCs and regulates TLR-activated atherosclerotic inflammation in hypercholesterolemic rats. *Mol. Cell. Biochem.* **2016**, *423*, 53–65. [CrossRef] [PubMed]
93. Kang, C.H.; Choi, Y.H.; Moon, S.K.; Kim, W.J.; Kim, G.Y. Quercetin inhibits lipopolysaccharide-induced nitric oxide production in BV2 microglial cells by suppressing the NF-kappaB pathway and activating the Nrf2-dependent HO-1 pathway. *Int. Immunopharmacol.* **2013**, *17*, 808–813. [CrossRef] [PubMed]
94. Sun, G.Y.; Chen, Z.; Jasmer, K.J.; Chuang, D.Y.; Gu, Z.; Hannink, M.; Simonyi, A. Quercetin Attenuates Inflammatory Responses in BV-2 Microglial Cells: Role of MAPKs on the Nrf2 Pathway and Induction of Heme Oxygenase-1. *PLoS ONE* **2015**, *10*, 0141509. [CrossRef] [PubMed]
95. Rahvar, M.; Owji, A.A.; Mashayekhi, F.J. Effect of quercetin on the brain-derived neurotrophic factor gene expression in the rat brain. *Bratisl. Lek. Listy* **2018**, *119*, 28–31. [CrossRef]
96. Hou, Y.; Aboukhatwa, M.A.; Lei, D.L.; Manaye, K.; Khan, I.; Luo, Y. Anti-depressant natural flavonols modulate BDNF and beta amyloid in neurons and hippocampus of double TgAD mice. *Neuropharmacology* **2010**, *58*, 911–920. [CrossRef]
97. Yao, R.-Q.; Qi, D.-S.; Yu, H.-L.; Liu, J.; Yang, L.-H.; Wu, X.-X. Quercetin Attenuates Cell Apoptosis in Focal Cerebral Ischemia Rat Brain Via Activation of BDNF–TrkB–PI3K/Akt Signaling Pathway. *Neurochem. Res.* **2012**, *37*, 2777–2786. [CrossRef]
98. Nakajima, K.; Niisato, N.; Marunaka, Y. Quercetin stimulates NGF-induced neurite outgrowth in PC12 cells via activation of Na(+)/K(+)/2Cl(-) cotransporter. *Cell. Physiol. Biochem. Int. J. Exp. Cell. Physiol. Biochem. Pharmacol.* **2011**, *28*, 147–156. [CrossRef]
99. Chan, G.K.L.; Hu, W.W.H.; Zheng, Z.X.; Huang, M.; Lin, Y.X.Y.; Wang, C.Y.; Gong, A.G.W.; Yang, X.Y.; Tsim, K.W.K.; Dong, T.T.X. Quercetin Potentiates the NGF-Induced Effects in Cultured PC 12 Cells: Identification by HerboChips Showing a Binding with NGF. *Evid.-Based Complement. Altern. Med.* **2018**, *2018*, 1502457. [CrossRef]
100. Ola, M.S.; Ahmed, M.M.; Shams, S.; Al-Rejaie, S.S. Neuroprotective effects of quercetin in diabetic rat retina. *Saudi J. Biol. Sci.* **2017**, *24*, 1186–1194. [CrossRef]
101. Testa, G.; Gamba, P.; Badilli, U.; Gargiulo, S.; Maina, M.; Guina, T.; Calfapietra, S.; Biasi, F.; Cavalli, R.; Poli, G.; et al. Loading into nanoparticles improves quercetin's efficacy in preventing neuroinflammation induced by oxysterols. *PLoS ONE* **2014**, *9*, e96795. [CrossRef] [PubMed]
102. Ioannis, B.; Afrodite, D.; Vasilios, P.; Despina, P. Phytochemicals and cognitive health: Are flavonoids doing the trick? *Biomed. Pharmacother.* **2019**, *109*, 1488–1497. [CrossRef]
103. Verghese, P.B.; Castellano, J.M.; Holtzman, D.M. Apolipoprotein E in Alzheimer's disease and other neurological disorders. *Lancet Neurol.* **2011**, *10*, 241–252. [CrossRef] [PubMed]
104. Boesch-Saadatmandi, C.; Niering, J.; Minihane, A.M.; Wiswedel, I.; Gardeman, A.; Wolffram, S.; Rimbach, G. Impact of apolipoprotein E genotype and dietary quercetin on paraoxonase 1 status in apoE3 and apoE4 transgenic mice. *Atherosclerosis* **2010**, *211*, 110–113. [CrossRef] [PubMed]

105. Egert, S.; Boesch-Saadatmandi, C.; Wolffram, S.; Rimbach, G.; Muller, M.J. Serum lipid and blood pressure responses to quercetin vary in overweight patients by apolipoprotein E genotype. *J. Nutr.* **2010**, *140*, 278–284. [CrossRef] [PubMed]
106. Zhang, X.; Hu, J.; Zhong, L.; Wang, N.; Yang, L.; Liu, C.C.; Li, H.; Wang, X.; Zhou, Y.; Zhang, Y.; et al. Quercetin stabilizes apolipoprotein E and reduces brain Abeta levels in amyloid model mice. *Neuropharmacology* **2016**, *108*, 179–192. [CrossRef]
107. Kulkarni, P.; Benzeroual, K. Neuroprotective effect of flavonoids, via up-regulating Nrf2-ARE pathway, in MPP+-induced PC12 cells, as a model of Parkinson's disease. *FASEB J.* **2015**, *29*, 621–623.
108. Liu, Y.-W.; Liu, X.-L.; Kong, L.; Zhang, M.-Y.; Chen, Y.-J.; Zhu, X.; Hao, Y.-C. Neuroprotection of quercetin on central neurons against chronic high glucose through enhancement of Nrf2/ARE/glyoxalase-1 pathway mediated by phosphorylation regulation. *Biomed. Pharmacother.* **2019**, *109*, 2145–2154. [CrossRef]
109. Bahar, E.; Kim, J.-Y.; Yoon, H. Quercetin Attenuates Manganese-Induced Neuroinflammation by Alleviating Oxidative Stress through Regulation of Apoptosis, iNOS/NF-κB and HO-1/Nrf2 Pathways. *Int. J. Mol. Sci.* **2017**, *18*, 1989. [CrossRef]
110. Wang, D.; Zhao, J.; Li, S.; Shen, G.; Hu, S. Quercetin attenuates domoic acid-induced cognitive deficits in mice. *Nutr. Neurosci.* **2018**, *21*, 123–131. [CrossRef]
111. Dong, F.; Wang, S.; Wang, Y.; Yang, X.; Jiang, J.; Wu, D.; Qu, X.; Fan, H.; Yao, R. Quercetin ameliorates learning and memory via the Nrf2-ARE signaling pathway in d-galactose-induced neurotoxicity in mice. *Biochem. Biophys. Res. Commun.* **2017**, *491*, 636–641. [CrossRef] [PubMed]
112. Dang, W. The controversial world of sirtuins. *Drug Discov. Today Technol.* **2014**, *12*, 9–17. [CrossRef] [PubMed]
113. Heger, V.; Tyni, J.; Hunyadi, A.; Horáková, L.; Lahtela-Kakkonen, M.; Rahnasto-Rilla, M. Quercetin based derivatives as sirtuin inhibitors. *Biomed. Pharmacother.* **2019**, *111*, 1326–1333. [CrossRef] [PubMed]
114. Herskovits, A.Z.; Guarente, L. Sirtuin deacetylases in neurodegenerative diseases of aging. *Cell Res.* **2013**, *23*, 746. [CrossRef]
115. Kim, D.; Nguyen, M.D.; Dobbin, M.M.; Fischer, A.; Sananbenesi, F.; Rodgers, J.T.; Delalle, I.; Baur, J.A.; Sui, G.; Armour, S.M.; et al. SIRT1 deacetylase protects against neurodegeneration in models for Alzheimer's disease and amyotrophic lateral sclerosis. *EMBO J.* **2007**, *26*, 3169–3179. [CrossRef]
116. Khan, R.I.; Nirzhor, S.S.R.; Akter, R. A Review of the Recent Advances Made with SIRT6 and its Implications on Aging Related Processes, Major Human Diseases, and Possible Therapeutic Targets. *Biomolecules* **2018**, *8*, 44. [CrossRef]
117. Peng, J.; Li, Q.; Li, K.; Zhu, L.; Lin, X.; Lin, X.; Shen, Q.; Li, G.; Xie, X. Quercetin Improves Glucose and Lipid Metabolism of Diabetic Rats: Involvement of Akt Signaling and SIRT1. *J. Diabetes Res.* **2017**, *2017*, 3417306. [CrossRef]
118. Hung, C.H.; Chan, S.H.; Chu, P.M.; Tsai, K.L. Quercetin is a potent anti-atherosclerotic compound by activation of SIRT1 signaling under oxLDL stimulation. *Mol. Nutr. Food Res.* **2015**, *59*, 1905–1917. [CrossRef]
119. Dong, J.; Zhang, X.; Zhang, L.; Bian, H.X.; Xu, N.; Bao, B.; Liu, J. Quercetin reduces obesity-associated ATM infiltration and inflammation in mice: A mechanism including AMPKalpha1/SIRT1. *J. Lipid Res.* **2014**, *55*, 363–374. [CrossRef]
120. Lazo-Gomez, R.; Tapia, R. Quercetin prevents spinal motor neuron degeneration induced by chronic excitotoxic stimulus by a sirtuin 1-dependent mechanism. *Transl. Neurodegener.* **2017**, *6*, 31. [CrossRef]
121. Fusi, J.; Bianchi, S.; Daniele, S.; Pellegrini, S.; Martini, C.; Galetta, F.; Giovannini, L.; Franzoni, F. An in vitro comparative study of the antioxidant activity and SIRT1 modulation of natural compounds. *Biomed. Pharmacother.* **2018**, *101*, 805–819. [CrossRef] [PubMed]
122. Ghosh, A.; Sarkar, S.; Mandal, A.K.; Das, N. Neuroprotective role of nanoencapsulated quercetin in combating ischemia-reperfusion induced neuronal damage in young and aged rats. *PLoS ONE* **2013**, *8*, e57735. [CrossRef] [PubMed]
123. Ahmad, N.; Ahmad, R.; Naqvi, A.A.; Alam, M.A.; Abdur Rub, R.; Ahmad, F.J. Enhancement of Quercetin Oral Bioavailability by Self-Nanoemulsifying Drug Delivery System and their Quantification Through Ultra High Performance Liquid Chromatography and Mass Spectrometry in Cerebral Ischemia. *Drug Res.* **2017**, *67*, 564–575. [CrossRef] [PubMed]

MDPI
St. Alban-Anlage 66
4052 Basel
Switzerland
Tel. +41 61 683 77 34
Fax +41 61 302 89 18
www.mdpi.com

Journal of Clinical Medicine Editorial Office
E-mail: jcm@mdpi.com
www.mdpi.com/journal/jcm